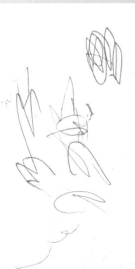

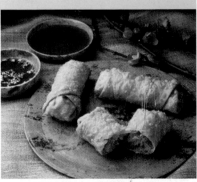

GREAT
TASTE FOR YOUR
HEALTHY LIFESTYLE
FROM BESTFOODS

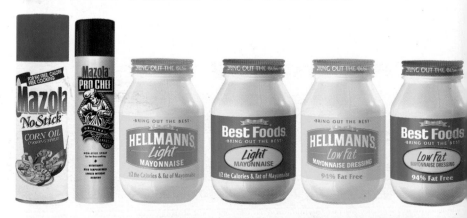

	POINTS®
Mazola No Stick® Cooking Spray, 1/3 second spray	0
Mazola® Pro Chef™ Cooking Spray, 1/3 second spray	0
Hellmann's® & Best Foods® Light Mayonnaise, 1 tablespoon	1
Hellmann's® & Best Foods® Low Fat Mayonnaise Dressing, 1 tablespoon	1
Hellmann's® & Best Foods® Citrus Splash™ Dressing, 2 tablespoons	2
Hellmann's® & Best Foods® Creamy Ranch Dressing, 2 tablespoons	4
Hellmann's® & Best Foods® Italian Dressing, 2 tablespoons	3
Hellmann's® & Best Foods® Honey Mustard, 1 teaspoon	0
Hellmann's® & Best Foods® Dijonnaise™, 1 teaspoon	0
Hellmann's® & Best Foods® Tartar Sauce, 2 tablespoons	2

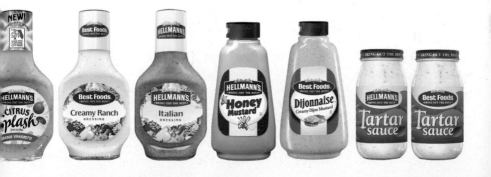

Introduction

Isn't it more fun when you do things with a friend? Whether it's going to the movies, heading to the mall, or taking a brisk walk around the neighborhood, you're more likely to be content when you're not doing things alone. Well, in your hands is one of the best friends you could have, whether you're menu planning, shopping, cooking, eating out, or tracking your progress on Winning Points – Weight Watchers *Complete Food Companion.*

Weight Watchers *Complete Food Companion* is easier than ever to use, convenient, and a wonderful tool to help you on your journey toward your weight-loss goals. You'll find *POINTS*® values for food products listed by brand, for general grocery items, and even for your own homemade recipes! (Don't cook? These can also be ordered in restaurants!)

Looking for the *POINTS* value of a food item from your local grocery or supermarket?
- Turn to the brand name section.
- Find the food category (they're listed alphabetically).
- Locate the brand (also listed alphabetically).
- Look through the list of foods to find your selection, along with the serving size and *POINTS* value.

Prefer a more general list of foods?

- Turn to the alphabetical general listing.
- Find your selection, along with the serving size and *POINTS* value.

Want to find the *POINTS* value for your favorite ethnic or regional food?

- Turn to the ethnic/regional foods section.
- Make your selection from the wide variety of different food styles.
- Find your favorite food listed alphabetically.

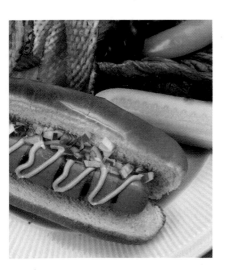

You can feel confident using the *Complete Food Companion* because the *POINTS* for all foods were calculated by Weight Watchers International, Inc. from the most current nutrition information provided by participating food companies at the time of publication.

However, since product formulations and nutrition information may change during the year, it's a good idea to read the nutrition labels on the foods you buy and to continue to use your *POINTS*finder® to check out the *POINTS* values.

The number of *POINTS* a food provides is based on a proprietary patented formula using calories, fat, and fiber. Be aware that *POINTS* values may vary from brand to brand. Additionally, *POINTS* values in the general listing may be different than for the branded products. This enables you to use the *POINTS* value that best reflects the version of the food you use. For example, beef stew is listed with different *POINTS* values in different places: twice in the general listing section – once as a homemade stew (with *POINTS* representing an average of recipes made at home or served in restaurants) and once as a non-specific store-bought product (with *POINTS* representing

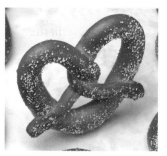 an average of several brands); and in the brand name section under various brands (with *POINTS* specific to the particular brands).

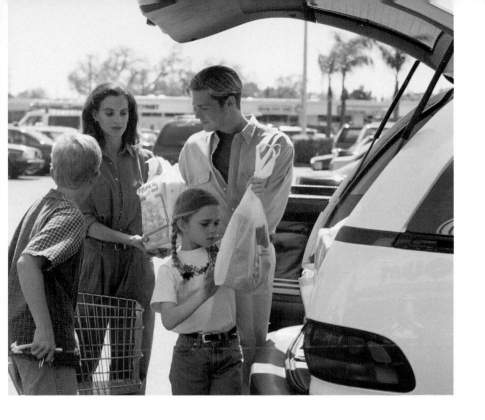

The differences in **POINTS** values for foods with more than one listing occur for many reasons. Different manufacturers may have different product formulations and/or different serving sizes, and homemade or restaurant recipes are often different than store-bought foods. For example, the ingredients in the beef stew for the specific brands are different than the average among several brands, and both are different from most homemade or restaurant versions. All, therefore, have different **POINTS** values.

POINT values for all foods in the *Complete Food Companion* represent products as purchased, unless otherwise stated. If "prepared" is noted in the listing, **POINTS** reflect the food when prepared according to package directions.

Weight Watchers *Complete Food Companion* – have some fun with this new friend. Take it with you, refer to it to comparison shop or just to get ideas, and let it be a guide in your weight-loss journey. Bon appétit!

Alphabetical General Listing of Foods

A

Adobo sauce
light, store-bought, ½ cup 5
regular, store-bought, 1 Tbsp 2
Alfredo sauce, regular, store-bought,
½ cup 10
Almond butter, 1 tsp 1
Almonds, 22 nuts 4
Ambrosia, ½ cup...................................2
Angel food cake, ¹⁄₁₆ of 10" tube
(2 oz)...2
Animal crackers, 13............................3
Antelope, cooked, 1 oz 1
Apple brown Betty, 1 cup 5
Apple cider, ½ cup (4 fl oz) 1
Apple crisp, ¾ cup 8
Apple juice, ½ cup (4 fl oz)...................1

B

Apples
baked, 1 large 7
candied, 1 large....................................10
caramel, 1 large 9
dried, ¼ cup..1
fresh, 1 large (8 oz) 2
fresh, 1 small (4 oz) 1
Applesauce, unsweetened, 1 cup...........1
Apricot nectar, ½ cup (4 fl oz) 1
Apricots
canned, unsweetened, 1 cup 2
dried, 6 halves (¾ oz) 1
fresh, 3 (4 oz)..1
Armadillo, cooked, 1 oz.........................1
Arrowroot, 1 tsp...................................0
Arroz con pollo, 3 oz chicken with
1½ cups rice 13
Artichoke hearts, cooked, 1 cup...........1
Artichokes
cooked, 1 medium 0
marinated, ½ cup 3
Arugula, 1 cup 0

Asparagus, cooked, 1 cup or 12 spears
(6½ oz)...0
Avocado, ¼ (2 oz) 2

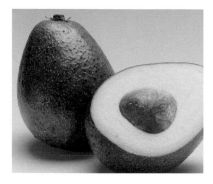

Baba au rhum, 1 8
Baba ganosh
¼ cup 3
store-bought, ¼ cup 3
Bacon
Canadian-style, cooked, 1 slice (1 oz) 1
cooked, crisp, 3 slices 3
reduced-fat, cooked, crisp, 3 slices 3
turkey, cooked, crisp, 3 slices 2
**Bacon, lettuce, and tomato
sandwich,** 1 12
Bacon bits, imitation, 1 tsp 0
Bacon fat, 1 Tbsp 3
Bagel
any type, 1 small or ½ large (2 oz)...........3
with cream cheese and lox, 1 large 12
Bagel chips
fat-free, 1 oz 2
regular, 1 oz...3
Bagel pizzas, mini, any type, 4 (3 oz) 4
Baked Alaska, ¹⁄₁₂ of 9" cake
(2" wedge) 5

Baking powder or soda, 1 tsp 0

Baklava
1 piece (2" square) 5
1 piece (2 oz) store-bought 5

Banana, 1 medium (6 oz) 2

Banana bread
with nuts, 1 slice (5" x ¾") 5
without nuts, 1 slice (5" x ¾") 5

Banana chips, 1 oz 3

Banana pudding, 1 cup........................7

Banana split, 3 scoops ice cream,
1 banana, 3 Tbsp syrup, and
½ cup whipped cream 19

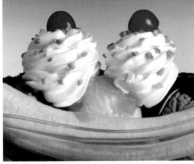

Bananas Foster, 2 scoops ice cream
with ½ banana and ⅓ cup sauce 16

Barbecue beef sandwich, frozen,
microwave, 1 (5 oz) 9

Barley
cooked, 1 cup...3
uncooked, ¼ cup 3

Bean and lentil stew
(Dal maharani), 1 cup 6

Bean dip, fat-free, ½ cup........................1

Beans
baked, ½ cup..5
baked, canned, ½ cup 2
baked, deli, ½ cup 3

baked, fast food, 1 serving 4
baked, vegetarian, canned, ½ cup 2

Beans, black
cooked, ½ cup 2
uncooked, 1 pound 31
refried, canned, ½ cup 1
refried, canned, low-fat or fat-free,
½ cup 1

Beans, black, and rice mix (prepared
according to package directions), 1 cup...4

Beans, cannellini, cooked, ½ cup 1

Beans, garbanzo
cooked, ½ cup 2
uncooked, 1 pound 35

Beans, green, cooked, 1 cup..................0

Beans, kidney
cooked, ½ cup 1
uncooked, 1 pound 30

Beans, lima
cooked, ½ cup 1
uncooked, 1 pound 30

Beans, navy
cooked, ½ cup 2
uncooked, 1 pound 30

Beans, pinto
cooked, ½ cup 2
uncooked, 1 pound 30

Beans, red, and rice, 1 cup 5

Beans, red, and rice mix (prepared
according to package directions), 1 cup...5

Beans, refried
½ cup 3
canned, ½ cup 2
fat-free, canned, ½ cup 2
with sausage, canned, ½ cup...................5

Beans, wax, cooked, 1 cup....................0

Beans, white
cooked, ½ cup 2
uncooked, 1 pound 30

Beans and franks, 1 cup 11

Bear, cooked, 1 oz...................................2

Béarnaise sauce
¼ cup 8
store-bought, ¼ cup 10

Beaver, cooked, 1 oz 1

Bechamel (white) sauce, ¼ cup..........4

Beef
ground, regular, cooked, 1 patty (3 oz) 6
ground, regular, cooked, ½ cup (2 oz).......4
ground, regular, uncooked, 1 pound 25
ground, lean, cooked, 1 patty (3 oz) 6
ground, lean, cooked, ½ cup (2 oz) 4
ground, lean, cooked (round or loin cuts
   with all visible fat trimmed), 1 slice or
   ½ cup cubed or shredded (2 oz) 3
ground, lean, uncooked, 1 pound...........22
orange-ginger, 1 cup 11
patty, country-fried, store-bought, 1
   (4 oz)..8
regular, cooked, 1 slice or ½ cup cubed
   or shredded (2 oz) 4
roast, open-faced sandwich with gravy, 1 ..9
tongue, cooked, 1 oz...............................2

Beef, sweet and sour, 1 cup..............12

Beefalo, cooked, 1 oz...........................1

Beef and broccoli
1 cup 4
frozen, 1 cup 5

Beef Bourguignon, 1½ cups 20

Beef broth and tomato juice, 1 cup
(8 fl oz)...2

Beef goulash, 1 cup 8

Beef in barbecue sauce, frozen,
¼ cup 3

Beef jerky or stick, 1 oz.....................3

Beef stew
1 cup 5
canned, 1 cup..6
frozen, 1 cup 3

Beef Stroganoff with noodles,
2 cups (1 cup Stroganoff with 1 cup
   noodles) 15

Beef Wellington, 1 slice
(3½" x 2½" x 1½"), 5 oz....................12

Beer
light, 1 can or bottle (12 fl oz) 2
non-alcoholic, 1 (12 fl oz).......................1
regular, 1 can or bottle (12 fl oz)..............3

Beets
cooked, 1 cup (6 oz) 0
pickled, ½ cup 1

Beignet
1 (2")..2
from mix, prepared, 1 3

Bialy, 1 (3 oz)..5

Biscotti
chocolate, 8 mini, 2 small, or 1 regular
   (1 oz)..3
fat-free, 8 mini, 2 small, or 1 regular
   (1 oz)..2
plain, 8 mini, 2 small, or 1 regular (1 oz) ..3

Biscuits
homemade, 1 small (2" diameter)............3
cheese, 1...5
refrigerated, baked, 1 small
   (2½" diameter) or ½ large 2

Bittermelon (balsam-pear pods)
cooked, 1 cup...0
uncooked, 1 cup 0

Blackberries, 1 cup (5 oz) 1

Black Russian, 1 (3 fl oz) 5

Blanquette of veal, 2 cups................13

Blintz
cheese, 1...5
cheese, frozen, 1 (2¼ oz).......................2
fruit, frozen, 1 (2¼ oz) 2
potato, frozen, 1 (2¼ oz) 2

Bloody Mary, 1 (5 fl oz) 2

Blueberries, 1 cup (5 oz)......................1

Bologna
  beef and pork, 1 slice (1 oz) 2
  turkey, 1 slice (1 oz) 1

Bolognese meat sauce, ½ cup 6

Borscht
  beet, 1 cup with 2 Tbsp sour cream.........4
  low-calorie, store-bought, 1 cup...............0
  store-bought, 1 cup 2

Boston brown bread, 1 slice
  (3¾" x ½"), 1½ oz.................................2

Boudin, 2 oz..2

Bouillabaisse, 2 cups..........................7

Boysenberries, 1 cup 1

Bran
  corn, uncooked, ¼ cup 0
  oat, uncooked, ¼ cup..............................1
  rice, uncooked, ¼ cup 2
  wheat, uncooked, 1 Tbsp.........................0
  wheat, uncooked, ¼ cup 0

Brandy, 1 jigger (1½ fl oz) 2

Bratwurst, 2 oz....................................5

Brazil nuts, 8 nuts (1 oz)......................5

Bread
  any type (white, wheat, rye, Italian,
    French, pumpernickel), 1 slice (1 oz).......2
  cocktail (party-style), any type, 2 slices
    (¾ oz) 1
  high-fiber (3 g or more dietary fiber
    per slice), 1 slice (1 oz) 1
  Indian (Navajo) fry, 1 (5" diameter) 6
  reduced-calorie, any type, 2 slices
    (1½ oz)...1

Bread crumbs
  dried, 3 Tbsp 1
  dried, 1 cup...9
  seasoned, 3 Tbsp 2

Breadfruit, uncooked, 1 cup 4

Breadsticks
  any type, 2 long (7½" x ½") or 4 short
    (5" x ½") or ¾ oz 1
  soft, 1 2

Brioche, 1 slice (1 oz)...........................3

Broccoli
  cooked, 1 cup or 4 spears.......................0
  uncooked, 1 cup 0

Broccoli rice casserole, 1 cup 5

Broccoli stir-fry, 1 cup 3

Brownie
  1 piece (2" square)..................................5
  fat-free, store-bought, 1 (1½ oz) 2
  low-fat, store-bought, 1 (1½ oz) 3

Brunswick stew, 1½ cups....................5

Bruschetta, 1 slice 3

Brussels sprouts
  cooked, 1 cup (5½ oz)............................0
  uncooked, 1 cup 0

Bubble and squeak, 1 cup 3

Buffalo, water, cooked, 1 oz..................1

Buffalo wings
  cooked, 3 9
  frozen (prepared without fat), 3...............4

Bulgur
  cooked, 1 cup...2
  uncooked, ¼ cup 2

Burgoo, 1 cup......................................4

Burritos
  bean, 1 large (8")...................................8
  bean, 1 small (6")...................................5
  bean, fast food, 1 6
  bean and cheese, reduced-fat,
    store-bought, 1 (5½ oz) 5
  bean and cheese, store-bought, 1 (5 oz)...6
  beef and bean, store-bought, 1 (5 oz) 8
  beef or chicken and cheese, reduced-fat,
    store-bought, 1 small or ½ large (4 oz) ...4
  beef with cheese, 1 (8")..........................8
  beef with cheese, 1 (6").........................5
  breakfast (egg, cheese & bacon, ham,
    or sausage), store-bought, 1 (3½ oz)......5
  chicken, store-bought, 1 (5 oz)................6

chicken with cheese, 1 (8") 7
chicken with cheese, 1 (6") 5

Butter
regular, 1 cup 51
regular or whipped, 1 tsp 1

Buttermilk, dry, ¼ cup.............................2

Buttermilk baking mix, 3 Tbsp 2

c

Cabbage, all varieties, including bok
choy, kai choi, won bok, makina,
Chinese, swamp, and mustard
cooked, 1 cup 0
uncooked, 1 cup 0
stuffed, 2 (2" x 2½") 6

Caesar salad, 3 cups..............................7

Cake mix, light, prepared, without icing,
1 slice (¹⁄₁₂ of 9" cake)...........................4

Cakes
fat-free, store-bought, 1 slice (3½ oz).......4
cupcake, creme-filled, store-bought, 1 4
snack, creme-filled, store-bought,
2 (2¼ oz) 6
sugar-free, store-bought, 1 slice (2½ oz) ...5
with icing, ¹⁄₁₂ of 9" layer cake or
3" square 12
with icing, store-bought, 1 slice (3 oz)......7

Calamari, fried, ½ cup 11

Calzone, 1 (5¼" x 6"), 7 oz 12

Candies
candy corn, 1 oz 2
caramels, 1 oz 2
chocolate, any type, 1 oz (2 assorted
pieces, ½ candy bar, or 2 Tbsp chips)......4
cotton candy, 1 (1½ oz)............................3
gumdrops, 1 oz..2
hard, 1 oz 2
jellybeans, 10 (1 oz) 2
licorice, 1 rope (43" long) 1
licorice, 1 oz 2
lollipop, 1 (1 oz) 2

mint, chocolate-covered, 1
(2¼" diameter) 3
sesame, 1 piece (2" x 1").........................2
taffy, 1 piece (½ oz) 1

Cannelloni, cheese
with meat sauce, 2 shells with
½ cup sauce...29
with tomato sauce, 2 shells with
½ cup sauce...14
with tomato sauce, frozen, 7 oz 6

Cannelloni, meat
with cream sauce, 2 shells with
½ cup sauce...17
with tomato sauce, 2 shells with
½ cup sauce...14

Cannelloni, spinach and cheese
with cream sauce, 2 shells with
½ cup sauce...15
with tomato sauce, 2 shells with
½ cup sauce...12

Cannoli, 1 (3½" long) 9

Cantaloupe
¼ (8 oz) 1
1 cup 1

Capers, 1 Tbsp 0

Capon, without bone, with skin, cooked,
1 oz..2

Caponata, 1 cup.....................................4

Caponate (eggplant appetizer),
store-bought, ¼ cup 2

Cappuccino, made with fat-free milk
grande, 1 (16 fl oz) 2
small, 1 (8 fl oz) 1
tall, 1 (12 fl oz)..2

Cappuccino, made with low-fat milk
grande, 1 (16 fl oz) 3
small, 1 (8 fl oz) 2
tall, 1 (12 fl oz)..3

Cappuccino, made with whole milk
grande, 1 (16 fl oz) 4

small, 1 (8 fl oz) 2

tall, 1 (12 fl oz)......................................3

Cappuccino, ready-made, from machine,
  any flavor, 1 cup......................................2

Cappuccino mix, any flavor, 4 tsp 2

Caraway seeds
  1 tsp......................................0
  1 Tbsp......................................0

Cardoon, 1 cup......................................0

Caribou, cooked, 1 oz 1

Carne asada, 4 oz................................10

Carob, unsweetened, 1 tsp......................0

Carrot and raisin salad, ½ cup 7

Carrot cake, with cream cheese icing,
  1/12 of 9" layer cake or 3" square 16

Carrot juice, canned, ½ cup..................1

Carrots, 1 cup......................................1

Carrots and parsnips, 1 cup................4

Casaba melon, 1 cup............................1

Cashew butter, without salt added,
  1 Tbsp 2

Cashews, dry roasted, without salt
  added, 14 (1 oz) 4

Cassoulet, 1 cup 11

Cauliflower
  cooked, 1 cup......................................0
  uncooked, 1 cup 0

Caviar or any type fish roe, 1 oz.......2

Caviar spread, store-bought, 2 Tbsp 3

Celeriac, 1 cup 0

Celery
  cooked, 1 cup......................................0
  uncooked, 1 cup 0

Cereal, hot
  cream of rice, cooked, 1 cup 2
  cream of wheat, cooked, 1 cup 2
  farina, cooked, 1 cup................................2

farina, uncooked, ¼ cup 3

grits, cooked, 1 cup..................................3

grits, uncooked, ¼ cup 3

oatmeal, cooked, 1 cup 3

oatmeal, flavored, cooked, 1 packet.........3

oatmeal, uncooked, 1 cup 6

Cereal, hot, in a cup, 1 (2 oz) 4

Cereal, ready-to-eat
  any type (other than those listed here),
    1 cup......................................2
  bran flakes, ¾ cup 1
  fortified, 1 cup......................................2
  frosted, 1 cup......................................3
  granola, ½ cup 4
  granola, homemade, ½ cup 6
  granola, low-fat, ½ cup......................................3
  nuggets, ½ cup......................................3
  puffed, 1 cup......................................1
  raisin bran, ¾ cup 1
  shredded wheat, 1 biscuit 1
  whole grain, 1 cup......................................2

Cereal bars
  fat-free, 1 (1½ oz)......................................2
  regular, 1 3

Ceviche, ½ cup 2

Challah bread, 1 slice (5" x 3" x ¾")....2

Chalupa (pork and bean dish),
  1 cup......................................6

Champagne, 1 small glass or ½ cup
  (4 fl oz)......................................2

Chapati, 1 piece (5" diameter) 2

Char shiu bao (roast pork bun), 1
  (2 oz)......................................4

Cheese, cottage
  fat-free, 1 cup......................................3
  fat-free, with fruit, 1 cup 4
  low-fat (1%), 1 cup..................................3
  low-fat (1%), with fruit, 1 cup 5
  reduced-fat (2%), 1 cup 4
  regular (4%), 1 cup..................................5
  regular, with fruit, 1 cup..........................6

C

Cheese, cream
fat-free, ¼ cup...1
light, 2 Tbsp 1
regular, 1 Tbsp 1
soy, 2 Tbsp 2
whipped, 2 Tbsp 2

Cheese, feta, ¼ cup crumbled 3

**Cheese, hard or semisoft, dairy
or soy**
fat-free, 1" cube, 4 Tbsp shredded, or
3 Tbsp grated (1 oz)...........................1
low-fat, 1" cube, 4 Tbsp shredded, or
3 Tbsp grated (1 oz)...........................2
regular, 1" cube, 4 Tbsp shredded, or
3 Tbsp grated (1 oz)...........................3
slice, fat-free, 1 (¾ oz) 1
slice, low-fat, 1 (¾ oz) 2
slice, regular, 1 (¾ oz) 2

Cheese, Neufchatel, 1 Tbsp 1

Cheese, pot, 1 cup 3

Cheese, ricotta
fat-free, 1 cup...4
part-skim, 1 cup 8
whole milk, 1 cup 11

Cheese and breadstick snack pack,
1 package (1 oz) 3

Cheese and pretzel snack pack,
1 package (1 oz) 3

Cheese ball, store-bought, 2 Tbsp 3

Cheeseburgers on buns
double, fast food, 1.............................12
double, with bacon, fast food, 1.............19
large, fast food, 1 15
microwave, frozen, 1 (4¾ oz) 9
small, fast food, 1 8
with bacon, microwave, frozen, 1..........11
without mayonnaise, lettuce, and
tomato, 1 11

Cheesecake
¹⁄₁₆ of 10" cake 10
fast food, 1 serving.................................7
frozen, 1 slice (4 oz)...............................9

Cheesecake with fruit topping
¹⁄₁₆ of 10" cake 10
fast food, 1 serving.................................8

Cheese puffs, hot, 2 (½ oz each) 2

Cheese sandwich
restaurant-type, grilled, 1 13
with bacon, grilled, 1 16

Cheese sauce
¼ cup 2
store-bought, ¼ cup 5

Cheese spread, American, process,
2 Tbsp (1 oz) 2

Cheese sticks, breaded (prepared
without fat), 2 (1 oz) 3

Cheese straws, 2 (2" long each), 2 oz ...2

Cheese twists or balls, 1½ cups 4

Chef's salad
fast food, 1 4
without dressing, 4 cups 6

Cherries
chocolate-covered, 2 (1 oz) 2
dried, ¼ cup 2
fresh, 1 cup 1
maraschino, 1 0

Chestnuts
European, roasted, 10 (3 oz)....................3
European, uncooked, 6 (2 oz) 2
water, 1 cup 1

Chicken (without skin and bone)
dark meat, cooked, 1 slice or ½ cup
cubed or shredded, 2 oz.......................3
dark meat, uncooked, 1 pound 13
giblets, cooked, chopped or diced, ½ cup ...3

white meat, cooked, 1 slice or ½ cup
  cubed or shredded, 2 oz........................2
white meat, uncooked, 1 pound.............11

Chicken, blackened, 1 breast (3 oz) 7

Chicken, canned, ½ cup (4 oz)..............4

Chicken, fried
  frozen, 3 oz..7
  skinless, frozen, 3 oz 5

Chicken, ginger, 1 cup 7

Chicken, orange, 1 cup 13

Chicken, sesame, 1 cup.......................9

Chicken, sweet and sour
  1 cup..10
  frozen, 1 cup 6

Chicken, Szechuan, frozen, 1 cup 5

Chicken, Tandori, without skin,
  1 breast and 1 thigh 9

Chicken a la king, 1 cup......................12

Chicken adobo, 1 thigh 6

Chicken and broccoli, 1 cup................2

Chicken and dumplings
  canned, 1 cup..5
  frozen, 1 cup 7

Chicken and meatball fricassee,
  2 cups 9

Chicken asopao, 1 cup with 1 piece
  chicken 8

Chicken breast
  barbecued, with skin (no bone),
    1 (4½ oz) 6
  cooked, with skin (no bone), 1 (3 oz) 4
  cooked, with skin and bone, 1 (4½ oz) 5
  cooked, without skin, 1 (4½ oz) 3
  cooked, without skin and bone, 1 (3 oz) ...3
  five spice, 1 breast (with skin and bone),
    4½ oz 7
  fried, with skin (with bone), 1 (4½ oz)....11

fried, with skin, fast food, 1 10
stuffed with long grain and wild rice,
  frozen, 1 (6 oz).....................................8
stuffed with vegetables and cheese,
  frozen, 1 (6 oz).....................................8

Chicken breast fillet
  breaded, frozen (prepared without fat),
    3 oz...4
  grilled, refrigerated, 3 oz 3

Chicken breast patty, breaded,
  fat-free (prepared without fat), 1
  (2½ oz)..2

Chicken cacciatore, 1 half breast or
  1 thigh and leg (6½ oz) 10

Chicken cordon bleu
  1 piece (5½ oz) 13
  frozen, 1 (6¾ oz)..................................10

Chicken drumstick
  barbecued with skin (with bone), 1
    (1½ oz)..2
  cooked with skin (no bone), 1...................2
  cooked with skin (with bone), 1 2
  cooked, without skin (no bone), 1 (1 oz) ...1
  cooked, without skin (with bone), 1
    (1½ oz)..1
  fried, with skin (with bone), 1 (1½ oz)......5
  fried, with skin, fast food, 1 4

Chicken in barbecue sauce, frozen,
  ¼ cup 3

Chicken in the pot, without skin,
  2 cups 10

Chicken Kiev
  1 serving (4" x 8") 18
  frozen, 1 (6 oz)....................................13

Chicken leg, five spice, 1 leg (thigh
  and drumstick), with skin and bone 9

Chicken macaroni salad, 1 cup...........6

Chicken marsala, 4 oz (no bone) 15

Chicken mole, 1 cup............................8

C

Chicken paprika, 1 breast or thigh
with ½ cup sauce 7

Chicken parmigiana
without sauce, 5½ oz..............................8
with sauce, 5 oz with ½ cup sauce.........10

Chicken parmigiana patty, 1 patty
with sauce (5 oz)...................................6

Chicken patty, fried, frozen, 1 (2½ oz)...4

Chicken pieces (nugget-style)
fat-free, frozen, 3 (3 oz) 2
fried, 6 (2" x ¾" each) 8
fried, fast food, 6...................................8
frozen, 6 (3 oz) 6

Chicken roll, 1 slice (1 oz) 1

Chicken salads
½ cup 6
grilled chicken, without dressing,
fast food, 1 4
Oriental, 2 cups 7
store-bought, ½ cup 5

Chicken salad sandwich
reduced-calorie bread, 1...........................8
regular bread, 1.....................................9

Chicken sandwich
fried, fast food, 1 12
grilled, fast food, 1 9
grilled, frozen, 1 (4¼ oz) 6

Chicken stew, canned, 1 cup.................4

Chicken tetrazzini, 1½ cups...............14

Chicken thigh
barbecued, with skin (with bone), 1
(3 oz)...5
cooked, with skin (no bone), 1 (2 oz) 4
cooked, with skin (with bone), 1 (3 oz).....4
cooked, without skin (no bone), 1 (2 oz)....3
cooked, without skin (with bone), 1
(3 oz)...3
fried, with skin (with bone), 1 (3 oz) 7
fried, with skin, fast food, 1....................8

Chicken tikka, 4 oz 5

Chicken wing
cooked, with skin (with bone), 1 (1½ oz) ...3
fried, with skin, fast food, 1.....................5

Chicken with cashews, 1 cup.............9

Chicken with dumplings
3 oz chicken with 2 dumplings
(with skin) 8
3 oz chicken with 2 dumplings
(without skin)..7

Chicory (curly endive), 1 cup.............0

Chiffon pie, ⅛ of 9" one-crust pie 9

Chili
bean, in a cup, 1 (2 oz) 3
low-fat, canned, 1 cup 5
turkey, with beans, canned, 1 cup 4
turkey, without beans, canned, 1 cup 3
vegetarian, low-fat or fat-free, canned,
1 cup..3
without beans, canned, 1 cup.................11
without beans, frozen, 1 cup 12

Chili con carne
with beans, 1 cup 8
without beans, 1 cup 8

Chili con queso
¼ cup 5
canned, ¼ cup.......................................2
frozen, ¼ cup 5

Chili dog on roll, 1 10

Chili mac, canned, 1 cup......................5

Chili relleños, 2................................18

Chili sauce
1 Tbsp...0
green, ¼ cup 1
red, ¼ cup..1

Chili with beans, canned, 1 cup...........6

Chimichangas
beef, 1 (3" x 3½") 11
beef or chicken, with beans, frozen,
1 (6½ oz)..8
chicken, 1 (3" x 3½") 9

Chinese vegetables
with beef, 1 cup......................................6
with chicken, 1 cup...............................5
with pork, 1 cup 7
with shrimp, 1 cup.................................4
with tofu, 1 cup.....................................4

Chitterlings, cooked, 1 oz 2

Chives, 1 Tbsp..0

Chocolate
drink, 1 cup..3
mousse, 1 cup 12
spread, 2 Tbsp.......................................4
syrup, 1 Tbsp...1

Cholent, 1 cup...4

Chop suey
beef, 1 cup 5
chicken, 1 cup 4
pork, 1 cup..4
vegetable, 1 cup 4

Chorizo, 1 link (5½" long), 3½ oz 12

Chow mein
beef, 1 cup 5
canned (beef, chicken, or pork), 1 cup 1
chicken, 1 cup 4
pork, 1 cup..5
noodles, ½ cup 3

Chutney, 2 Tbsp.....................................1

Cinnamon bun, 1 large (4 oz) 6

Cioppino, 2 cups 13

Clam juice, canned, ½ cup 0

Clam sauce
red, ½ cup...3
red, store-bought, ½ cup 2
white, ½ cup...5
white, store-bought, ½ cup....................3

Clam-tomato juice, 1 cup (8 fl oz) 2

Clementines, 2 small (3 oz each)...........1

Club sandwich, 1 15

Club soda, 1 can or bottle (12 fl oz) 0

Cobbler, fruit
any type, 1 cup 10
frozen, 4½ oz 6

Cobb salad (without dressing), 3 cups ...10

Cocoa, unsweetened, 1 tsp 0

Cocoa, hot, instant
fat-free, 6 fl oz.......................................1
no sugar added, 6 fl oz 1
regular, 6 fl oz..2

Coconut, packaged, shredded
1 tsp...0
1 cup...8

Coconut cream, canned, ¼ cup
(2 fl oz)..15

Coconut custard pie, ⅛ of 9"
one-crust pie 9

Coconut juice, 1 can (12 fl oz) 3

Coconut milk
canned, ¼ cup (2 fl oz) 3
light, ¼ cup (2 fl oz) 1

Coconut rice
Indian, 1 cup 5
Thai, 1 cup 19

Coconut shrimp, 4 jumbo...................16

Coffee
black, without sugar, 1 cup (8 fl oz) 0
decaffeinated, black, without sugar,
1 cup (8 fl oz) 0

Coffee cake
3" square or 1⁄12 of 9" tube....................8
fat-free, store-bought, 2 oz....................3
store-bought, 2 oz 6

Coffee drink
Jamaican, store-bought, 1 cup (8 fl oz) 2
with milk, canned, 1 (10 fl oz) 4

Coffee mix, flavored
sugar-free, prepared, 1 cup (8 fl oz)..........1
with sugar, prepared, 1 cup (8 fl oz).........1

Coffee substitute or cereal
beverage powder, 1 tsp 0

Colcannon, 1 cup 7

Coleslaw
½ cup 4
store-bought, ½ cup 4

Cookies
amaretti, 1 (1" diameter) 2
any type, packaged (other than those
listed here), 2 small (1 oz) 3
bar, 1 (2" square) 3
fig bar, 2 2
fortune, 1 1
from refrigerated dough, baked, 2 3
fruit bar, 2 2
gingerbread, 1 (2" diameter) 2
gingersnaps, 2 (½ oz) 1
macaroons, 2 2
reduced-calorie, store-bought, 2 (1 oz) 2
sugar-free, store-bought, 2 (1 oz) 2
vanilla wafers, 3 2
vanilla wafers, reduced-fat, 3 1
Viennese wafers, filled with chocolate
cream, store-bought, 1 oz 4

Coq au vin, 2 cups 13

Coquilles St. Jacques, 2 shells 8

Corn
baby (ears), 1 cup 1
breaded, frozen (prepared without fat),
6 (3 oz) 4
cream-style, 1 cup 2
grilled, 1 ear, with butter 4
kernels, cooked, 1 cup 2
on the cob, 1 small ear (5") 1

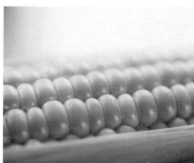

Corn bread
1 piece (2" square) 3
Mexican, 1 piece (1/12 of 10" round) or
3⅓ oz 7

Corn bread dressing, 1 cup 8

Corn casserole, ½ cup 8

Corn chips, 10 large or 30 small (1 oz) ...4

Corn dog, frozen, 1 (2¾ oz) 5

Corned beef, canned, 1 slice (2 oz) 4

Cornflake crumbs, ½ cup 3

Corn nuts, ½ cup (1½ oz) 4

Corn pudding, home-prepared, 1 cup 7

Cornish hen
cooked, with skin, ½ hen 9
cooked, without skin, ½ hen 3

Cornmeal
cooked, ¼ cup 4
uncooked, 2 Tbsp (½ oz) 1

Cornmeal mix, self-rising, 2 Tbsp
(¾ oz) 1

Couscous (semolina)
cooked, 1 cup 3
uncooked, ¼ cup 3

Couscous in a cup, 1 (2 oz) 4

Cowpeas, cooked, ½ cup 1

Crabapple, 1 cup slices 2

Crab cakes, 2 (2¼ oz each or
3" round) 4

Crab puffs, 6 (1½" rounds) 5

Crab Rangoon
1 serving, large (4½") or 5 mini 5
frozen, 8 (5¼ oz) 11

Cracker meal, ¼ cup 2

Crackers
any type (other than those listed here)
1 oz 3
cheese squares, mini, reduced-fat, 1 oz 3
cheese squares, mini, regular, 1 oz 3

fat-free, 7 (¾ oz) 1
oyster, 1 cup...4
saltines, 6 2
snack, 1 oz...3
snack, with filling (cheese, wheat,
   rye, toast, or wafer crackers with
   cheese, peanut butter, or cream
   cheese filling), 6 5

Cranberries
dried, ¼ cup (1½ oz)..............................2
fresh, 1½ cups (5 oz) 1

Cranberry juice cocktail
½ cup (4 fl oz)...1
low-calorie, 1 cup (8 fl oz).......................1

Cranberry sauce, canned, ¼ cup...........2

Crawfish pie, 1 slice, (⅛ of 9" pie) 13

Cream
clotted (English double Devon cream),
   2 Tbsp 4
half and half, 2 Tbsp 1
light, 2 Tbsp 2
sour, fat-free, ¼ cup 1
sour, light, 3 Tbsp 1
sour, regular, 1 Tbsp 1
soy, 1 oz 1
whipped (no sugar added), homemade,
   ¼ cup 3
whipped, aerosol, ¼ cup 1
whipped, dairy or nondairy, frozen,
   ¼ cup 1
whipping, heavy, 2 Tbsp 3
whipping, light, 2 Tbsp............................3

Creamed chipped beef, 1 cup...........11

Creamed chipped chicken, 1 cup.....11

Creamed chipped turkey, 1 cup.......11

Creamer
fat-free, liquid, flavored, 2 Tbsp 1
nondairy, liquid, 2 Tbsp 1
nondairy, powder, 1 Tbsp........................1

Cream pie
with fruit, ⅛ of 9" one-crust pie 9
without fruit, ⅛ of 9" one-crust pie 9
with or without fruit, frozen, 1 slice
   (4¾ oz) 10

Cream puff, 1 (2 oz).............................7

Creme brulee, ¾ cup 11

Creme caramel, 1 cup..........................7

Creme fraiche, 2 Tbsp 3

Creole
chicken, without rice, 1 cup 6
shrimp, store-bought, 1 cup.....................5
shrimp, without rice, 1 cup 4

Crepes
1 (6" diameter) 2
chicken, 2...12
seafood, 2...11
Suzette, 2..10

Crispbreads, ¾ oz (1 wafer or 5 thin
   wafers) 1

Croissants
chocolate-filled, 1 (5" long), 3¾ oz 6
plain, 1 (5" long), 1¾ oz 5

Croque monsieur, 1..............................11

Croquettes
beef, 2 (2½ oz each) 10
chicken, 2 (2½ oz each)...........................9

Croutons
homemade, ½ cup 3
packaged, fat free, ½ cup........................2
packaged, regular, ½ cup 3

Cruller
French, glazed, 1 (3" diameter)................4
glazed, 1 (4" diameter)............................6
glazed, 1 long twist (approximately
   5¼" x 2½" x 1½" high).........................9

Crumpet, 1 (3" diameter).....................3

Cucumber, 1 cup 0

Currants
dried, ¼ cup 2
fresh, 1 cup 1

Curry
beef, 1 cup 10
Bengali fish, 1 fillet (4½ oz) and
  1 cup vegetables 10
chicken, 1 cup 10
goat, 4 oz 5
green chicken (Gaeng Kheow Wan Gai),
  1 cup...7
lamb, 1 cup 10
Mussaman beef, 1 cup 19

Custard, 1 cup 8

D

Daikon, cooked, 1 cup 0

Daiquiri, 1 (3 fl oz) 3

Daiquiri mix, ½ cup (4 fl oz) 3

Dairy shake, reduced-calorie, 1 packet ...2

Danish
fast food, 1 8
store-bought, 1 (2¼ oz) 6

Date-nut bread, 1 slice (5" x ½")........5

Dates
dried, ¼ cup (5) 2
fresh, 2 (¾ oz).......................................1

Dhansak, 1 cup 6

Dip
any type, 2 Tbsp 2
artichoke, baked, ¼ cup 6
spinach, ¼ cup 5

Dolma
4 4
store-bought, 4......................................3

Donair, 4 oz meat with onion, tomato
  and 2 Tbsp sauce................................14

Donair sauce, 2 Tbsp 2

Doro wat, 1 cup 7

Doughnut holes, yeast, glazed, 2 3

Doughnuts
any type, store-bought, 1 (2 oz) 5
cake-type, 1 (3" diameter)......................6
cake-type, sugared or glazed, 1
  (3" diameter) 6
cake-type, with icing, 1 (3" diameter) 7
holes, yeast, glazed, 2 3
mini, chocolate-covered, store-bought,
  3-4 doughnuts (2 oz) 7
mini, powdered sugar-covered, store-
  bought, 3-4 doughnuts (2 oz)...............6
with creme filling, 1 (3½" x 2½" oval).....8
yeast, plain or glazed, 1 (3" diameter) 6
yeast, with jelly filling, 1
  (3½" x 2½" oval) 7

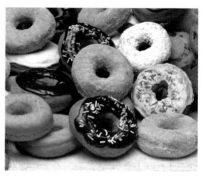

Duck
a l'orange, ¼ duck with 2 Tbsp sauce.....19
domestic, with skin, cooked, ¼ duck
  (3½ oz without bone) 13
domestic, without skin, cooked, ¼ duck
  (3½ oz without bone) 5
sauce, 1 Tbsp...1
with fruit sauce, ¼ duck with skin
  and ½ cup sauce 13

Dumplings
beef or pork, fried, 4 11
beef or pork, steamed, 4 6
chicken, fried, 4 9
chicken, steamed, 4 4
shrimp, fried, 4 9
shrimp, steamed, 4 4

E

Eclair, 1 9

Egg and cheese sandwich, fast food,
1 8

Egg foo yung
beef, 1 (3" diameter) 4
chicken, 1 (3" diameter) 4
pork, 1 (3" diameter) 5
shrimp, 1 (3" diameter) 4

Eggnog
homemade, with liquor, ½ cup 4
homemade, without liquor, ½ cup 4
reduced-calorie, store-bought
(without liquor), ½ cup 3
store-bought (without liquor), ½ cup........5

Eggplant, cooked, 1 cup 0

Eggplant parmigiana
frozen, 5 oz 4
without sauce, 1 serving (3" x 4") 11
with sauce, 1 serving (3" x 4"), with
½ cup Italian tomato sauce 13

Egg rolls
beef, 1 (4½" long) 5
chicken, 1 (4½" long) 4
chicken, store-bought, 1 (3 oz) 3
pork, 1 (4½" long) 5
pork, store-bought, 1 (3 oz) 3
shrimp, 1 (4½" long) 4
shrimp, store-bought, 1 (3 oz) 3
vegetable, store-bought, 1 (3 oz) 3

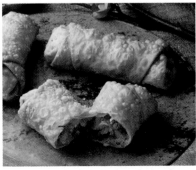

Egg roll snacks
pork or shrimp, store-bought, 3 oz 3
vegetable, store-bought, 3 oz 3

Egg roll wrapper, 1 1

Eggs
deviled, 2 stuffed halves 4
fried, 1 large 2
scrambled, 2 or ½ cup 5
substitute, fat-free, ¼ cup 1
substitute, regular, ¼ cup 2
white, 1 0
whites, 3 1
whole, 1 2

Egg salad, ½ cup 8

Egg salad sandwich, 1 11

Eggs Benedict, 2 English muffin
halves with 2 eggs and ¼ cup
Hollandaise sauce...............................16

Elderberries, 1 cup 1

Elk, cooked, 1 oz 1

Empanadas, 2 (3" diameter) 5

Emu, cooked, 1 oz 1

Enchiladas
beef, 2 12
cheese, 2 10
chicken, 2 9
frozen, beef, cheese, or chicken,
1 (4¼ oz) 4
meals, frozen, beef, cheese, or chicken
(2 enchiladas, beans, and rice), 1
(11½ oz) 7
pork, 2 12
sour cream, 1 8

Enchilada sauce, canned, ½ cup 1

Endive, 1 cup.......................................0

English muffins
light, 1 1
regular, 1 (2 oz) 2

Escargots, 6 snails with 2 Tbsp butter 7

Escarole, 1 cup (2 oz)............................0

Etouffee
crawfish, 1 cup....................................20
crawfish or shrimp, store-bought, 1 cup ...8
shrimp, 1 cup 9

Etouffee mix, 2 Tbsp 1

Fadge, 1 cup..3

Fajita kit, beef or chicken, frozen,
prepared, 2 fajitas (7½ oz) 5

Fajitas
beef, 2 11
chicken, 2...8
pork, 2 13
shrimp, 2..8

Falafel in pita, 1 large pita with
4 falafel patties 13

Falafel patties
4 (2" diameter each) 10
from mix, prepared, 2 patties....................4

**Fennel (anise, sweet anise, or
finocchio),** 1 cup 0

Fettuccine Alfredo
1 cup..16
frozen, 1 cup 7

**Fettuccine with broccoli and
chicken in Alfredo sauce,** frozen,
1 cup..9

Fiddlefern (fiddlehead greens),
1 cup..0

Figs
dried, 1 1
fresh, 1 0

Fillo dough, frozen, 1½ sheets (1 oz)......2

Fish
anchovies, canned in oil, drained, 6..........1
baked, stuffed, 1 serving 8
bass, striped, cooked, 1 fillet (6 oz) 5

blackened, 1 fillet (6 oz) **12**
bluefish, cooked, 1 fillet (6 oz)................6
carp, cooked, 1 fillet (6 oz) 7
catfish, cooked, 1 fillet (6 oz)..................6
cod, cooked, 1 fillet (6 oz) 4
dried, 1 oz...2
eel, cooked, 1 oz....................................2
flounder, cooked, 1 fillet (6 oz)................4
fried, 1 fillet (6 oz)...............................**12**
grouper, cooked, 1 fillet (6 oz) 4
haddock, cooked, 1 fillet (6 oz)................4
halibut, cooked, 1 fillet (6 oz) 5
herring, cooked, 1 oz..............................1
mackerel, canned, ½ cup........................3
mackerel, cooked, 1 fillet (6 oz) 8
mahimahi (dolphinfish), cooked, 1 fillet
(6 oz)...4
perch, cooked, 6 oz................................4
pike, cooked, 1 fillet (6 oz)......................4
pollock, cooked, 6 oz 4
pompano, cooked, 6 oz 9
rockfish, cooked, 1 fillet (6 oz) 4
salmon, canned, drained, ½ cup (4 oz) 4
salmon, cooked, 1 fillet (6 oz)..................7
salmon, grilled, frozen, 3 oz.....................2
salmon, smoked, 1 oz 1
sardines, canned in oil, drained, 5 3
smelt, cooked, 1 oz 1
snapper, cooked, 1 fillet (6 oz) 4
sole, cooked, 1 fillet (6 oz)......................4
stuffed, frozen, 1 (5 oz) 5
swordfish, cooked, 1 steak (6 oz) 4
trout, cooked, 1 fillet (6 oz) 8
trout, rainbow, cooked, 1 fillet (6 oz)........6
tuna, canned in oil, drained, ½ cup 5
tuna, canned in water, drained, ½ cup......3
tuna, cooked, 1 fillet (6 oz).....................6
tuna, grilled, frozen, 1 oz.........................2
whitefish, smoked, 2 oz...........................1
whiting, cooked, 6 oz 4

Fish amandine, 1 fillet (6 oz) **13**
Fish and brewis, 1 cup......................**13**

Fish and cheese sandwich, fried, fast food, 1 13

Fish and chips, 5 oz fish fillet with 20 chips (French fries).........................15

Fish fillets
battered (prepared without fat), frozen, 1 (3 oz)..5
breaded (prepared without fat), frozen, 2 (3¾ oz)..7
grilled, with garlic butter, frozen, 1 (3¾ oz) 3
grilled, with lemon pepper, frozen, 1 (3¾ oz) 3
light, breaded (prepared without fat), frozen, 3¾ oz..3

Fish fillet sandwich, frozen, 1 (4½ oz) 8

Fish portions, breaded or battered, prepared from minced fish (prepared without fat), frozen, 3 oz......................5

Fish sticks, breaded, frozen, 4 (2½ oz) 4

Fish Veronique, 1 fillet (6 oz) 11

Flan, ¾ cup 8

Flanken, 2 slices (4 oz).........................8

Flatbreads, ¾ oz 1

Flautas
beef, 1 (6" x 1¼") 12
chicken, 1 (6" x 1¼") 10
pork, 1 (6" x 1¼").................................11

Flax seed, 1 Tbsp.................................1

Flour
potato, 1 tsp 0
potato, ¼ cup...2
soy, ¼ cup 2
white, 1 cup 9
white, 3 Tbsp...1
white, 1 tsp...0
whole wheat, 1 cup 8
whole wheat, 3 Tbsp...............................1
whole wheat, 1 tsp.................................0

Focaccia bread
1 piece (10" diameter)..........................25
any type, store-bought, 2 oz 3

Fondue, cheese, ½ cup fondue with 2 oz bread 12

Frankfurter rolls
light, 1 (1½ oz)......................................2
reduced-calorie, 1 1
regular, 1 (2 oz) 3

Frankfurters
beef or pork, fat-free, 1 (1¾ oz)............1
beef or pork, light, 1 (1¾ oz)..................2
beef or pork, regular, 1 (2 oz) 5
beef or pork, with cheese, 1 (2 oz)...........5
chicken, 1 (2 oz) 4
turkey, 1 (2 oz) 3
turkey, fat-free, 1 (1½ oz) 1
turkey, light, 1 (2 oz).............................3

F

Franks in blankets, frozen, 6 (3 oz) 9

French fries
fast food, 1 small serving 6
fast food, 1 medium serving.................10
fast food, 1 large serving 13
frozen, baked, 15 (3 oz) 2
homemade, 20 (each 4½" long) 10

French toast
2 slices 7
frozen, baked, 2 slices (4 oz)...................5

French toast sticks
fast food, 5 pieces 12
frozen, 3 (2½ oz) 6

Fritters
corn, 3 (2½" x 2" each) 5
vegetable, 1 cup 10

Frog legs, fried, 2 4

Fromage frais (soft cheese with fruit), 3½ oz...3

Frosting
store-bought, reduced-fat, 2 Tbsp 3
store-bought, regular, 2 Tbsp 3

Fruit
candied, 2 Tbsp 1
dried, mixed, ¼ cup 2
spreadable, 1½ Tbsp 1

Fruit butter, 1 Tbsp....................................1

Fruitcake, 1 slice (2½" x 1¾" x ½") or 2 oz...4

Fruit cocktail, unsweetened, canned, 1 cup...2

Fruit compote, ½ cup..........................4

Fruit drink mix, powdered, prepared, 1 cup...2

Fruit-flavored pieces, 1 package.........2

Fruit-flavored rolls
1 large..1
1 small 1

Fruit ice, ½ cup 3

Fruit juice, combined, ½ cup..................1

Fruit juice bars
1 1
no sugar added, frozen, 2 (2 oz each) 1

Fruit juice cup, frozen, 1 cup 3

Fruit salad, 1 cup..................................2

Fudge, plain, 1 piece (1" x 2") or 1 oz.....3

Funnel cake, ½ (8" diameter) 12

Garlic bread
1 slice (1 oz) 5
frozen, 1 piece (1½ oz)............................4

Gefilte fish, 1 piece (1½ oz) 1

Gelatin
fruit-flavored, ½ cup 2
fruit-flavored, sugar-free, ½ cup 0

Gelatin fruit mold, ½ cup....................2

General Tso's chicken, 1 cup.............15

Giardeniera (vegetable medley, without olives, packed in vinegar), 5 pieces (1 oz).......................................0

Gin, 1 jigger (1½ fl oz) 2

Gin and tonic, 1 (6 fl oz)........................3

Gin gimlet, 1 (2½ fl oz) 2

Gingerbread, 1 piece (3" square) 9

Gizzard, chicken, cooked, 1 oz................1

Gnocchi
any type, frozen, 1 cup 7
cheese, 1 cup 11
potato, 1 cup 4
potato, dry, 1 cup 3
potato, refrigerated, 1 cup......................5
spinach, 1 cup 12

Goat, cooked, 1 oz....................................1

Gobo (burdock), ½ cup 1

Goose
with skin, cooked, 2 oz............................4
without skin, cooked, 2 oz.......................3

Gooseberries, 1 cup 1

Gordita, beef, 1 (3" diameter) 10

Gourd, white, flowered, 1 cup 0

Graham cracker crumbs, 2 Tbsp 1

Graham crackers
2 (2½" square)..1
chocolate-coated, 2 (2½" square) 3
mini, any variety, ¾ oz 2

Granola bars
chocolate-covered, 1 4
reduced-calorie, 1 (1 oz)......................2
regular, 1 3

Grapefruit
juice, ½ cup..1
sections, 1 cup....................................2
whole, 1 small (8 oz)...........................1
whole, 1 large (16 oz) 2

Grape juice, ½ cup..............................2

Grape leaves, 1 cup 0

Grapes, 1 cup 1

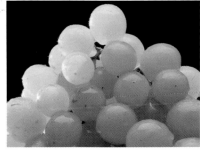

Gravy
beef, canned, ¼ cup.............................1
brown, ¼ cup 2
chicken, canned, ¼ cup 1
cream, ¼ cup 4
fat-free, canned, ½ cup 1
giblet, ¼ cup 2
sausage, ¼ cup...................................4
sausage, canned, ¼ cup 2
turkey, canned, 1 cup 1

Gravy and salisbury steak, frozen,
1 steak with gravy (4¾ oz) 4

Gravy and sliced beef
canned, ½ cup....................................6
frozen, 2 slices with gravy (4¾ oz) 2

Gravy and sliced turkey, frozen,
2 slices with gravy (4¾ oz) 2

Greek salad
with dressing, 3 cups 9
without dressing, 3 cups 2

Green bean casserole, 1 cup...............5

Green papaya, 1 cup...........................1

Green rice, 1 cup 8

Greens
beet, 1 cup...0
chard, 1 cup 0
collard, 1 cup 0
dandelion, 1 cup..................................0
kale, 1 cup 0
mustard, 1 cup 0
turnip, 1 cup 0
seasoned with bacon or salt pork, 1 cup....4

Green tea ice cream, ½ cup 3

Grinder sandwich, 1 (6")....................6

Guacamole
¼ cup 2
store-bought, ¼ cup 2

Guava, 1 cup 1

Guinea hen, cooked, 1 oz 1

Gum, chewing, with sugar or sugarless,
1 piece 0

Gumbo
chicken, 1 cup 6
seafood, 1 cup.....................................5
seafood, with rice, store-bought, 1 cup.....5
with rice mix, ¼ cup 3

Gumbo base (seasoning mix),
1½ Tbsp...1

Gyro, 1 (6") 15

Halvah
1 piece (2" x 1¾" x 1")..........................5
store-bought, 1½ oz 6

G

H

Ham
cooked, lean, 1 slice or ½ cup cubed
   or shredded (2 oz) 2
cooked, regular, 1 slice or ½ cup cubed
   or shredded (2 oz) 3
glazed with pineapple, 4 oz ham with
   ½ pineapple slice 6

Ham and cheese sandwich,
   restaurant-style, grilled, 1....................15

Hamantaschen, 1 piece (3" diameter) ...3

Hamburger buns
1 (2 oz)...3
light, 1..2
reduced-calorie, 1 1

Hamburger dinner in a box,
   prepared, 1 cup 7

Hamburgers on buns
large, fast food, 1 13
microwave, frozen, 1 small (1½ oz)..........3
small, fast food, 1 6
without mayonnaise, lettuce, and
   tomato, 1 9

Haroset, 1 cup.......................................4

Hash
corned beef, canned, 1 cup...................10
roast beef, canned, 1 cup 9

Hazelnut and chocolate spread,
   1 Tbsp 2

Hazelnuts, 20 nuts (1 oz shelled)............4

Heart
beef, cooked, 1 oz...................................1
chicken, cooked, 1 oz 1

Hearts of palm (palmetto), 1 cup......0

Hero sandwich, 1 (6")........................6

Herring
chopped, ¼ cup......................................4
fillets, store-bought, ¼ cup......................3
in cream sauce, ¼ cup 3
in wine sauce, ½ cup 2
pickled, ½ cup.......................................2
salad, store-bought, ¼ cup......................3

Highball, 1 (6 fl oz)..............................3

Hoagie sandwich, 1 (6")......................6

Hollandaise sauce
¼ cup 8
store-bought, ¼ cup 4

Hominy, whole, cooked, 1 cup.................2

Honey
1 Tbsp..1
1 cup...20

Honeybun, glazed, 1 (4" x 3" oval)......6

Honey cake, 1 slice (5" x 3" x 1") 7

Honeydew melon
⅛ (6 oz)..1
1 cup..1

Honey roll, 1 5

Horse, cooked, 1 oz 1

Horseradish, prepared, 1 Tbsp 0

Horseradish sauce, store-bought,
   2 Tbsp 3

Horseradish tree leaves, cooked,
   1 cup...0

Hot chocolate
homemade, with whipped topping,
   1 cup...7
homemade, without whipped topping,
   1 cup...6

Hot dogs (see Frankfurters)

Hot dog sauce, ¼ cup 1

Huevos rancheros, 2 eggs on
   2 tortillas...14

Hummus
   ¼ cup..3
   store-bought, ¼ cup 2

Hunan beef, 1 cup 9

Hush puppies
   2...4
   frozen (prepared without fat), 3 (2 oz) 2

Hush puppy mix, ¼ cup 3

Ice cream
   fat free, no sugar added, 1 scoop or
     ½ cup...2
   fat-free, sweetened with sugar, 1 scoop
     or ½ cup..2
   fried, 1 scoop or ½ cup 11
   light, no sugar added, 1 scoop or
     ½ cup (4 fl oz).....................................2
   light, sweetened with sugar, 1 scoop
     or ½ cup..3
   premium, 1 scoop or ½ cup....................7
   regular, 1 scoop or ½ cup.......................4

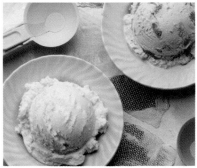

Ice cream bars
   chocolate-covered, 1 (3 fl oz) 5
   chocolate-covered with crisp rice,
     no sugar added, 1 (1½ oz) 3
   chocolate-covered with crisp rice,
     sweetened with sugar, 1 (2 oz).............5

Ice cream cone, plain or sugar, 1 small...1

Ice cream sandwich
   1 4
   reduced-calorie, 1 4

Ice cream soda, 12 fl oz.......................8

Ice cream sundae, ½ cup ice cream
   with syrup, nuts, and whipped topping...8

Ice cream sundae cone, 1 (3½ oz) 8

Ice pop, fruit-flavored
   1 (1¾ fl oz)..1
   frozen, 1¾ fl oz.......................................1

Imperial roll, 1 (4½" long)....................4

Instant breakfast powder
   1 envelope...3
   prepared with reduced-fat (2%) milk, 1....5
   prepared with fat-free milk, 1 4
   prepared with whole milk, 1...................6

Irish brown stew, 1 cup......................7

Irish coffee, 6 fl oz with 2 Tbsp
   whipped cream 4

Irish soda bread, ¹⁄₁₂ of 8" round loaf
   (3½ oz)..5

Italian ice, restaurant-prepared, ½ cup ...1

Italian toast snacks, store-bought, 4
   (1 oz)...3

Jackfruit, uncooked, ½ cup 1

Jalapeño bread, 1 slice (1½ oz) 2

Jalapeño poppers, 1 4

Jalapeños, stuffed (prepared without
   fat), store-bought, 2 (2 oz) 4

Jam, 1 Tbsp 1

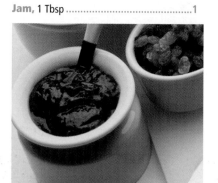

Jamaican rice and peas, 1 cup 6

Jambalaya
chicken, with rice, 1½ cups......................9
fish, with rice, 1½ cups 7

Jambalaya mix, ¼ cup 3

Jelly, 1 Tbsp 1

Jerk chicken breast, 1 large breast
(without skin).....................................5

Jerusalem artichokes (sunchokes),
1 cup...2

Jicama, 1 cup 1

K

Kabobs
beef or lamb, 2.......................................8
chicken, 2...8
fish, 2 6

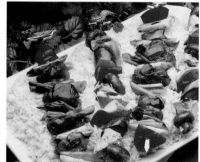

Kasha (buckwheat groats)
cooked, 1 cup..3
uncooked, ¼ cup 2

Kasha varnishkes, 1 cup......................4

Kashmiri (lamb meatballs), 6
(3½ oz)..11

Kataifi, 1 piece (2" long).......................5

Ketchup
¼ cup 1
1 Tbsp..0

Key lime pie, ⅛ of 9" one-crust pie 12

Kheer, ½ cup...5

Kibbe
baked, 3 pieces (1½" squares).................3
uncooked, ½ cup 4

Kidney
beef, cooked, 1 oz...................................1
pork, cooked, 1 oz 1

Kielbasa, 1 oz 2

Kim Chee, ½ cup 0

King ranch chicken casserole,
1 cup...8

Kishke, 1 small piece.............................4

Kiwi fruit, 1 (4 oz) 1

Knish
potato, 1 (3½" square) 6
potato, store-bought, 1 (4½ oz) 4

Knockwurst, 2 oz 5

Kohlrabi
cooked, 1 cup..1
uncooked, 1 cup 0

Korma
chicken, 1 cup 14
lamb, 1 cup 15
vegetable, 1 cup 11

Kreplachs
boiled, 2 pieces (4" x 3" x 3" each).........5
fried, 2 pieces (4" x 3" x 3" each) 7
frozen, 4 (3 oz) 4

Kugel

lukschen, 1 piece (3" x 3 ¼")..................7

noodle, store-bought, ½ cup....................3

potato, 1 piece (3" x 3 ¼").....................3

potato, store-bought, ½ cup 4

Kumquats, 5 (3 oz)...............................0

Kung Pao

beef, 1 cup 10

chicken, 1 cup 8

pork, 1 cup..9

sauce, 2 Tbsp..1

shrimp, 1 cup 9

Ladyfingers, store-bought, 1 large or
2 small (½ oz) 1

Lamb

ground, cooked, ½ cup (2 oz) 4

lean (leg and loin cuts with all visible
fat trimmed), cooked, 1 slice, 1 chop,
or ½ cup cubed or shredded (2 oz) 3

regular, cooked, 1 slice, 1 chop, or ½ cup
cubed or shredded (2 oz) 4

Lamb biryani, 1 cup 12

Lamb stew, 1 cup 5

Lambs quarters, cooked, 1 cup.............1

Lard, 1 Tbsp 3

Lasagna

cheese, with tomato sauce, frozen,
1 (10 oz)...8

chicken, frozen, 1 cup 5

noodles, uncooked, 2½ (2 oz) 4

vegetable, frozen, 1 cup 5

vegetarian, with cheese, 1 serving 10

vegetarian, with cheese and spinach,
1 serving...9

with meat, 1 cup 6

with meat sauce, frozen, 1 cup 6

Latte

made with fat-free milk, grande, 1
(16 fl oz)...3

made with fat-free milk, small, 1
(8 fl oz)...2

made with fat-free milk, tall, 1 (12 fl oz)....2

made with low-fat milk, grande, 1
(16 fl oz)...5

made with low-fat milk, small, 1 (8 fl oz)....3

made with low-fat milk, tall, 1 (12 fl oz) 4

made with whole milk, grande, 1
(16 fl oz)...6

made with whole milk, small, 1 (8 fl oz)...3

made with whole milk, tall, 1 (12 fl oz) 5

Lavash, ¼ of 10" cracker (2¼ oz)............6

Leeks

cooked, 1 cup 0

uncooked, 1 cup 0

Lemon, 1 0

Lemon grass chicken, 1 cup 8

Lemonade, 1 cup 2

Lentils

cooked, ½ cup 2

uncooked, 1 pound 30

Lettuce

iceberg, 1 cup..0

romaine, 1 cup 0

Limeade, 1 cup.....................................2

Linguini

with red clam sauce, 1 cup linguini
with ½ cup sauce 6

with white clam sauce, 1 cup linguini
with ½ cup sauce 8

Liqueurs, any type, 1 jigger (1½ fl oz) 4

Liver

beef, cooked, ½ cup (2 oz) or 1 slice 2

chicken, cooked, ½ cup (2 oz) 2

chopped, ¼ cup.....................................5

with bacon, 2 slices (4 oz) 9

with onions, 2 slices (4 oz) 7

L

Liver pâté, 1 slice (4¼" x 1½" x ½") 3

Liverwurst, 1 oz 3

Lobster
Cantonese, 1 cup 9
Newburg, 1 cup 11
roll sandwich, 1 5
salad, ½ cup......................................4
salad sandwich, 1 8
steamed, 1 (1¼ pound lobster or
    4½ oz lobster meat) 3
thermidor, 1 cup 16

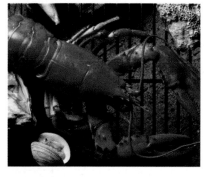

Lo mein
beef, 1 cup 8
chicken, 1 cup 8
pork, 1 cup..8
shrimp, 1 cup 8

Loganberries, 1 cup 1

Loquats, 10.....................................1

Lotus root, cooked, 1 cup 1

Luncheon meat
canned, 2 oz 5
fat-free, 2 oz 1
lean (3 g fat or less per oz), 1 slice
   (1 oz)..1
light, canned, 2 oz 3
regular (4 g fat or more per oz), 1 slice
   (1 oz)..2

Macadamia nuts, shelled, 12 (1 oz) 5

Macaroni
cooked, 1 cup......................................3
uncooked, 1 pound 34
uncooked, 1 cup 7

Macaroni and cheese
1 cup...9
frozen, 1 cup.......................................6
package mix, prepared, 1 cup.................9
in a cup, 1 (2 oz) 5

Macaroni salad
½ cup...6
store-bought, ½ cup 5

Mandarin orange
1 large or 2 small (6 oz) 1
unsweetened, canned, 1 cup 2

Mandelbrot, 2 slices (3" x 2" x ½") 3

Mango
1 (8 oz)...2
1 cup 2

Manhattan, 1 (2 fl oz) 3

Manicotti
cheese, with tomato sauce, frozen, 1
   (10 oz)...8
cheese, without sauce, frozen, 2 (5½ oz) ..6
shells, uncooked, 2 (1 oz) 2
with meat sauce, 2 shells with ½ cup
   sauce...15
with tomato sauce, 2 shells with
   ½ cup sauce.....................................12

Margarine
fat-free, 4 Tbsp 1
reduced-calorie, 2 tsp...........................1
regular, 1 cup 50
regular, 1 tsp......................................1

Margarita, 1 (4 fl oz)..........................5

Margarita mix, ½ cup 3

Marinara sauce
½ cup 3
store-bought, ½ cup 2

M

Marmalade, 1 Tbsp 1

Marshmallow, 2 medium (½ oz)............1

Marshmallow créme, store-bought,
2 Tbsp 1

Martini, 1 (2 fl oz) 3

Marzipan, 1 (1 oz)...............................3

Matzo, 1 board 2

Matzo brie, ¼ of 10" round or 1 cup 6

Matzo farfel, store-bought, ¼ cup.........1

Matzo meal
3 Tbsp..2
1 tsp...0

Mayonnaise
commercial and homemade, 1 tsp 1
fat-free, 4 Tbsp 1
reduced-calorie, 2 tsp...........................1

**Meal replacement/supplement bar
for weight loss,** 1 (1 oz)...................3

**Meal replacement/supplement
drink,** 1 cup (8 fl oz) 5

**Meal replacement/supplement
drink for weight loss** (prepared from
powder using fat-free milk, or canned),
1 cup.......................................3

Meat, ground
cooked, 1 patty (3 oz) 6
lean, cooked, 1 patty (3 oz) 6

Meatballs
without sauce, 2 (each 1¼" diameter) ...10
without sauce, frozen, 6 (3 oz)................6
with sauce, 2 meatballs and
½ cup Italian tomato sauce.................13

Meat loaf, 1 slice (⅝" thick) 6

Meat sauce, ½ cup 5

Meat spread, canned, ¼ cup.................3

Melba toast, 4 slices or 6 rounds
(¾ oz) 1

Melon balls, 1 cup 1

**Menudo (beef tripe and hominy
stew)**
1 cup......................................6
canned, 1 cup...........................4

Mexican coffee, 6 fl oz with 2 Tbsp
whipped cream 3

Mexican seven-layer dip, ½ cup 3

Mexican wedding cookies, 2
each 1½" wide) 2

Milk
buttermilk, fat-free, low-fat (1%), or
reduced-fat (2%), 1 cup 2
chocolate, low-fat, 1 cup 3
chocolate, reduced-fat, 1 cup...................4
chocolate, regular, 1 cup 4
evaporated, fat-free, ½ cup 2
evaporated, low-fat, ½ cup......................2
evaporated, whole, ½ cup 3
fat-free, 1 cup...................................2
goat, 1 cup......................................4
instant nonfat dry powder, ⅓ cup 2
low-fat (½% or 1%) or light, 1 cup 2
reduced-fat (2%), 1 cup 3
sweetened condensed, ½ cup................11
whole, 1 cup 4

Milk shake, any flavor, fast food,
1 (10 fl oz)................................9

Millet
cooked, 1 cup.....................................4
uncooked, ¼ cup 3

Mimosa, 1 (6 fl oz)...............................2

Mincemeat, store-bought, ¼ cup 3

Mincemeat pie
with meat, ⅛ of 9" two-crust pie...........14
without meat, ⅛ of 9" two-crust pie......14

Mince pie, frozen, 1 slice (4¼ oz) 7

Miso, 1 tsp...0

Molasses
1 Tbsp.......................................1
blackstrap, 1 Tbsp...................................1

M

Mole poblano, ¼ cup 4

Mole sauce
store-bought, brown, 2 Tbsp...................5
store-bought, green, 2 Tbsp.....................4

Mongolian beef, 1 cup.........................8

Moo goo gai pan, 1 cup 7

Moose, cooked, 1 oz.............................1

Moo shoo pork, ½ cup with
2 pancakes...10

Mornay sauce, ¼ cup 4

Moussaka, 1 piece (3" x 4") 12

Mozzarella
breaded, frozen (prepared without fat),
2 pieces (1 oz)....................................3
fried, 2 slices (2¾" x 1" x ½" each) 10

Muffins
any type (other than those listed here),
1 large (3" diameter)...........................6
any type, fast food, 1 6
any type, store-bought, 1 large (4 oz).....10
breakfast (egg and cheese with sausage,
ham, or Canadian bacon on English
muffin), frozen, 1 (4½ oz)......................7
fat-free, store-bought, 1 small or
½ large (2 oz) 2
mini, any type, store-bought, 2 (2 oz).......6

Muffuletta, 1 (6").............................20

Mulberries, 1 cup 1

**Mushroom gravy and charbroiled
beef patty,** frozen, 1 patty with gravy
(5¾ oz) 4

Mushrooms
breaded (prepared without fat), 7 (3 oz)...3
dried, 4 large or 16 small 1
dried, reconstituted, 1 cup.....................1
fresh, 1 cup 0
marinated, ½ cup 3
stuffed, 4 3

Mussels Mariniere, 4 mussels with
3 Tbsp sauce 7

Mustard, 1 tsp....................................0

Naan, 1 piece (7" x 8" diameter).............4

Nachos
beef, 4 13
cheese, 4..8
cheese and bean, 4................................9
chicken, 4..11
with cheese sauce, ½ cup tortilla chips
with ¼ cup cheese sauce 5

Nam Prik, 1 Tbsp 1

Napoleon, 1 piece (4½" x 2" x 1½")....13

Nebeyaki udon, 2 cups 8

Nectar, any type, ½ cup 1

Nectarine, 1 (2½" diameter).................1

Noodles
cellophane, cooked, 1 cup 3
cellophane, uncooked, 2 oz 4
egg, cooked, 1 cup.................................3
egg, uncooked, 1 cup..............................3
Oriental (bean thread), cooked, 1 cup 4

Noodles and sauce mix, prepared,
½ cup 3

Nuoc cham, 1 Tbsp................................0

POINTS

Nuts
mixed, shelled, 1 oz 4
wheat-based, 1 oz 5

Oat milk, any flavor, 1 cup 2

Oil
vegetable, 1 tsp.....................................1
vegetable, 1 cup 58

Okra
breaded, frozen (prepared without fat),
  ¾ cup...2
cooked, 1 cup.......................................0
fried, 1 cup..8

Old fashioned, 1 (2 fl oz).....................3

Olives
10 small (1 oz) 1
6 large (1 oz) 1

Olive spread, store-bought, 1 Tbsp 2

Omelets
cheese, 1 (2-egg) 8
ham and cheese, 1 (2-egg) 9
herb or plain, 1 (2-egg) 6
vegetable, 1 (2-egg)..............................7

Onion, blooming, battered and fried,
  ¼ (16" diameter) 6

Onion rings
breaded, frozen (prepared without fat),
  10 large rings (3-4" diameter)...............7
fast food, 1 medium serving (8-9 onion
  rings)...10
fried, 4 (4" diameter each) 6

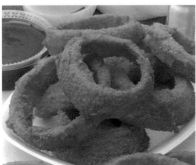

POINTS

Onions
cooked, 1 cup..1
uncooked, 1 cup 0

Opossum, cooked, 1 oz 1

Orange
1 (5 oz)..1
juice, ½ cup...1
orange-grapefruit juice, ½ cup 1
sections, 1 cup..1

Osso bucco, 6 oz veal with
  ¼ cup sauce......................................13

Ostrich, cooked, 1 oz..............................1

Oyster pie, 1 slice (⅛ of 9" pie) 9

Oyster po' boy, 1 (6")........................17

Oysters Rockefeller, 4 5

Pad Thai, 1 cup....................................7

Paella, 1 cup.......................................7

Pakora, vegetable, 1 (2" x 3") or
  1¾ oz...3

Pancake and sausage on a stick,
  1 (2 oz)...5

Pancakes
any type, from mix, 1 (4" diameter) 1
any type, frozen, 1 (4" diameter) 2
Chinese, 3 2
fast food, without margarine and syrup,
  3 6
homemade, 1 (4" diameter) 3
mini, frozen, without syrup, 6 (2¼ oz) 3

Panettone, 1/12 of 9" tube or 1½ oz 6

Panini
chicken, 1...11
ham and cheese, 1................................11
vegetable, 1 10

Papaya
fresh, ½ (8 oz)......................................1
fresh, 1 cup 1

O

P

35

Paprikash, ½ cup chicken mixture
with ½ cup sauce 9

Paratha, 1 (4" triangle) 4

Parsley, 1 cup 0

Parsnips
cooked, 1 cup (5½ oz)..............................2
uncooked, 1 cup 1

Passion fruit, 3 0

Passover sponge cake, ½₂ of 9" tube...3

Pasta
cooked, 1 cup..3
uncooked, 1½ oz 3
uncooked, 1 cup 7
uncooked, 1 pound 34
whole wheat, cooked, 1 cup 3
whole wheat, uncooked, 2 oz 4

Pasta e fagioli, 1 cup 8

Pasta primavera
2 cups..6
with cream sauce, 1 cup pasta with
¾ cup sauce 12

Pasta salad
½ cup 3
packaged (prepared according to
directions), ½ cup 4
store-bought, ½ cup 3

Pasta sauce
bottled, any type, ½ cup.........................2
bottled, any type, reduced-fat, ½ cup 1

Pasta shells, stuffed with ricotta
cheese, without sauce, frozen,
2-3 pieces (5¼ oz) 6

Pastitsio, 1 piece (3¼" x 3")...............11

Pastrami
beef, 1 slice (1 oz)....................................3
turkey, 1 slice (1 oz) 1

Pâté
fish, store-bought, 2 oz 3
meat, store-bought, ¼ cup (2 oz)............5

Peaches
canned, unsweetened, 1 cup 2
fresh, 1 (6 oz)...1

Peach melba, ½ cup ice cream with
2 peach halves and raspberry sauce.......8

Peanut brittle
1 oz...4
store-bought, 4 pieces (1 oz) 3

Peanut butter
1 Tbsp...2
reduced-fat, 1 Tbsp 2

Peanuts
40 (1 oz) 4
chocolate-covered, 1 oz 3
honey, reduced-fat, ¼ cup 2

Peanut sauce
2 Tbsp...4
Thai, canned, 2 Tbsp 2

Pears
canned, unsweetened, 1 cup 2
fresh, 1 (6 oz)...1
poached, 1 pear with 2 Tbsp whipped
cream 4

Peas
black-eyed, cooked, ½ cup 1
black-eyed, uncooked, 1 pound..............30
chick, cooked, ½ cup 2
chick, dry, 1 pound.................................35
green, cooked, 1 cup 2
snow (Chinese pea pods), 1 cup 0
split, cooked, ½ cup 2
split, uncooked, 1 pound 31
sugar snap, 1 cup 0

Pecans, 14 halves (1 oz) 5

Peking duck, 2 oz duck with 1 piece
duck skin and 3 pancakes 11

Penne a la vodka, 1 cup pasta with
½ cup sauce...7

Peppers
bell, 1 0
bell, 1 cup 0

P

stuffed with beef, in tomato sauce,
    frozen, 1 (7 oz) 4
stuffed with beef and rice, 1 6

Pepper steak, 6 oz 13

Pepperoni, 1 oz 4

Persimmon, 1 (6 oz) 2

Pesto sauce
    2 Tbsp..3
    store-bought, 2 Tbsp 3

Petite marmite, 2 cups 7

Petit fours, 2 (1¾" x 1½" x 1" each) 3

Pheasant, cooked, 1 oz 2

Philly cheese steak sandwich, 1 13

Phyllo dough, frozen, 1½ sheets (1 oz) ..2

Picadillo, 1 cup 10

Pickles
    dill, 1 cup or 1 medium 0
    sweet, 2 large, 4 midgets, 1½ spears,
        1 large gherkin, or 1 oz........................1

Pico de gallo, ½ cup.............................0

Pie crusts
    any type, ⅛ of 9" one-crust pie 5
    any type, ⅛ of 9" two-crust pie 7
    any type, frozen, 1 slice (⅛ of 9" crust) 2
    any type, refrigerated, ⅛ of 9" crust 2
    graham cracker, ⅛ of 9" crust 5

Pie fillings
    canned, fruit, ⅓ cup 2
    fruit, light, ⅓ cup 1

Pierogies
    cabbage, 3 (each 3½")............................7
    cheese, 3 (each 3½") 7
    meat, 3 (each 3½") 8
    potato, 3 (each 3½") 7
    potato and cheese or onion, low-fat,
        frozen, 3 (4½ oz) 4
    potato and cheese, frozen, 3 (4 oz) 4

Pies
    custard, ⅛ of 9" one-crust pie 8
    fruit, any type, frozen, 1 slice
        (2½" x 1¾" x ½") 8
    fruit, fast food, 1 7
    fruit, one-crust, 1 slice (⅛ of 9" pie) 6
    fruit, two-crust, 1 slice (⅛ of 9" pie) 9
    individual, 1 (5" x 3¾").........................9
    meringue, 1 slice (⅛ of 9" pie)..............10
    meringue, any type, frozen, 1 slice (5 oz) ..7
    pecan, ⅛ of 9" one-crust pie 11
    pecan, frozen, 1 slice (4½ oz) 10
    pumpkin, ⅛ of 9" one-crust pie 8
    pumpkin, frozen, 1 slice (5 oz) 6
    rhubarb, ⅛ of 9" two-crust pie 11

Pigeon, cooked, 1 oz 1

Pigs' feet, pickled, store-bought, 2 oz 3

Pigs in blankets, 2 (1 oz) 6

Pimiento-cheese spread
    reduced-fat, store-bought, 2 Tbsp 2
    regular, store-bought, 2 Tbsp 3

Pimientos, 1 cup 1

Piña colada, 1 (5 fl oz) 6

Piña colada mix, ½ cup 4

Pineapple
    fresh, ¼ (12 oz)....................................1
    fresh, 1 cup 1
    chunks, canned, unsweetened, 1 cup 2
    juice, ½ cup (4 fl oz) 1

Pineapple upside down cake,
    1 slice (⅛ of 10" skillet cake) 10

Pine nuts (pignolias), 1 oz 4

Pistachios, shelled, 40 nuts (1 oz) 4

Pita, any type, 1 small or ½ large (1 oz) ...1

Pizza
    Canadian style bacon, frozen, 1 slice
        (5 oz)..7
    cheese, deep dish, restaurant-type, 1 slice
        (⅛ of 12", ⅒ of 14", or ⅟₁₂ of 16") 5

P

cheese, deep dish, restaurant-type, 1 slice
(⅛ of 14", ⅒ of 16", or 1/12 of 18") 7

cheese, deep dish, restaurant-type,
1 slice (⅛ of 18") 10

cheese, frozen, 1 slice (5 oz) 8

cheese, single serving, fast food, 1 14

cheese, thin crust, restaurant-type, 1 slice
(⅛ of 12", ⅒ of 14", or 1/12 of 16") 4

cheese, thin crust, restaurant-type, 1 slice
(⅛ of 14", ⅒ of 16", or 1/12 of 18") 5

cheese, thin crust, restaurant-type,
1 slice (⅛ of 18") 9

hamburger, frozen, 1 slice (5 oz) 8

meat and vegetable, thin crust, 1 slice
(⅛ of 12", ⅒ of 14", or 1/12 of 16") 4

meat and vegetable, thin crust, 1 slice
(⅛ of 14", ⅒ of 16", or 1/12 of 18") 5

meat and vegetable, thin crust, 1 slice
(⅛ of 18") 9

one-meat topping, deep dish, restaurant-
type, 1 slice (⅛ of 12", ⅒ of 14", or
1/12 of 16") 6

one-meat topping, deep dish, restaurant-
type, 1 slice (⅛ of 14", ⅒ of 16", or
1/12 of 18") 8

one-meat topping, deep dish, restaurant-
type, 1 slice (⅛ of 18") 11

one-meat topping, thin crust, restaurant-
type, 1 slice (⅛ of 12", ⅒ of 14", or
1/12 of 16") 5

one-meat topping, thin crust, restaurant-
type, 1 slice (⅛ of 14", ⅒ of 16", or
1/12 of 18") 6

one-meat topping, thin crust, restaurant-
type, 1 slice (⅛ of 18") 10

pepperoni, frozen, 1 slice (5 oz) 8

sausage, frozen, 1 slice (5 oz) 8

single serving, cheese, 1 (7 oz) 13

single serving, pepperoni, frozen, 1
(7 oz)..14

single serving, sausage, frozen, 1 (7 oz) ...14

single serving, supreme, frozen, 1
(7 oz)..14

supreme, frozen, 1 slice (5 oz) 8

vegetable, frozen, 1 slice (5 oz)................6

Pizza crust dough, refrigerated, frozen
or ready-made, 1 oz..............................2

Pizza pieces, frozen (prepared without
fat), 6 (3 oz)..5

Pizza sauce, store-bought, ¼ cup 1

Plantain
1 cup..3
fried, 1 cup..4

Plums, 2 (4 oz) 1

Pocket sandwich, frozen, 1 (4½ oz) 8

Poi, ½ cup (4 oz) 3

Polenta, ¼ cup 4

Pomegranates, 1 (3⅜" diameter) 2

Pomelo (pummelo), 1 3

Poor boy sandwich, 1 (6") 6

Popcorn
buttered, popped, 3 cups with
2 Tbsp butter......................................7
butter-flavored, popped, 3 cups 4
light, butter-flavored, popped, 3 cups 2
light, caramel-coated, popped, 3 cups 6
light, cheese-flavored, popped, 3 cups......3
light, microwave-popped, 3 cups 1
light, plain, popped, 3 cups 2
movie, without butter, 3 cups 3
plain, air-popped, 3 cups 1
plain, microwave-popped, 3 cups.............3
plain, oil-popped, 3 cups 3
plain, popped, packaged, 3 cups 4
popped, caramel-coated, 3 cups 8
popped, cheese-flavor, 3 cups 3
reduced-fat (94% fat-free), microwave-
popped, 5 cups....................................1

Popcorn cakes
mini, 6 1
other than butter-flavored, 1 (½ oz) 1
plain or butter-flavored, 2 1

Popovers, 2 (3" diameter or
1½ oz each) 4

Poppy seeds
1 tsp..0
1 Tbsp..1

Pork
lean (leg and loin cuts with all visible
fat trimmed), cooked, 1 slice, 1 chop, or
½ cup cubed or shredded (2 oz) **3**
regular, cooked, 1 slice, 1 chop, or
½ cup cubed or shredded (2 oz) **5**
with cashews, 1 cup **10**

Pork, barbecue, 1 cup **8**

Pork, sweet and sour, 1 cup **12**

Pork and beans, canned, ½ cup **2**

Pork and broccoli, 1 cup **3**

Pork in barbecue sauce, frozen,
¼ cup **2**

Pork rinds, 1 oz **4**

Portuguese sweet bread, ⅛ loaf........**5**

Potato chips
baked, 1 oz **2**
fat-free (made with Olean), 1 oz **1**
reduced-calorie, 14 chips (1 oz) **3**
regular, 14 chips (1 oz).............................**4**

Potatoes
baked, stuffed with cheese sauce and
bacon, fast food, 1..............................**11**
baked, stuffed with sour cream and
chives, fast food, 1.............................**10**
baked, stuffed with vegetables and
cheese, fast food, 1............................**11**
garlic, mashed, ½ cup **4**
hash brown, 1 cup **5**
hash brown, fast food, ½ cup **4**
hash brown patty, frozen (prepared
without fat), 1 cup...............................**8**
hash brown patty, frozen (prepared
without fat), 1 ....**1**
home fried, 1 cup **4**
mashed, ½ cup.......................................**2**
mashed, frozen, prepared, ⅔ cup **2**
mashed, in a cup, 1 (1½ oz) **3**
scalloped, ½ cup....................................**4**
shoestring, canned, 1 cup........................**6**
stuffed with cheese, frozen, 1 (5½ oz) **4**
stuffed with sour cream and chives,
frozen, 1 (5½ oz) **4**

sweet, candied, ½ cup **3**
sweet, canned, in syrup, 1 cup **3**
sweet, cooked, 1 cup or 8 oz **3**
sweet, uncooked, 1 large (10 oz) **3**
white or red, cooked, 1 large (8 oz)..........**3**
white or red, cooked, 1 cup **3**
white or red, cooked, 1 small
(2" diameter) **1**
white or red, uncooked, 10 oz **3**

Potatoes au gratin, 1 cup **12**

Potatoes O'Brien
frozen (prepared without fat), 1 cup **1**
home-prepared, 1 cup..............................**3**

Potato flakes, uncooked, ⅓ cup **1**

Potato latkes, 2 (3½" diameter) **5**

Potato mix, flavored, prepared, ½ cup....**3**

Potato pancakes
1 ....**2**
frozen, 1 (2 oz)..**1**
mix, 3 Tbsp **1**

Potato puffs (appetizer pastry),
frozen, 2 (2 oz)......................................**4**

Potato salad
½ cup **7**
German, ½ cup..**2**
hot, with ham, 1 cup................................**6**
store-bought, ½ cup **4**

Potato skins
frozen, 2 (4 oz)..**5**
with cheese, bacon, and sour cream, 2 .....**9**

Potato tots, frozen (prepared without
fat), 9 (3 oz)..**4**

Pot pies
any type, 4" square or 8½ oz **20**
any type, fast food, 1 ....**17**
beef, chicken, or turkey, frozen, 1 (7 oz) ...**11**

**Pot stickers (filled wontons),
pork or vegetable,** frozen, 1 large
or 2 small (1½ oz) **2**

Pound cake
1 slice (5" x 3" x 1") 8
store-bought, 1 slice (2½ oz) 6

Poutine, 20 French fries with 2 oz
cheese and ½ cup sauce 7

Pozole, 1 cup 4

Praline, 1 (2½" diameter) or 1½ oz.........5

Preserves, 1 Tbsp 1

Pretzels
1 hard, 1 Bavarian, 2 rods, 45 sticks,
7 regular twists, 15 small twists, or
¾ oz 2
soft, 1 (2½ oz) 3
soft, Philadelphia, 1 (4½" x 4"), 2½ oz 3

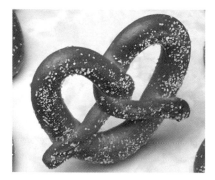

Prickly pear (cactus pear), 1 (5 oz) 0

Profiterole, 1 oz 2

Prune juice, ½ cup (4 fl oz)....................2

Prunes, 2 (¾ oz) 1

Puddings
any flavor, 1 cup 7
bread, 1 cup..9
Indian, 1 cup 12
plum, ½ cup with 1 Tbsp sauce..............12
ready-made, ½ cup 3
ready-made, reduced-calorie, ½ cup 2
reduced-calorie (made with fat-free or
low-fat [½ or 1%] milk), 1 cup 2
rice, 1 cup 7

tapioca, 1 cup 6
Yorkshire, 1 piece (4" square).................6

Puff pastry, frozen, baked, 1 oz 4

Pumpkin
canned, 1 cup...1
fresh, cooked, 1 cup...............................0

Pumpkin bread, 1 slice (¾" thick) 7

Pumpkin leaves, cooked, 1 cup 0

Pumpkin seeds
1 tsp..1
1 Tbsp..1

Puris, 1 (4" diameter) 2

Quail, cooked, 1 oz 2

Quenelles, 8 (2½" x 1½" x ¾")...........14

Quesadillas
beef, 1 (½ of 6" diameter).....................7
cheese, 1 (½ of 6" diameter) 5
chicken, 1 (½ of 6" diameter) 6
vegetable, 1 (½ of 6" diameter)..............6

Quiches
appetizer, frozen, any type, 2 (1½ oz) 3
crab, frozen, 5 oz 11
Lorraine, ⅛ of 9" pie.............................12
Lorraine, frozen, 5½ oz.........................10
vegetable, ⅛ of 9" pie 9
vegetable, frozen, 5 oz 9

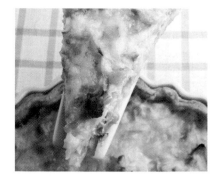

Q

Quince, 1 1
Quinoa, 2 Tbsp 1

Rabbit, cooked, 1 oz................................1
Raccoon, cooked, 1 oz 2
Radishes, 1 cup 0
Raisins,
¼ cup 2
chocolate-covered, 1 oz 2
Raita, ½ cup 1
Raspberries, 1½ cups 1

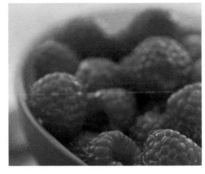

Ratatouille, 1 cup 5
Ravioli
beef, breaded, frozen, 6 (4 oz) 5
beef, in meat sauce, canned, 1 cup..........5
beef or chicken, without sauce, frozen,
1 cup...4
cheese, breaded, frozen, 6 (4 oz)..............7
cheese, with tomato sauce, 8 pieces or
1 cup with ½ cup sauce 16
cheese, without sauce, 8 pieces or
1 cup...13
cheese, without sauce, frozen, 1 cup 6
meat, with tomato sauce, 8 pieces or
1 cup with ½ cup sauce 14
meat, without sauce, 8 pieces or 1 cup....12

Red snapper Veracruz, 6 oz cooked
fillet with ¾ cup sauce 11
Relish, any type, 1 tsp............................0
Remoulade sauce, 1 Tbsp 2
Reuben sandwich, 1 17
Rhubarb
frozen, cooked, with sugar, 1 cup.............5
uncooked, diced, 1 cup............................0
Rice
brown, cooked, 1 cup...............................4
brown, uncooked, 1 cup.........................13
dirty, 1 cup...9
dirty, mix (prepared without fat), 1 cup 3
fried, plain, 1 cup....................................8
fried, with beef, 1 cup 8
fried, with chicken, 1 cup 8
fried, with chicken or pork, frozen,
½ cup..2
fried, with pork, 1 cup.............................8
fried, with shrimp, 1 cup 8
Spanish, canned, 1 cup 3
Spanish, cooked, 1 cup............................5
white, cooked, 1 cup 4
white, uncooked, 1 cup 13
wild, cooked, 1 cup 3
wild, uncooked, 1 cup 11
Rice (crisp) and marshmallow
treat, store-bought, 1 small (¾ oz) 2
Rice cakes
other than plain, 1 (½ oz)........................1
plain, 2 regular or 6 mini.........................1
Rice crackers, 8 (½ oz) 1
Rice drinks
1 cup...3
chocolate, 1 cup 4
fat-free, 1 cup..2
Rice mix, flavored, any type, prepared,
½ cup 3
Rice noodles, packaged, ½ cup 3
Rice pilaf, 1 cup 7

R

Risotto, ½ cup 4

Roast beef sandwich, fast food, 1 8

Rocky mountain oysters, 2 slices
   (1 oz each)...10

Rolls
   crescent dinner, store-bought, 1 (1 oz)......2
   dinner, 1 (2 oz) 3
   hard, 1 (2 oz) 3
   high-fiber (3 g or more dietary fiber
    per roll), 1 (2 oz) 2

Roux, store-bought, 1 Tbsp......................5

Rugalach, 1 piece (2½" x 1¼") or 1 oz...3

Rum, 1 jigger (1½ fl oz)............................2

Runza, 1 8

Rutabaga, cooked, 1 cup 1

S

Sachertorte, ⅟₁₆ of 9" cake....................8

Saganaki, 1 piece (1" x 2" x ½" thick) ...6

Saimin, 1 cup 2

Salad dressings
   fat-free (except Italian), 2 Tbsp 1
   fat-free, Italian, 2 Tbsp 0
   reduced-calorie (except Italian), 2 Tbsp 2
   reduced-calorie, Italian, 2 Tbsp 1
   regular, 2 Tbsp.......................................4

Salad Niçoise
   with dressing, 4 cups 13
   without dressing, 4 cups 5

Salads
   mixed greens, 1 cup.................................0
   side, without dressing, fast food, 1 cup 0
   three-bean, ½ cup 5
   three-bean, canned, ½ cup 1

Salami, beef or pork, 1 slice (1 oz)......3

**Salmon salad, kippered (with
   mayonnaise),** store-bought, 2 oz 5

Salsa
   1 cup 0
   black beans and corn, ½ cup 1

Salsa con queso, store-bought, 2 Tbsp ..2

Salsify (oyster plant), cooked, 1 cup ...1

Samosa, 1 (2½" x 2½" x 3" triangle)......3

Sandwich spread, pork or beef,
   2 Tbsp 2

Sangria, 4 fl oz......................................2

**Sashimi (except salmon or
   mackerel),** 4 pieces 1

Sashimi, salmon or mackerel,
   4 pieces...2

Satay, 2 skewers with ¼ cup sauce..........9

Sauces
   barbecue, 1 Tbsp 0
   barbecue, ¼ cup 1
   black bean, 1 tsp 0
   cocktail, ¼ cup..1
   hoisin, ready-to-serve, 1 tsp.....................0
   oyster, 1 tsp 0
   plum, 1 Tbsp 1
   soy, 1 Tbsp 0
   Spanish, ½ cup 1
   steak, 1 Tbsp 0
   sweet and sour, 2 Tbsp............................1
   taco, 1 Tbsp...0
   tartar, 1 Tbsp 2
   tartar, fat-free, ¼ cup 1
   teriyaki, ¼ cup..1
   teriyaki, 1 Tbsp 0
   white, medium, ¼ cup..............................2
   white, thick, ¼ cup 3
   white, thin, ¼ cup...................................2
   Worcestershire, 1 Tbsp 0

Sauerbraten, 3 oz beef with
   2 Tbsp gravy 6

Sauerkraut, 1 cup..................................0

Sausage biscuits
  fast food, 1 12
  frozen, 1 large or 2 small (2 oz) 7

Sausage in brioche, 1 slice
  (2" thick) 15

Sausages
  beef or pork, cooked, 1 link or patty
  (1 oz)..3
  low-fat (1 g fat or less per oz), 2 oz 2
  mini, 6 (2 oz).......................................5

Scallions, 1 cup 0

Schave, canned, 1 cup 0

Schmaltz, 1 Tbsp 3

Schnapps, any flavor, 1 jigger
  (1½ fl oz) 4

Scone, 1 (4" x 4" x 5½") or 2½ oz 5

Scotch, 1 jigger (1½ fl oz) 2

Scrapple, 1 slice (4½" x ¾" x ⅜"
  thick) or 2 oz 3

Screwdriver, 1 (6 fl oz) 4

Seafood cakes (Haw Mok Thalay),
  ¾ cup...8

Seafood salad, store-bought, ½ cup 6

Seal, cooked, 1 oz 1

Seitan mix, 2 Tbsp 1

Seitan slices, 2 slices (2 oz)....................1

Seltzer, plain or flavored,
  unsweetened, 1 can or bottle (12 fl oz) ..0

Sesame noodles, 1 cup 7

Sesame seeds
  1 tsp...0
  1 Tbsp...1

Sesame sticks, store-bought, ⅓ cup 4

Shabu shabu, 4 oz beef, 2 oz tofu, and
  1½ cups vegetables 8

Shallots, uncooked, 1 cup 2

Shark, cooked, 1 steak (6 oz) 5

Sharon fruit, 3 oz.................................1

Shellfish
  abalone, cooked, 3 oz 2
  abalone, fried, 3 oz 4
  clams, baked, 6....................................7
  clams, canned, ½ cup 3
  clams, cooked, ½ cup 2
  clams, fried, 1 cup...............................10
  clams, fried, frozen (prepared without
    fat), 3 oz 6
  clams, stuffed, frozen (prepared
    without fat), 1 (3 oz) 2
  crab, deviled, ½ cup 4
  crab, imitation, ½ cup 2
  crab, stuffed, frozen, 1 (3 oz) 3
  crabmeat, canned, ½ cup 3
  crabmeat, cooked, ½ cup 1
  crayfish, cooked, ½ cup or 16 (2 oz)........1
  lobster, cooked, ½ cup..........................1
  mussels, cooked, ½ cup 2
  oysters, canned, ½ cup 2
  oysters, cooked, 6 medium (2 oz) 2
  oysters, fried, 10 7
  oysters, uncooked, 6 medium..................1
  scallops, cooked, ½ cup (2 oz) 1
  scallops, fried, 20 (3½ oz)......................7
  scallops, fried, frozen (prepared
    without fat), 3¼ oz 5
  shellfish, canned, any type (meat only),
    drained, ½ cup 2
  shrimp, canned, ½ cup 2
  shrimp, cooked, 2 oz 1
  shrimp, sweet and sour, 1 cup...............10
  squid, fried, 3 oz 4

Shells, stuffed with cheese, no sauce,
  frozen, 2 (4½ oz) 6

Shepherd's pie, 1 cup 9

Sherbet, ½ cup....................................2

Sherry, dry or sweet, ½ cup (4 fl oz) ...3

S

Shish kebob, 2 small skewers 10

Shortcakes, store-bought, 2 (1 oz each) ...4

Shortening, 1 cup 54

Shrimp
 barbecued, 4 large shrimp with ¼ cup
  sauce...**11**
 broiled, stuffed, 6 large **14**
 butterfly, breaded, frozen (prepared
  without fat), 3½ oz...............................**6**
 fried, 10 ....**8**
 fried, stuffed, 6 large **9**
 popcorn, breaded, frozen (prepared
  without fat), 1 cup................................**5**

Shrimp and broccoli, 1 cup **2**

Shrimp Cantonese, 1 cup **9**

Shrimp po' boy, 1 (6") **22**

Shrimp puffs, 6 (1½" rounds) **5**

Shrimp remoulade, 6 small shrimp
 with ¼ cup remoulade sauce.................**9**

Shrimp salad, ½ cup...........................**4**

Shrimp salad sandwich, 1 ....**9**

Shrimp scampi, 9 medium shrimp
 (3 oz)...**11**

Shrimp toast, 1 piece **2**

Singapore sling, 1 (6 fl oz) **4**

Sloppy Joe, 1.......................................**8**

Sloppy Joe sauce, store-bought,
 ¼ cup **1**

Smoothie, 1 cup...................................**2**

Snack mixes
 Oriental, low-fat, store-bought, ½ cup......**2**
 reduced-fat, store-bought, ½ cup **3**
 store-bought, ½ cup **4**

Sofrito sauce, ½ cup **6**

Soft drinks
 diet, any flavor, 1 can or bottle (12 fl oz) ...**0**
 sweetened with sugar, any flavor, 1 can
  or bottle (12 fl oz) **3**

Sopaipillas, 2 (4" x 3" each) **2**

Sorbet, 1 scoop or ½ cup **2**

Souffles
 cheese, 1 cup **7**
 fruit, ½ cup..**4**

Soup mixes
 beef noodle soup mix in a cup, 1 ....**4**
 chicken noodle, prepared, 1 cup...............**1**
 onion mix, 1 cup prepared or
  ¼ envelope **1**
 Oriental mix in a cup, 1 (1 oz) **2**
 ramen noodle soup mix, 1 (3 oz) **8**
 ramen noodle soup mix, low-fat,
  1 (3 oz)..**6**
 vegetable mix, prepared, 1 cup................**1**

Soups
 asparagus crab, 1 cup **2**
 avgolemono, 1 cup **4**
 bean and bacon, canned (made
  with water), 1 cup **3**
 bean and ham, canned (made
  with water), 1 cup **3**
 beef, canned (made with water),
  1 cup..**2**
 beef vegetable, canned
  (made with water), 1 cup......................**1**
 black bean, 1 cup **2**
 black bean, canned (made with
  water), 1 cup.......................................**2**
 black bean, canned, condensed,
  made with water, 1 cup **1**
 black bean soup in a cup, 1 (2 oz) **3**
 bouillon, any type, 1 cup **0**
 broccoli cheese, 1 cup **7**
 broccoli cheese, canned (made with
  fat-free milk), 1 cup **3**
 broccoli cheese, canned (made with
  low-fat [2%] milk), 1 cup **4**
 broccoli cheese, canned (made with
  whole milk), 1 cup................................**4**
 broccoli cheese, low-fat, canned
  (made with fat-free or low-fat milk),
  1 cup..**2**

broth, any type, 1 cup 0

cabbage, 1 cup 1

cheddar cheese, 1 cup...............................9

cheddar cheese, canned (made with
fat-free milk), 1 cup 4

cheddar cheese, canned (made with
low-fat milk), 1 cup 4

cheddar cheese, canned (made with
whole milk), 1 cup 5

chicken and stars, canned (made with
water), 1 cup..1

chicken noodle, 1 cup 3

chicken noodle, canned, condensed,
(made with water), 1 cup 2

chicken noodle in a cup, 1 (1 oz)..............2

chicken vegetable in a cup, 1 (1 oz) 2

chicken with matzo balls, 1 cup soup
with 2 (1½") matzo balls 3

chicken without matzo balls (broth
only), 1 cup..0

chicken with rice, canned (made with
water), 1 cup..2

chicken with rice, canned, condensed,
(made with water), 1 cup 1

chicken with wild rice, canned (made
with water), 1 cup 2

corn chowder, made with fat-free or
low-fat milk, 1 cup 4

corn chowder, made with whole milk,
1 cup...5

corn chowder in a cup, 1 (1 oz) 3

cream of broccoli, 1 cup..........................6

cream of broccoli, canned (made with
fat-free milk), 1 cup 3

cream of broccoli, canned (made with
low-fat milk), 1 cup 3

cream of broccoli, canned (made with
whole milk), 1 cup 4

cream of broccoli, low-fat, canned
(made with fat-free milk), 1 cup 3

cream of broccoli, low-fat, canned
(made with low-fat milk), 1 cup.............3

cream of celery, canned (made with
fat-free milk), 1 cup 3

cream of celery, canned (made with
low-fat milk), 1 cup 3

cream of celery, canned (made with
whole milk), 1 cup.................................4

cream of celery, canned, condensed,
1 can (10¾ oz).....................................5

cream of celery, low-fat, canned
(made with fat-free milk), 1 cup 2

cream of celery, low-fat, canned
(made with low-fat milk), 1 cup.............3

cream of chicken, canned (made with
fat-free milk), 1 cup 4

cream of chicken, canned (made with
low-fat milk), 1 cup 4

cream of chicken, canned (made with
whole milk), 1 cup.................................5

cream of chicken, canned, condensed,
1 can (10¾ oz).....................................7

cream of chicken, low-fat, canned
(made with fat-free milk), 1 cup 3

cream of chicken, low-fat, canned
(made with low-fat milk), 1 cup.............3

cream of mushroom, 1 cup......................8

cream of mushroom, canned (made
with fat-free milk), 1 cup 3

cream of mushroom, canned (made
with low-fat milk), 1 cup.......................3

cream of mushroom, canned (made
with whole milk), 1 cup 4

cream of mushroom, canned, condensed,
1 can (10¾ oz).....................................8

cream of mushroom, low-fat, canned
(made with fat-free milk), 1 cup 2

cream of mushroom, low-fat, canned
(made with low-fat milk), 1 cup.............3

cream of potato, 1 cup............................2

cream of potato, canned (made with
fat-free milk), 1 cup 3

cream of potato, canned (made with
low-fat milk), 1 cup 4

cream of potato, canned (made with
whole milk), 1 cup.................................4

egg drop, 1 cup 1

escarole, canned, ready-to-serve, 1 cup 1

S

French onion au gratin, 1 cup 6
gazpacho, 1 cup.......................................4
gazpacho, canned (made with water),
  1 cup..1
gazpacho, canned, ready-to-serve, 1 cup....1
hot and sour, 1 cup 2
lentil, 1 cup 3
lentil in a cup, 1 (2 oz) 3
lentil with ham, canned, ready-to-serve,
  1 cup..3
lobster bisque, 1 cup...............................5
lobster bisque, canned (made with
  fat-free milk), 1 cup 2
lobster bisque, canned (made with
  low-fat milk), 1 cup 2
lobster bisque, canned (made with
  whole milk), 1 cup 3
Manhattan clam chowder, 1 cup..............5
Manhattan clam chowder, canned,
  condensed (made with water), 1 cup 1
matzo ball, canned, 1 cup 2
minestrone, 1 cup 4
minestrone, low-fat, canned (made
  with water), 1 cup 2
minestrone in a cup, 1 (1½ oz) 2
miso, 1 cup 2
mulligatawny, 1 cup................................5
mushroom barley, 1 cup 5
New England clam chowder, 1 cup 5
New England clam chowder, canned
  (made with fat-free milk), 1 cup 3
New England clam chowder, canned
  (made with low-fat milk), 1 cup.............3
New England clam chowder, canned
  (made with whole milk), 1 cup 4
New England clam chowder, low-fat,
  canned (made with fat-free milk),
  1 cup..2
New England clam chowder, low-fat,
  canned (made with low-fat milk),
  1 cup..2
oxtail, 1 cup 1
oyster stew, canned (made with fat-free
  milk), 1 cup 3

oyster stew, canned (made with low-fat
  milk), 1 cup..3
oyster stew, canned (made with whole
  milk), 1 cup..4
pasta with vegetables, canned (made
  with water), 1 cup 2
Persian noodle, store-bought, 1 cup 3
Persian pomegranate, store-bought,
  1 cup..4
potato, frozen, 1 (7½ oz)..........................2
potato leek in a cup, 1 (1 oz)...................2
pozole (pork and hominy), canned,
  1 cup..3
ramen in a cup, low-fat, 1 (2 oz)..............3
red beans and rice in a cup, 1 (2 oz) 3
Scotch broth, 1 cup..................................5
shark fin, 1 cup 2
split pea, frozen, 1 (7½ oz).......................2
split pea in a cup, 1 (2 oz) 3
split pea, with ham, canned, condensed
  (made with water), 1 cup.......................4
Thai chicken coconut, 1 cup.....................8
Thai coconut ginger, canned, 1 cup 3
tomato, 1 cup..2
tomato, canned (made with fat-free
  milk), 1 cup 2
tomato, canned (made with low-fat
  milk), 1 cup 2
tomato, canned (made with water),
  1 cup..1
tomato, canned (made with whole
  milk), 1 cup..3
tortilla, 1 cup...6
turkey noodle, canned, condensed
  (made with water), 1 cup 1
turtle, 1 cup 3
vegetable, 1 cup 2
vegetable, canned, condensed
  (made with water), 1 cup 3
vegetable beef, canned, condensed
  (made with water), 1 cup 1
vegetarian vegetable in a cup, 1 (2 oz).....3
Vietnamese beef noodle, 1 cup 2
wonton, 1 cup with 4 wontons................4
yogurt and cucumber, 1 cup 2

S

Soursop (guanabana), ½ cup pulp 1

Souvlaki, 1 large skewer or 2 small
skewers 10

Souvlaki sandwich, 1 7

Soybean nuts, ¼ cup...........................3

Soybeans
cooked, ½ cup 3
uncooked, 1 pound 45

Soy beverage drink
1 cup..3
reduced-fat, 1 cup 2

Soy milk
1 cup..3
fat-free, 1 cup..2

Soy yogurt
flavored, ¾ cup 3
plain, ¾ cup 3

Spaetzle, ½ cup.....................................4

Spaghetti
cooked, 1 cup 3
uncooked, 1½ oz 3
whole wheat, cooked, 1 cup 3
whole wheat, uncooked, 2 oz 4

Spaghetti Bolognese, 1 cup spaghetti
with ½ cup sauce 9

Spaghetti carbonara, 1 cup 10

Spaghetti in tomato sauce
with cheese, canned, 1 cup.....................3
with meatballs, canned, 1 cup 5

Spaghetti sauce
bottled, any type, ½ cup.........................2
bottled, any type, reduced-fat, ½ cup 1

Spaghetti with garlic and oil,
1 cup..7

Spaghetti with marinara sauce,
1 cup spaghetti with ½ cup sauce 6

**Spaghetti with meatballs and
tomato sauce,** 1 cup spaghetti,
2 meatballs and ½ cup sauce 16

Spaghetti with meat sauce,
1 cup spaghetti with ½ cup sauce 9

Spanakopita
1 (3" square) 9
frozen, 2 pieces (1 oz each) 4

Spareribs
barbecued, 4 (each 4" long)..................8
Chinese, barbecued, 2 (each 4" long).......4

Spinach
cooked, 1 cup..0
uncooked, 1 cup 0

Spinach salad, with dressing, 2 cups 7

Spinach souffle, homemade, 1 cup 6

Sponge cake, 1/12 of 9" tube 4

Spoon bread, ½ cup 4

Sports drink, 1 cup..............................1

**Spring roll dipping sauce,
Vietnamese,** 2 Tbsp...........................0

Spring rolls
with beef, chicken, pork, or shrimp, fried,
1 (4½" long) 4
Vietnamese, 1..2

Sprinkles, any type, 1 Tbsp...................1

Sprouts
alfalfa, 1 cup 0
bean, 1 cup 0

Spumoni, ½ cup 6

Squab, cooked, 1 oz 1

Squash
spaghetti, cooked, 1 cup 0
summer, cooked, 1 cup...........................0
winter, cooked, 1 cup 1

Squash leaves, 1 cup 0

Squid, cooked, 3 oz 2

Squirrel, cooked, 1 oz 1

Starfruit (carambola), 1 large
(4½" long) 0

S

Steaks

au poivre, 6 oz steak with 1 Tbsp
sauce..15

blackened, 6 oz 16

chicken fried, 6 oz with ¼ cup cream
gravy..15

lean, cooked (round or loin cuts
with all visible fat trimmed), 1 small
(4 oz)..5

regular, cooked, 1 small (4 oz) 7

Salisbury, 6 oz 12

Steak sandwich, frozen, 1 (2 oz)...........5

**Stir-fry beef with garlic or black
bean sauce,** 1 cup 8

Stir-fry chicken, frozen (prepared
without fat), 1 cup...................................3

**Stir-fry chicken with garlic or
black bean sauce,** 1 cup 7

**Stir-fry pork with garlic or black
bean sauce,** 1 cup 8

**Stir-fry shrimp with garlic or black
bean sauce,** 1 cup 7

Strawberries, fresh, 1½ cups 1

Strawberry shortcake, 1/12 of 9" cake
or 1 filled individual shortcake..............7

Stromboli, 1 slice (1" thick) or 2 oz.......4

Strudel, any type, 1 piece (5½" x 2")......8

Stuffing

½ cup 4

bread, from mix, prepared, ½ cup 4

Submarine sandwich, 1 (6")...............6

Succotash, cooked, 1 cup.....................4

Sugar

brown, 1 cup...17

brown, 1 Tbsp 1

white, 1 cup 15

white, 1 Tbsp..1

Suimono, 1 cup 1

Sukiyaki, 2½ cups 12

Summer squash casserole, 1 cup.......9

Sunflower seeds

1 tsp...0

1 Tbsp..1

Sunomono, ½ cup 1

Sushi

California roll, 4 pieces (1" high x 1¾"
diameter or 1 oz each)........................3

maki, 4 pieces 2

nigiri, 4 pieces 2

nori maki, 4 pieces 2

Swedish meatballs, 6 (1" diameter) 8

Swedish meatballs with noodles,
frozen, 1 cup..7

Sweet and sour beverage mix,
½ cup 2

Sweetbreads, cooked, 1 oz 1

Sweet potato leaves, cooked, 1 cup....0

Sweet potato pie, 1 slice
(⅛ of 9" pie)......................................11

Sweet rolls

1 large (4 oz) 5

store-bought, 1 (2¾" square).................5

Sweet rolls, pecan-swirl,
store-bought, 2 (2 oz) 5

Sweetsop (sugar apple)

½ (2⅞" diameter) 1

⅓ cup 1

Syrup, pancake
low-calorie, 2 Tbsp...................................1
regular, 1 Tbsp.......................................1

Tabouli
½ cup 4
from mix, prepared, ½ cup 2

Tacos
beef, 1 5
breakfast, 1 5
chicken, 1 4
fish, 1 4
hard, dinner kit in a box, prepared, 2 7
hard, fast food, 1 5
pork, 1 4
soft, fast food, 1 5
soft, kit in a box, prepared, 1 9

Taco salad
with shell, without dressing, fast food,
    1 15
without shell and dressing, fast food, 1 8

Taco salad shells
large, store-bought, 1..............................5
small, store-bought, 2 (1½ oz) 5

Taco shells, store-bought, 1 large
(6½" diameter), 2 small (4½" diameter),
4 miniature (3" diameter), or ¾ oz 2

Tahini
2 Tbsp...2
canned, 2 Tbsp 5

Tamale pie, 1 cup 11

Tamales
beef, canned, 2 (1 oz)..............................5
beef, frozen, 3 small or 1 large (4¾ oz)....7
chicken, canned, 2 (4 oz) 3
chicken, frozen, 3 small or 1 large (6 oz) ..6
pork, frozen, 3 small or 1 large (4½ oz)....7
with sauce, 2 (4" x 2") 10

Tamarinds, 10 (3" x 1") 1

Tamari sauce, 1 Tbsp.............................0

Tangelo, 1 large 1

Tangerine, 1 large or 2 small (6 oz)........1

Tangerine juice, ½ cup..........................1

Tapioca, uncooked, 1 tsp 0

Taquitos, frozen, 2.................................3

Taro, cooked, 1 cup 3

Taro leaves, cooked, 1 cup 0

Tarte aux fruits
⅛ of 9" tart 7
4" tart...10

Tart shell
1 (4" diameter) 6
store-bought, 1 (4" diameter)...................6

Tea
black, decaffeinated or regular, without
    sugar, 1 cup 0
decaffeinated or regular, sweetened, 1 2

Tempeh (fermented soybean
cake), ¼ cup 1

Tempura
shrimp, 4 jumbo 12
vegetable, 1 cup 8

Tempura batter mix, ¼ cup 2

Teppan yaki, 1½ cups.........................10

Tequila, 1 jigger (1½ fl oz)....................2

Teriyaki
beef, 2 slices (4 oz) 7
chicken, 2 slices (4 oz) 6
fish, 4 oz...5

Texas trash (cereal and nut mix),
1 cup..8

Textured vegetable protein, dry,
⅓ cup 1

Thai beef salad, 1 cup 14

Thai chicken with basil, 1 breast
(no skin or bone), 3 oz..........................5

Thai coffee or tea, 1 cup....................6

Thai crisp noodles, 1 cup 11

Thai curry paste, 1 Tbsp 1

Thai paste, 2 Tbsp...............................2

Thai seafood salad, 2 cups................10

Tirami-su, 1 piece (2¼" square) 9

Toaster pastry
low-fat, 1 (1¾ oz) 4
regular, any type, 1 (1¾ oz)...................5

Tofu
firm, ⅓ cup, ⅕ block, or 3 oz 2
frozen, ½ cup 5
low-fat, ⅓ cup, ⅕ block, or 3 oz..............1
soft, ⅓ cup, ⅕ block, or 3 oz...................1

**Tomato and mozzarella salad
    without dressing,** 1 large tomato
    with 2¼ oz cheese 6

Tomatoes
canned, 1 cup...0
dried (not packed in oil), ¼ cup 0
dried, packed in oil, drained, ¼ cup..........1
fresh, 1 cup 0
green, fried, 2 slices (1½" thick) 4

Tomato juice, canned, 1 cup 0

Tomato paste
canned, ½ cup..1
canned, 2 Tbsp 0

Tomato puree, canned, ½ cup...............0

Tomato sauce, canned, ½ cup...............0

Tomato sauce, Italian, ½ cup...............3

Tom yum kung, 1 cup 2

Tonkatsu, ¾ cup 12

Toppings
fruit, 1 Tbsp...1
fudge, fat-free, 1 Tbsp 1
fudge, regular, 1 Tbsp............................1
whipped, dairy or nondairy, light or
    fat-free, aerosol or frozen, ⅓ cup...........1

Tortellini
beef, chicken, or pork without sauce,
    frozen, 1 cup 5

cheese, without sauce, 10 (⅔ cup) 3
cheese, without sauce, frozen, 1 cup 6
meat, without sauce, 10 (⅔ cup) 3
mushroom, without sauce, frozen, 1 cup ...6
sausage, without sauce, frozen, 1 cup 7

Tortiere (Canadian meat pie), 1 slice
    (⅛ of 9" pie)...9

Tortilla chips
12 (1 oz)...3
baked, low-fat, 12 (1 oz) 2
reduced-fat, 12 (1 oz) 2

Tortillas
corn, 2 (4" diameter), 1 (6" diameter),
    ½ (10" diameter), or 1 oz 1
flour, 2 (4" diameter), 1 (6" diameter),
    ½ (10" diameter), or 1 oz 2

Tortoni, 1 serving 7

Tostadas
beef, 1 10
chicken, 1..8
with beans and cheese, fast food, 1 5

Tostada shells, store-bought, 2 (1 oz)....2

Trail mix
¼ cup 4
tropical, ¼ cup 3
with chocolate chips, ¼ cup 5

Trifle, 1 cup 5

Tuna dinner in a box, prepared,
    1 cup..7

Tuna macaroni salad, 1 cup 5

Tuna melt sandwich, 1 9

Tuna noodle casserole, 1 cup 14

Tuna salad, ½ cup................................7

Tuna salad sandwich, 1 10

Turkey
canned, ½ cup..4
cooked, dark meat, without skin, 1 slice
    or ½ cup cubed or shredded (2 oz) 3
cooked, white meat, without skin, 1 slice
    or ½ cup cubed or shredded (2 oz) 2

T

ground, cooked, 1 patty (3 oz) 5
ground, cooked, ½ cup 3
ground, lean, cooked, 1 patty (3 oz) 4
ground, lean, cooked, ½ cup (2 oz) 3
ground, lean, uncooked, 1 pound 16
ground, regular, uncooked, 1 pound 20

Turkey and gravy, frozen, 1 cup 4

Turkey breast, with skin, cooked,
    1 slice (2 oz) 2

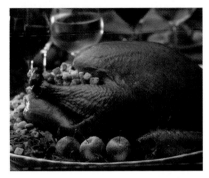

Turkey burger, frozen, 1 5

Turkey croquette, breaded, frozen, 1
    (with gravy), 3½ oz 3

Turkey leg (thigh and drumstick)
    with skin, cooked, 1 27
    with skin, cooked, 1 slice (2 oz) 3

Turkey macaroni salad, 1 cup 5

Turkey roll, 1 slice (1 oz) 1

Turkey tetrazzini, 1½ cups 9

Turnips, cooked, 1 cup 0

Turnover
    fruit, any type, 1 (3" x 1½") 4
    fruit, any type, fast food, 1 7

Tyropitas, frozen, 2 4

Tzimmes, vegetable, ¾ cup 2

Veal
    cooked, lean, 1 slice, 1 chop, or
        ½ cup cubed or shredded (2 oz) 3
    cooked, regular, 1 slice, 1 chop, or
        ½ cup cubed or shredded (2 oz) 4

Veal cutlet, breaded, fried, 4 oz 10

Veal marsala, 4 oz 11

Veal parmigiana
    without sauce, 5½ oz 10
    with sauce, 5 oz with ½ cup tomato
        sauce 12

Veal piccata, 2 slices (4 oz) 11

Veal scaloppine, 2 pieces (3" x 5") or
    4½ oz 12

Veal with peppers, 5 oz 11

Vegetable juice, mixed, 1 cup 0

Vegetables
    creamed (except creamed corn), 1 cup ...10
    fried, 1 cup..6
    in sauce, frozen, 1 cup 1
    mixed, drained, ½ cup...............................0
    packed in oil, drained, 1 cup 3
    pot roasted with pan drippings, 1 cup 3
    sautéed, 1 cup...6

**Vegetarian breakfast links
    (sausage-type),** 2 (1½ oz)................2

**Vegetarian breakfast patty
    (sausage-type),** 1 (1 oz) 1

Vegetarian breakfast strips, 4
    (1 oz)..3

Vegetarian burgers
    black bean, frozen, 1 (1½ oz) 2
    fat-free, 1 (2¾ oz) 1
    regular, 1 (2¾ oz) 2

Vegetarian chicken patty, frozen,
    1 (3 oz)...2

**Vegetarian chicken pieces
    (nugget-style),** frozen, 4 (2¾ oz) 2

V

Vegetarian deli slices, frozen, 3 (2¾ oz) 1

Vegetarian frankfurter
fat-free, frozen, 1 small or ½ large (2½ oz) 1
regular, frozen, 1 small or ½ large (3 oz) ..1

Vegetarian ground "meat", frozen, ½ cup 1

Vegetarian sausage, frozen, 1½ oz 2

Vegetarian topping (made with soy), 2 Tbsp 1

Venison, cooked, 1 oz 1

Vichyssoise, 1 cup 5

Vienna sausage
beef and pork, canned, 3 (each 2" long), 1¾ oz...4
chicken, canned, 3 (½ oz) 3

Vietnamese beef balls (Thit bo vien), 6 (1½ oz) 2

Vindaloo
chicken, 1 cup 8
pork, 1 cup...9

Vinegar, 1 Tbsp......................................0

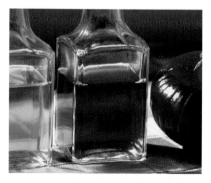

Vitello Tonnato, 2 slices veal (4 oz) with ½ cup sauce 20

Vodka, 1 jigger (1½ fl oz) 2

Vodka gimlet, 1 serving (2½ fl oz) 3

Waffles
any type, 1 (7" square) 6
any type, frozen, 1 (4" round or square), or 1¼ oz...2
any type, made from mix, 1 (4" round or square) 2
Belgian, frozen, 1 (1 oz) 2
low-fat, any type, frozen, 2 (4" round or square) 3
mini, frozen, 4 (1¾ oz)............................2
sticks, frozen, 1 large or 2 small (2 oz) 3

Waldorf salad, ½ cup 6

Walnuts, 1 oz (14 halves) 5

Watercress, 1 cup 0

Watermelon, 1 cup or 2" slice..............1

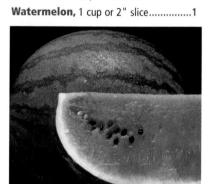

Water or mineral water, 1 cup 0

Wax gourd (Chinese winter melon), 1 cup 1

Whale, cooked, 1 oz 1

Wheat germ, 3 Tbsp 1

Whiskey, 1 jigger (1½ fl oz) 2

Whiskey sour, 3 fl oz 3

Whitefish and pike
large, store-bought, 1 (1¼ oz) 2
small, store-bought, 2 (1 oz)....................2

Whitefish salad, store-bought, 1½ oz....5

W

Wine

1 small glass or ½ cup (4 fl oz) 2
dessert, dry, 2 fl oz 1
dessert, sweet, 2 fl oz 2
light, 4 fl oz..1
non-alcoholic, 4 fl oz 0

Wine cooler, 8 fl oz...............................3

Wine sauce, ¼ cup 3

Wine spritzer, 8 fl oz 2

Wontons

boiled, 6 4
fried, 6...10

Wonton skins (wrappers), 5

(3½" squares) 2

Yakitori, 1 skewer with 3 Tbsp sauce 6

Yams

cooked, 1 large (8 oz) 3
cooked, 1 cup...3
patty, frozen, 1 (4 oz)..............................1
sweet, canned, in syrup, 1 cup 3
uncooked, 1 large (10 oz)......................3

Yeast, 1 tsp..0

Yogurt

fat-free, flavored (vanilla, lemon, coffee),
sweetened with sugar, 1 cup 3
fat-free, fruit-flavored, sweetened with
sugar, 1 cup 4
fat-free, plain, sweetened with sugar,
1 cup...3

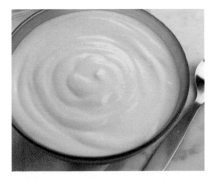

frozen, fat-free, no sugar added,
1 scoop or ½ cup....................................2
frozen, fat-free, sweetened with sugar,
1 scoop or ½ cup....................................2
frozen, low-fat, 1 scoop or ½ cup 3
light (artificially sweetened), 1 cup 2
low-fat, plain, 1 cup.................................3
low-fat, sweetened with sugar, flavored
(vanilla, lemon, coffee), 1 cup.................4
low-fat, sweetened with sugar,
fruit-flavored, 1 cup................................5
plain, 1 cup 4

Yogurt and cucumber salad, ¼ cup ...1

Yogurt bar, chocolate-covered,
frozen, 1 5

Yogurt-covered pretzels, 7 (8 oz).......3

Yogurt-covered raisins, 2 oz 3

Yogurt drink, 1 cup 5

Yosenabe, 2 cups 8

Zabaglione, ½ cup 6

Zeppole, 1 (4" diameter).......................5

Ziti

baked, with meat, 1 cup.........................9
baked, without meat, 1 cup....................6

Zucchini

breaded, frozen (prepared without fat),
6 pieces (8 oz)......................................4
cooked, 1 cup...0
uncooked, 1 cup 0

Zucchini bread, 1 slice (¾" thick) 13

Zuppa di pesce, 2 cups......................12

Zuppa Inglese, 1⁄16 of 10" cake 7

Zwieback, 3 (8 oz)................................2

General Listing of Ethnic/ Regional Foods

Cajun Foods

Bananas Foster, 2 scoops ice cream
with ½ banana and ⅓ cup sauce 16

Beans, red, and rice, 1 cup 5

Beignet, 1 (2") 2

Boudin, 2 oz 2

Chicken, blackened, 1 breast (3 oz) 7

Crawfish pie, 1 slice (⅛ of 9" pie) 13

Creole
chicken, without rice, 1 cup 6
shrimp, without rice, 1 cup 4

Etouffee
crawfish, 1 cup 20
shrimp, 1 cup 9

Fish, blackened, 1 fillet (6 oz) 12

Green rice, 1 cup 8

Gumbo
chicken, 1 cup 6
seafood, 1 cup..5

Jambalaya
chicken, with rice, 1½ cups......................9
fish, with rice, 1½ cups 7

Muffuletta, 1 (6")...............................20

Oyster pie, 1 slice (⅛ of 9" pie) 9

Oyster po' boy, 1 (6") 17

Praline, 1 (2½" diameter) or 1½ oz.........5

Remoulade sauce, 1 Tbsp 2

Rice, dirty, 1 cup 9

Shrimp, barbecued, 4 large shrimp
with ¼ cup sauce 11

Shrimp po' boy, 1 (6") 22

Shrimp remoulade, 6 small shrimp
with ¼ cup remoulade sauce.................9

Soup, turtle, 1 cup................................3

Steak, blackened, 6 oz 16

Canadian Foods

Donair, 4 oz meat with onion, tomato,
and 2 Tbsp sauce..................................14

Donair sauce, 2 Tbsp 2

Fish & brewis, 1 cup............................13

Poutine, 20 French fries with 2 oz
cheese and ½ cup sauce 7

Tortiere (Canadian meat pie),
1 slice (⅛ of 9" pie)...............................9

Caribbean Foods

Chicken asopao, 1 cup with 1 piece
chicken 8

Curry, goat, 4 oz...................................5

Jamaican rice and peas, 1 cup 6

Jerk chicken breast, 1 large breast
(without skin)...5

Plantain, fried, 1 cup 4

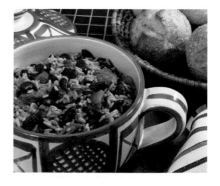

Chinese Foods

Beef, orange-ginger, 1 cup................11

Beef and broccoli, 1 cup.....................4

Black bean sauce, 1 tsp.....................0

Broccoli stir-fry, 1 cup.........................3

Char shiu bao (roast pork bun),
  1 (2 oz)..4

Chicken, orange, 1 cup 13

Chicken and broccoli, 1 cup...............2

Chicken breast, five spice, 1 breast
  (with skin and bone), 4½ oz.................7

Chicken leg, five spice, 1 leg (thigh
  and drumstick), with skin and bone 9

Chicken with cashews, 1 cup..............9

Chinese vegetables
  with beef, 1 cup.....................................6
  with chicken, 1 cup................................5
  with pork, 1 cup 7
  with shrimp, 1 cup.................................4
  with tofu, 1 cup......................................4

Chop suey
  beef, 1 cup..5
  chicken, 1 cup 4
  pork, 1 cup...4
  vegetable, 1 cup 4

Chow mein
  beef, 1 cup...5
  chicken, 1 cup 4
  pork, 1 cup..5

Chow mein noodles, ½ cup.................3

Crab Rangoon, 1 large (4½") or 5 mini..5

Duck sauce, 1 Tbsp 1

Dumplings
  beef or pork, fried, 4 11
  beef or pork, steamed, 4 6
  chicken, fried, 4 9
  chicken, steamed, 4 4
  shrimp, fried, 4 9
  shrimp, steamed, 4 4

Egg foo yung
  beef, 1 (3" diameter) 4
  chicken, 1 (3" diameter)..........................4
  pork, 1 (3" diameter)...............................5
  shrimp, 1 (3" diameter)............................4

Egg rolls
  beef, 1 (4½" long) 5
  chicken, 1 (4½" long) 4
  pork, 1 (4½" long)....................................5
  shrimp, 1 (4½" long)................................4

Egg roll wrapper, 1 1

General Tso's chicken, 1 cup.............15

Hunan beef, 1 cup 9

Kung Pao
  beef, 1 cup...10
  chicken, 1 cup..8
  pork, 1 cup..9
  shrimp, 1 cup 9

Kung Pao sauce, 2 Tbsp 1

Lobster Cantonese, 1 cup 9

Lo Mein
  beef, 1 cup...8
  chicken, 1 cup 8
  pork, 1 cup..8
  shrimp, 1 cup 8

Mongolian beef, 1 cup........................8

Moo goo gai pan, 1 cup 7

Moo shoo pork, ½ cup with
  2 pancakes...10

Oyster sauce, 1 tsp..............................0

Pancakes, Chinese, 3...........................2

Peking duck, 2 oz duck with 1 piece
  duck skin and 3 pancakes 11

Plum sauce, 1 Tbsp 1

Pork and broccoli, 1 cup 3

Pork with cashews, 1 cup 10

Rice, fried
  plain,1 cup..8
  with beef, 1 cup......................................8

Rice, fried (con't) POINTS

with chicken, 1 cup 8
with pork, 1 cup 8
with shrimp, 1 cup 8

Sesame chicken, 1 cup 9

Sesame noodles, 1 cup 7

Shrimp and broccoli, 1 cup 2

Shrimp Cantonese, 1 cup 9

Shrimp toast, 1 piece 2

Soups
egg drop, 1 cup 1
hot and sour, 1 cup 2
wonton, 1 cup with 4 wontons 4

Soy sauce, 1 Tbsp................................0

Spareribs, Chinese barbecued,
2 (each 4" long).....................................4

**Spring roll, with beef, chicken,
pork or shrimp (fried),** 1
(4½" long)...4

Stir-fry
beef with garlic or black bean sauce,
1 cup...8
chicken with garlic or black bean
sauce, 1 cup 7
pork with garlic or black bean
sauce, 1 cup 8
shrimp with garlic or black bean
sauce, 1 cup 7

Sweet and sour
beef, 1 cup 12
chicken, 1 cup 10
pork, 1 cup...12
shrimp, 1 cup 10

Sweet and sour sauce, 2 Tbsp 1

Wontons
boiled, 6 4
fried, 6..10

Wonton skins (wrappers), 5
(3½" squares) 2

English/Irish Foods

Beef Wellington, 1 slice
(3½" x 2½" x 1½"), 5 oz....................12

Bubble and squeak, 1 cup...................3

Carrots and parsnips, 1 cup................4

Colcannon, 1 cup 7

Crumpet, 1 (3" diameter)......................3

Fadge, 1 cup 3

Fish and chips, 5 oz fish fillet with
20 chips (French fries).........................15

Fruitcake, 1 slice (2½" x 1¾" x ½")
or 2 oz...4

Irish brown stew, 1 cup.......................7

Irish coffee, 6 fl oz with 2 Tbsp
whipped cream 4

Irish soda bread, 1/12 of 8" round loaf
(3½ oz)...5

Popovers, 2 (3" diameter) or
1½ oz each 4

Puddings
bread, 1 cup...9
plum, ½ cup with 1 Tbsp sauce..............12
Yorkshire, 1 piece (4" square).................6

Scone, 1 (4" x 4" x 5½") or 2½ oz..........5

Shepherd's pie, 1 cup 9

Trifle, 1 cup 5

French Foods

Baba au rhum, 1 8

Béarnaise sauce, ¼ cup 8

Bechamel (white) sauce, ¼ cup..........4

Beef Bourguignon, 1½ cups 20

Blanquette of veal, 2 cups...............13

Bouillabaisse, 2 cups...........................7

Brioche, 1 slice (1 oz) 3

Cassoulet, 1 cup 11

Chicken cordon bleu, 1 piece
(5½ oz) 13

Chocolate mousse, 1 cup 12

Coq au vin, 2 cups 13

Coquilles St. Jacques, 2 shells 8

Cream puff, 1 (2 oz)..............................7

Creme caramel, 1 cup 7

Creme fraiche, 2 Tbsp 3

Crepes
1 (6" diameter) 2
chicken, 2..12
seafood, 2..11
Suzette, 2..10

Croissants
chocolate-filled,1 (5" long), 3¾ oz 6
plain,1 (5" long), 1¾ oz..............................5

Croque monsieur, 1 11

Croquettes
beef, 2 (2½ oz each) 10
chicken, 2 (2½ oz each)..........................9

Duck a l'orange, ¼ duck with 2 Tbsp
sauce..19

Eclair, 1 9

Escargots, 6 snails with 2 Tbsp butter.....7

Fish amandine, 1 fillet (6 oz) 13

Fish Veronique, 1 fillet (6 oz) 11

Fondue, cheese, ½ cup fondue with
2 oz bread 12

Frog legs, fried, 2 4

Hollandaise sauce, ¼ cup 8

Liver pâté, 1 slice (4¼" x 1½" x ½") 3

Mornay sauce, ¼ cup 4

Mussels Mariniere, 4 mussels with
3 Tbsp sauce 7

Napoleon, 1 piece (4½" x 2" x 1½")....13

Oysters Rockefeller, 4 5

Peach melba, ½ cup ice cream with
2 peach halves and raspberry sauce.......8

Petit fours, 2 (1¾" x 1½" x 1" each) 3

Petite marmite, 2 cups 7

Potatoes au gratin, 1 cup 12

Profiterole, 1 small serving (1 oz) 2

Quenelles, 8 (2½" x 1½" x ¾")...........14

Quiches
Lorraine, ⅛ of 9" pie.............................12
vegetable, ⅛ of 9" pie 9

Ratatouille, 1 cup..................................5

Salad Niçoise
with dressing, 4 cups 13
without dressing, 4 cups 5

Sausage in brioche, 1 slice
(2" thick) 15

Sorbet, 1 scoop or ½ cup 2

Souffles
cheese, 1 cup 7
fruit, ½ cup 4

Soup, French onion au gratin, 1 cup...6

Steak au poivre, 6 oz steak with
1 Tbsp sauce 15

Tarte aux fruits
⅛ of 9" tart 7
4" tart 10

Vichyssoise, 1 cup 5

German Foods

Potato salad, German, ½ cup 2

Sachertorte, ⅟₁₆ of 9" cake....................8

Sauerbraten, 3 oz beef with 2 Tbsp
gravy 6

Spaetzle, ½ cup......................................4

Strudel, any type, 1 piece (5½" x 2")......8

Hispanic Foods

Arroz con pollo, 3 oz chicken with
1½ cups rice 13

Beans, refried, ½ cup 3

Breakfast taco, 1 5

Burritos
bean, 1 large (8") 8
bean, 1 small (6") 5
beef with cheese, 1 (8") 8
beef with cheese, 1 (6") 5
chicken with cheese, 1 (8") 7
chicken with cheese, 1 (6") 5

Carne asada, 4 oz...............................10

Ceviche, ½ cup 2

Chalupa (pork and bean dish),
1 cup...6

Chicken adobo, 1 thigh 6

Chicken mole, 1 cup............................8

Chili con carne
with beans, 1 cup 8
without beans, 1 cup 8

Chili con queso, ¼ cup......................5

Chili relleños, 2...................................18

Chili sauce
green, ¼ cup 1
red, ¼ cup...1

Chimichangas
beef, 1 (3" x 3½") 11
chicken, 1 (3" x 3½") 9

Chorizo, 1 link (5½" long), 3½ oz 12

Empanadas, 2 (3" diameter)..................5

Enchiladas
beef, 2 12
cheese, 2..10
chicken, 2...9
pork, 2 12
sour cream, 1 8

Fajitas
beef, 2 11
chicken, 2...8
pork, 2 13
shrimp, 2..8

Flan, ¾ cup..8

Flautas
beef, 1 (6" x 1¼") 12
chicken, 1 (6" x 1¼") 10
pork, 1 (6" x 1¼")................................11

Gazpacho, 1 cup 4

Gordita, beef, 1 (3" diameter) 10

Guacamole, ¼ cup 2

Huevos rancheros, 2 eggs on
2 tortillas...14

Ice cream, fried, 1 scoop or ½ cup........11

Jalapeño poppers, 1 4

Menudo, 1 cup 6

Mexican coffee, 6 fl oz with 2 Tbsp
whipped cream 3

Mexican corn bread, 1 piece
(1/12 of 10" round) or 3⅓ oz 7

Mexican seven-layer dip, ½ cup 3

Mexican wedding cookies, 2
(each 1½" wide) 2

Mole poblano, ¼ cup 4

Nachos
beef, 4 13
cheese, 4..8
cheese and bean, 4..............................9
chicken, 4...11

Nachos with cheese sauce, ½ cup
tortilla chips with ¼ cup cheese sauce ...5

Paella, 1 cup..7

Picadillo, 1 cup 10

Pico de gallo, ½ cup.............................0

Portuguese sweet bread, ⅛ loaf........5

Pozole, 1 cup 4

Quesadillas
beef, 1 (½ of 6" diameter)......................7
cheese, 1 (½ of 6" diameter) 5
chicken, 1 (½ of 6" diameter) 6
vegetable, 1 (½ of 6" diameter)..............6

Red snapper Veracruz, 6 oz cooked
fillet with ¾ cup sauce 11

Salsa, black beans and corn, ½ cup...1

Sangria, 4 fl oz.....................................2

Sofrito sauce, ½ cup 6

Sopaipillas, 2 (4" x 3" each) 2

Soups
black bean, 1 cup 2
tortilla, 1 cup...6

Spanish rice, 1 cup 5

Spanish sauce, ½ cup 1

Tacos
beef, 1 5
chicken, 1..4
fish, 1 4
pork, 1 4

Taco salad
with shell, without dressing, fast food, 1 ..15
without shell and dressing, fast food, 1 8

Tamale pie, 1 cup 11

Tamales with sauce, 2 (4" x 2")........10

Tostadas
beef, 1 10
chicken, 1..8

Tortilla chips, 12 (1 oz)........................3

Tortillas
corn, 2 (4" diameter), 1 (6" diameter),
½ (10" diameter), or 1 oz 1
flour, 2 (4" diameter), 1 (6" diameter),
½ (10" diameter), or 1 oz 2

Indian Foods

**Bean and lentil stew
(Dal maharani),** 1 cup 6

Chapati, 1 (5" diameter) 2

Chicken tikka, 4 oz 5

Coconut rice, Indian, 1 cup 5

Curry
beef, 1 cup 10
Bengali fish, 1 fillet (4½ oz) and
1 cup vegetables 10
chicken, 1 cup 10
lamb, 1 cup 10

Dhansak, 1 cup 6

Fritters, vegetable, 1 cup..................10

Kashmiri (lamb meatballs), 6
(3½ oz)..11

Kheer, ½ cup...5

Korma
chicken, 1 cup 14
lamb, 1 cup 15
vegetable, 1 cup 11

Lamb biryani, 1 cup 12

Naan, 1 piece (7" x 8" diameter)............4

Pakora, vegetable, 1 (2" x 3") or
1¾ oz...3

Paratha, 1 (4" triangle) 4

Puris, 1 (4" diameter) 2

Raita, ½ cup 1

Samosa, 1 (2½" x 2½" x 3" triangle)......3

Soup, mulligatawny, 1 cup 5

Tandori chicken, without skin,
1 breast and 1 thigh 9

Vindaloo
chicken, 1 cup 8
pork, 1 cup...9

HISPANIC

INDIAN

Italian Foods

Artichokes, marinated, ½ cup 3

Biscotti, plain, 8 mini, 2 small, or
1 regular (1 oz) 3

Bolognese meat sauce, ½ cup 6

Bruschetta, 1 slice 3

Caesar salad, 3 cups...........................7

Calamari, fried, ½ cup 11

Calzone, 1 (5¼" x 6"), 7 oz 12

Cannelloni, cheese
with meat sauce, 2 shells with
½ cup sauce......................................29
with tomato sauce, 2 shells with
½ cup sauce......................................14

Cannelloni, meat
with cream sauce, 2 shells with
½ cup sauce......................................17
with tomato sauce, 2 shells with
½ cup sauce......................................14

Cannelloni, spinach and cheese
with cream sauce, 2 shells with
½ cup sauce......................................15
with tomato sauce, 2 shells with
½ cup sauce......................................12

Cannoli, 1 (3½" long) 9

Caponata, 1 cup...................................4

Cappuccino
made with fat-free milk, 1 grande
(16 fl oz)..2
made with fat-free milk, 1 small (8 fl oz)...1
made with fat-free milk, 1 tall (12 fl oz) ...2
made with low-fat milk, 1 grande
(16 fl oz)..3
made with low-fat milk, 1 small (8 fl oz) ..2
made with low-fat milk, 1 tall (12 fl oz) ...3
made with whole milk, 1 grande
(16 fl oz)..4
made with whole milk, 1 small (8 fl oz)....2
made with whole milk, 1 tall (12 fl oz) 3

Chicken cacciatore, 1 half breast
or 1 thigh and leg (6½ oz) 10

Chicken marsala, 1 serving, without
bone (4 oz) 15

Chicken parmigiana
without sauce, 5½ oz.............................8
with sauce, 5 oz with ½ cup sauce.........10

Chicken tetrazzini, 1½ cups...............14

Cioppino, 2 cups 13

Clams
baked, 6..7
fried, 1 cup...10

Clam sauce
red, ½ cup..3
white, ½ cup 5

Cookies, amaretti, 1 (1" diameter).......2

Eggplant parmigiana
without sauce, 1 serving (3" x 4") 11
with sauce, 1 serving (3" x 4") with
½ cup Italian tomato sauce 13

Fettuccine Alfredo, 1 cup.................16

Garlic bread, 1 slice (1 oz) 5

Gnocchi
cheese, 1 cup 11
potato, 1 cup...4
spinach, 1 cup 12

Lasagna
with meat, 1 cup 6
vegetarian, with cheese, 1 serving 10
vegetarian, with cheese and spinach,
1 serving...9

Linguini
with red clam sauce, 1 cup linguini
with ½ cup sauce 6
with white clam sauce, 1 cup linguini
with ½ cup sauce 8

Manicotti
with meat sauce, 2 shells with
½ cup sauce......................................15
with tomato sauce, 2 shells with
½ cup sauce......................................12

Marinara sauce, ½ cup 3

Meat sauce, ½ cup 5

Meatballs
without sauce, 2 (each 1¼" diameter) ...10
with sauce, 2 meatballs and ½ cup
Italian tomato sauce............................13

Mozzarella, fried, 2 slices
(2¾" x 1" x ½" each) 10

Mushrooms, marinated, ½ cup...........3

Osso bucco, 6 oz veal with ¼ cup
sauce..13

Panettone, ¹⁄₁₂ of 9" tube or 1½ oz 6

Panini
chicken, 1..11
ham and cheese, 1...............................11
vegetable, 1 10

Pasta, 1 cup cooked.............................3

Pasta e fagioli, 1 cup 8

Pasta primavera
2 cups..6
with cream sauce, 1 cup pasta with
¾ cup sauce 12

Penne a la vodka, 1 cup pasta with
½ cup sauce..7

Pesto sauce, 2 Tbsp 3

Pizza, cheese, deep dish
1 slice (⅛ of 12", ¹⁄₁₀ of 14", or
¹⁄₁₂ of 16")..5
1 slice (⅛ of 14", ¹⁄₁₀ of 16", or
¹⁄₁₂ of 18")..7
1 slice (⅛ of 18") 10

Pizza, cheese, thin crust
1 slice (⅛ of 12", ¹⁄₁₀ of 14", or
¹⁄₁₂ of 16")..4
1 slice (⅛ of 14", ¹⁄₁₀ of 16", or
¹⁄₁₂ of 18")..5
1 slice (⅛ of 18") 9

**Pizza, meat and vegetable,
thin crust**
1 slice (⅛ of 12", ¹⁄₁₀ of 14", or
¹⁄₁₂ of 16")..4
1 slice (⅛ of 14", ¹⁄₁₀ of 16", or
¹⁄₁₂ of 18")..5
1 slice (⅛ of 18") 9

Pizza, one-meat topping, deep dish
1 slice (⅛ of 12", ¹⁄₁₀ of 14", or
¹⁄₁₂ of 16")..6
1 slice (⅛ of 14", ¹⁄₁₀ of 16", or
¹⁄₁₂ of 18")..8
1 slice (⅛ of 18") 11

Pizza, one-meat topping, thin crust
1 slice (⅛ of 12", ¹⁄₁₀ of 14", or
¹⁄₁₂ of 16")..5
1 slice (⅛ of 14", ¹⁄₁₀ of 16", or
¹⁄₁₂ of 18")..6
1 slice (⅛ of 18") 10

Ravioli, cheese
with tomato sauce, 8 pieces or 1 cup
with ½ cup sauce 16
without sauce, 8 pieces or 1 cup...........13

Ravioli, meat
with tomato sauce, 8 pieces or 1 cup
with ½ cup sauce 14
without sauce, 8 pieces or 1 cup...........12

Risotto, ½ cup 4

Shrimp scampi, 9 medium shrimp
(3 oz)..11

Soups
lentil, 1 cup 3
minestrone, 1 cup 4

Spaghetti Bolognese, 1 cup
spaghetti with ½ cup sauce...................9

Spaghetti carbonara, 1 cup 10

Spaghetti
with garlic and oil, 1 cup........................7
with marinara sauce, 1 cup spaghetti
with ½ cup sauce 6

Spaghetti (con't)   POINTS

with meat sauce, 1 cup spaghetti with
½ cup sauce...9
with meatballs and tomato sauce,
1 cup spaghetti, 2 meatballs and
½ cup sauce...16

Spumoni, ½ cup 6

Stromboli, 1 slice (1" thick) or 2 oz........4

Tirami-su, 1 piece (2¼" square) 9

**Tomato and mozzarella salad
without dressing,** 1 large tomato
with 2¼ oz cheese 6

Tomato sauce, Italian, ½ cup..............3

Tortellini
cheese, without sauce, 10 (⅔ cup) 3
meat, without sauce,10 (⅔ cup) 3

Tortoni, 1 serving 7

Turkey tetrazzini, 1½ cups...................9

Veal
marsala, 4 oz 11
parmigiana, without sauce, 5½ oz 10
parmigiana, with sauce, 5 oz with
½ cup tomato sauce 12
piccata, 2 slices (4 oz)...........................11
scaloppine, 2 pieces (3" x 5") or 4½ oz ..12
with peppers, 5 oz 11

Vitello Tonnato, 2 slices veal (4 oz)
with ½ cup sauce 20

Zabaglione, ½ cup 6

Zeppole, 1 (4" diameter).......................5

Ziti, baked
with meat, 1 cup 9
without meat, 1 cup 6

Zuppa di pesce, 2 cups.......................12

Zuppa Inglese, ¹⁄₁₆ of 10" cake 7

POINTS

Japanese Foods

Green tea ice cream, ½ cup 3

Nebeyaki udon, 2 cups 8

**Sashimi (except salmon or
mackerel),** 4 pieces 1

Sashimi, salmon or mackerel,
4 pieces...2

Shabu shabu, 4 oz beef, 2 oz tofu,
and 1½ cups vegetables 8

Soup, miso, 1 cup 2

Suimono, 1 cup 1

Sukiyaki, 2½ cups................................12

Sunomono, ½ cup..................................1

Sushi
California roll, 4 pieces (1" high x 1¾"
diameter) or 1 oz each.........................3
maki, 4 pieces 2
nigiri, 4 pieces 2
nori maki, 4 pieces 2

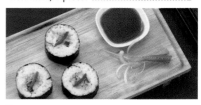

Tempura
shrimp, 4 jumbo 12
vegetable, 1 cup 8

Teppan yaki, 1½ cups.........................10

Teriyaki
beef, 2 slices (4 oz) 7
chicken, 2 slices (4 oz) 6
fish, 4 oz...5

Teriyaki sauce, 1 Tbsp.........................0

Tonkatsu, ¾ cup 12

Yakitori, 1 skewer with 3 Tbsp sauce 6

Yosenabe, 2 cups 8

Jewish Foods

Bagel, any type, 1 small or ½ large
(2 oz)..3
Bagel, with cream cheese and lox,
1 large..12

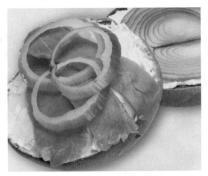

Beets, pickled, ½ cup 1
Bialy, 1 (3 oz).....................................5
Blintz, cheese, 1 5
Borscht, beet, 1 cup with 2 Tbsp
sour cream..4
Cabbage, stuffed, 2 (2" x 2½") 6
Challah bread, 1 slice (5" x 3" x ¾")....2
Chicken and meatball fricassee,
2 cups 9
Chicken in the pot, without skin,
2 cups 10
Cholent, 1 cup.....................................4
Flanken, 2 slices (4 oz).........................8
Fruit compote, ½ cup............................4
Hamantaschen, 1 piece (3" diameter) ...3
Haroset, 1 cup......................................4

Herring
cooked, 1 oz..1
chopped, ¼ cup..4
in cream sauce, ¼ cup 3
pickled, ½ cup 2
Honey cake, 1 slice (5" x 3" x 1") 7
Kasha varnishkes, 1 cup.....................4
Kishke, 1 small piece.............................4
Knish, potato, 1 (3½" square)...............6
Kreplachs
boiled, 2 pieces (4" x 3" x 3" each).........5
fried, 2 pieces (4" x 3" x 3" each)...........7
Kugel
lukschen, 1 piece (3" x 3¼")...................7
potato, 1 piece (3" x 3¼") 3
Liver, chopped, ¼ cup 5
Mandelbrot, 2 slices (3" x 2" x ½") 3
Matzo, 1 board 2
Matzo brie, ¼ of 10" round or 1 cup 6
Passover sponge cake, 1⁄12 of 9" tube..3
Potato latkes, 2 (3½" diameter) 5
Rugalach, 1 piece (2½" x 1¼") or 1 oz...3
Schmaltz, 1 Tbsp 3
Soups
cabbage, 1 cup 1
chicken, with matzo balls, 1 cup soup
with 2 (1½") matzo balls 3
chicken, without matzo balls
(broth only), 1 cup...............................0
mushroom barley, 1 cup 5
Sponge cake, 1⁄12 of 9" tube 4
Tzimmes, vegetable, ¾ cup 2

JEWISH

Middle Eastern Foods

Baba ganosh, ¼ cup 3

Baklava, 1 piece (2" square) 5

Dolma, 4 4

Falafel in pita, 1 large pita with
    4 falafel patties 13

Falafel patties, 4 (2" diameter each) ..10

Greek salad
    with dressing, 3 cups 9
    without dressing, 3 cups 2

Gyro, 1 (6") 15

Halvah, 1 piece (2" x 1¾" x 1) 5

Hummus, ¼ cup 3

Kataifi, 1 piece (2" long) 5

Kibbe
    baked, 3 pieces (1½" squares) 3
    uncooked, ½ cup 4

Lavash, ¼ of 10" cracker (2¼ oz) 6

Moussaka, 1 piece (3" x 4") 12

Pastitsio, 1 piece (3¼" x 3") 11

Pita, any type, 1 small or ½ large (1 oz)..1

Rice pilaf, 1 cup 7

Saganaki, 1 piece (1" x 2" x ½" thick) ...6

Sesame candy, 1 piece (2" x 1") 2

Shish kebob, 2 small skewers 10

Soups
    avgolemono, 1 cup 4
    yogurt and cucumber, 1 cup 2

Souvlaki, 1 large skewer or 2 small
    skewers 10

Souvlaki sandwich, 1 7

Spanakopita, 1 (3" square) 9

Tabouli, ½ cup.......................................4

Tahini, 2 Tbsp 2

Yogurt and cucumber salad, ¼ cup ...1

Thai Foods

Ginger chicken, 1 cup 7

**Green chicken curry (Gaeng
    Kheow Wan Gai),** 1 cup...................7

Mussaman beef curry, 1 cup.............19

Nam Prik, 1 Tbsp...................................1

Pad Thai, 1 cup......................................7

Peanut sauce, 2 Tbsp............................4

Satay, 2 skewers with ¼ cup sauce..........9

Seafood cakes (Haw Mok Thalay),
    ¾ cup..8

Thai beef salad, 1 cup 14

Thai chicken coconut soup, 1 cup......8

Thai chicken with basil, 1 breast
    (without skin or bone), 3 oz 5

Thai coconut rice, 1 cup 19

Thai coffee or tea, 1 cup....................6

Thai crisp noodles, 1 cup 11

Thai curry paste, 1 Tbsp 1

Thai paste, 2 Tbsp................................2

Thai seafood salad, 2 cups...............10

Tom yum kung, 1 cup 2

Vietnamese Foods

Imperial roll, 1 (4½" long)....................4

Lemon grass chicken, 1 cup 8

Nuoc cham, 1 Tbsp................................0

Soups
    asparagus crab, 1 cup 2
    Vietnamese beef noodle, 1 cup 2

**Vietnamese beef balls
    (Thit bo vien),** 6 (1½ oz) 2

Vietnamese spring roll, 1 2

**Vietnamese spring roll dipping
    sauce,** 2 Tbsp.....................................0

Foods Listed by Brand Name

POINTS

Alfalfa seeds
Tropical Fruit & Nut Alfalfa seeds
  30 g 0

Alfredo sauce
Classico
  Alfredo di roma – alfredo, ¼ cup 3
  Alfredo di sorrento – roasted garlic
  alfredo, ¼ cup 3
Di Giorno
  Alfredo sauce, ¼ cup 5
  Light alfredo sauce, ¼ cup......................4
Five Brothers
  Alfredo & mushroom, ¼ cup...................2
  Creamy alfredo, ¼ cup 3
Progresso Alfredo (authentic), ½ cup.......5
Ragu Cheese Creations
  Classic alfredo, ¼ cup 3
  Lite Parmesan alfredo, ¼ cup..................2

Almonds
Dole
  Blanched slivered, ⅓ cup........................4
  Blanched whole, ¼ cup 4
  Chopped natural, ¼ cup 4
  Sliced natural, ⅓ cup 4
  Whole natural, ¼ cup 4
Tropical Nut & Fruit
  Almonds roasted/salted, 1 oz 4
  Honey roast almonds, ¼ cup 5
  Raw almonds, 1 oz 4
  Roasted almonds, 1 oz 4
  Sliced almonds, 1 oz 4
  Slivered almonds, 1 oz 4
  Smoked almonds, 1 oz 4

Apples
Boston Markets Cinnamon apples,
  1 serving (255 g) 9
Del Monte Fruit Pleasures Pie
  spiced apples in naturaly-flavored sauce,
  ½ cup 1
Del Monte Fruit Rageous Amazing
  cinnamon apples, 4-oz cup 2
Dole Apple, 1 1

POINTS

Knouse Canned sliced apples, ½ cup........1
Stouffer's Escalloped apples, 6 oz 3
Tropical Nut & Fruit
  Apple snack with cinnamon, 30 g 2
  Natural apple rings, 40 g........................2
  Natural apples, diced, 40 g.....................2
  Sulphured apple, diced, 40 g..................2
  Sulphured apple rings, 40 g....................2

Apple juice
Apple Time Original apple juice, 8 fl oz ...2
Indian Summer Apple juice, premium
  with vitamin c added, 8 fl oz 2
Knouse
  Apple juice with calcium and vitamin c,
  8 fl oz..2
  Premium apple juice, 8 fl oz....................2
Lucky Leaf Old fashioned apple juice,
  8 fl oz 2
Minute Maid Apple juice, 8 fl oz 2
Minute Maid Premium
  Apple juice with vitamin c and calcium
  added, 1 drink box (200 ml) 2
  Apple juice with vitamin c and calcium
  added, 8 fl oz 2
Musselman's Natural apple juice, 1 cup ...2
Payaso Apple juice, 1 bottle (8.45 fl oz) 2
Snapple Snapple farms apple juice,
  12 fl oz 4
Tropicana Season's Best
  Apple juice, 1 carton (6 fl oz).................2
  Apple juice, 1 bottle (7 fl oz) 2
  Apple juice, 8 fl oz 2
  Apple juice, 10 fl oz 3
  Apple juice, 1 can (12 fl oz) 3
Wilderness
  Apple juice, 8 fl oz 2
  Apple juice with vitamin c added,
  8 fl oz..2
  Apple juice, premium, with vitamin c
  added, 8 fl oz 2
  Natural apple juice, 8 fl oz......................2

Applesauce
Apple Time
Original apple sauce in 23 oz glass,
½ cup 1
Original apple sauce in single serve cups,
1 serving (4-oz unit) 1
Knouse Apple sauce, ½ cup 1
Lucky Leaf Natural apple sauce in
23 oz glass, ½ cup 1
Musselman's
Apple sauce, ½ cup 1
Natural apple sauce in 23 oz glass,
½ cup 1
Natural apple sauce in single serve cups,
1 serving (4-oz unit) 1
Wilderness
Applesauce, unsweetened, ½ cup 1
Old Fashioned Applesauce, ½ cup 1

Apricots
Del Monte
Almond flavored apricot halves in light
syrup, ½ cup..2
Lite unpeeled apricot halves, ½ cup 1
Unpeeled apricot halves in heavy syrup,
½ cup 2
Del Monte Orchard Select Unpeeled
apricot halves in light syrup, ½ cup.........1
Dole Apricots, ½ cup 0
EXPRESSnacks Apricot, 1 (2.75 oz) 3
Sunsweet Dried apricots, 1½ oz 1
Tropical Nut & Fruit
Austrialian apricots, 3 oz 6
California apricots, 40 g 2
Turkish apricots, 5 pieces (40 g) 1
Unsulphured turk apricots, 5 pieces 1

Artichokes
Progresso
Artichoke hearts (in brine), 2 pieces
(82 g) 0
Artichoke hearts (marinated), 2 pieces
with liquid (32g)....................................2

Asparagus
Del Monte
Cuts & tips, asparagus early green,
½ cup 0
Spears, asparagus extra long, ½ cup 0
Spears, asparagus tender young, ½ cup 0
Tips, asparagus hand selected, ½ cup 0
Green Giant
Asparagus spears, canned, 4½ oz..............0
Cut spears asparagus, 50% less sodium,
canned, ½ cup.......................................0
Cut spears asparagus, canned, ½ cup 0
Extra long asparagus spears, canned,
4½ oz 0
Green Giant Harvest Fresh
Asparagus cuts, frozen, ⅔ cup 0
Hanover The Gold Line Petite
asparagus spears, 8 spears 0
LeSueur Extra large asparagus spears,
canned, 4½ oz.......................................0

Avocados
Brooks Lite avocado, ⅛ cup 1
Chiquita Avocado, California,
⅕ medium (30 g)...................................1

B

Bacon
Betty Crocker Bac Os chips or bits,
1½ Tbsp...1
Boar's Head
Canadian style bacon, 2 oz.......................2
Domestic bacon, 2 slices (12 g)................2
Imported naturally smoked sliced bacon,
2 slices (12 g)..2
Pancetta, ½ oz 1
Farmland
Butcher's cut extra thick sliced bacon,
2 slices 2
Canadian style bacon, 2 oz.......................1
Hickory smoked bacon, 2 slices (15 g) 2
Lower sodium hickory smoked bacon,
2 slices (15 g).......................................2

Bacon, Farmland (con't)   POINTS

Thick sliced hickory smoked bacon,
2 slices (15 g).................................2
Thick sliced peppered bacon, 1 slice
(11 g) 2

Hormel

Bacon bits, 1 Tbsp.............................1
Bacon pieces, 1 Tbsp 1
Bacon, fully cooked, 2½ slices (14 g) 2
Canadian style bacon, 2 oz......................2
Microwave bacon, cooked, 4 slices
(15 g) 2

Hormel Black Label

Bacon, cooked, 2 slices (15 g) 2
Center cut bacon, cooked, 3 slices (15 g)....2
Low salt bacon, cooked, 2 slices (15 g) 2

Hormel Old Smokehouse Bacon,

cooked, 2 slices (15 g)............................2

Hormel Range Brand Bacon, cooked,

2 slices (21 g)......................................3

Hormel Red Label Bacon, cooked,

2 slices (15 g)......................................2

Louis Rich Bacon, turkey, cooked,

1 slice (14 g) 1

Oscar Mayer

Bacon bits, real, 1 Tbsp 1
Bacon pieces, real, 1 Tbsp........................1
Bacon, ⅛" thick cut, cooked, 1 slice
(12 g) 2
Bacon, center cut, cooked, 2 slices (12 g) ...2
Bacon, cooked, 1 slice (14 g) 2
Bacon, lower sodium, cooked, 2 slices
(14 g) 2

Bagels

Cobblestone Mill Plain bagels, 1

(85 g)...4

Otis Spunkmeyer

Blueberry, 1 (85 g) 4
Cinnamon raisin, 1 (85 g) 4
Onion, 1 (85 g) 4
Plain, 1 (85 g)....................................4

Bagel chips

Burns & Ricker

Garlic bagel chips, 3 pieces (29 g).............3
Plain bagel chips, 3 pieces (29 g) 3

POINTS

Seasalt bagel chips, 3 pieces (29 g)...........3
Sesame bagel chips, 3 pieces (29 g) 3

New York Style

Cinnamon raisin bagel chips, 3 pieces
(29 ml)..3
Garlic bagel chips, 3 pieces (29 ml) 3
Plain bagel chips, 3 pieces (29 ml) 3
Seasalt bagel chips, 3 pieces (29 ml) 3
Sesame bagel chips, 3 pieces (29 ml) 3

Tropical Nut & Fruit

Cinnamon bagel chips, 28 (31 g)..............3
Hot & spicy bagel chips, 28 (31 g)............3
Plain bagel chips, 28 (31 g) 3
Rye bagel chips, 28 (31g) 3

Bagel pizza

Ore-Ida Bagel Bites

Cheese & pepperoni, 4 pieces (88 g) 4
Cheese & sausage, 4 pieces (88 g) 4
Cheeseburger, 4 pieces (88 g) 5
Four meat, 4 pieces (88 g) 4
Mozzarella cheese, 4 pieces (88 g) 4
Sausage & pepperoni, 4 pieces (88 g)........4
Supreme, 4 pieces (88 g) 4
Three cheese, 4 pieces (88 g) 4

Baking mix

Bisquick

Original baking mix, ⅓ cup....................4
Reduced fat baking mix, ⅓ cup................3
Sweet baking mix, ⅓ cup 4

Bananas

Chiquita Banana, 1 medium (126 g) 1

Dole Banana, 1.................................2

Banana chips

Tropical Nut & Fruit

Banana chips, 1 oz................................3
Unsulfured unsweetened banana chip,
35 pieces (40 g)...............................2

Barbecue sauce

Heinz

Buffalo wing BBQ sauce, 2 Tbsp................0
Hickory smoke BBQ sauce, 2 Tbsp 1
Mesquite BBQ sauce, 2 Tbsp....................1
Original BBQ sauce, 2 Tbsp......................1

Heinz Thick & Rich

Cajun style barbecue sauce, 2 Tbsp 1
Chunky barbecue sauce, 2 Tbsp 1
Hawaiian barbecue sauce, 2 Tbsp..............1
Honey mustard barbeque sauce, 2 Tbsp.....1

House of Tsang Hong Kong barbecue
    sauce, 1 tsp................0

Kraft

Char-grill, 2 Tbsp 1
Extra rich original, 2 Tbsp 1
Hickory smoke, 2 Tbsp 1
Hickory smoke onion bits, 2 Tbsp 1
Honey, 2 Tbsp 1
Honey hickory, 2 Tbsp...............................1
Honey mustard, 2 Tbsp..............................1
Hot, 2 Tbsp 1
Hot hickory smoke, 2 Tbsp 1
Kansas City style, 2 Tbsp 1
Mesquite smoke, 2 Tbsp 1
Molasses, 2 Tbsp.......................................1
Onion bits, 2 Tbsp.....................................1
Original, 2 Tbsp 1
Roasted garlic, 2 Tbsp 1
Spicy honey, 2 Tbsp...................................1
Teriyaki, 2 Tbsp...1

Kraft Thick 'N Spicy

Brown sugar, 2 Tbsp..................................1
Hickory bacon, 2 Tbsp...............................1
Hickory smoke, 2 Tbsp 1
Honey, 2 Tbsp 1
Honey mustard, 2 Tbsp..............................1
Kansas City style, 2 Tbsp 1
Mesquite smoke, 2 Tbsp 1
Original, 2 Tbsp 1

Lea & Perrins Barbecue sauce, original,
    2 Tbsp...1

Naturally Fresh

Bar-b-que sauce, 2 Tbsp 1
Messquite BBQ sauce, 2 Tbsp 1

Beans

B&G Maple flavor baked beans, ½ cup 2
Chi-Chi's Pinto beans, ½ cup 1

Del Monte

Cut beans, ½ cup...0
Cut, Italian beans, ½ cup............................0
Cut, no salt added beans, ½ cup 0
French style beans, ½ cup...........................0
French style, no salt added beans,
    ½ cup...0
Green lima beans, ½ cup 1
Seasoned French style beans, ½ cup..........0
Whole beans, ½ cup.....................................0

Faraon

Black beans, canned, ½ cup........................1
Black beans, uncooked, ¼ cup 1
Garbanzo beans, canned, ½ cup 1
Garbanzo beans, uncooked, ¼ cup 2
Great northern beans, uncooked, ¼ cup 1
Lima beans, uncooked, ¼ cup 1
Mexican habas, uncooked, ¼ cup...............3
Pink beans, uncooked, ¼ cup......................1
Pinto beans, canned, ½ cup 1
Pinto beans, uncooked, ¼ cup.....................1
Red kidney beans, uncooked, ¼ cup 1
Small red beans, uncooked, ¼ cup 2
Small white beans, uncooked, ¼ cup 1
White kidney beans, uncooked, ¼ cup.......2

Green Giant

Baby lima beans, frozen, ⅔ cup 2
Black beans, canned, ½ cup........................1
Butter beans, canned, ½ cup.......................1
Cut green beans, canned, ½ cup 0
Cut green beans, frozen, ¾ cup 0
Dark red kidney beans, canned, ½ cup 1
French style green beans, canned,
    ½ cup...0
Garbanzo beans, canned, ½ cup 2
Great northern beans, canned, ½ cup........1
Kitchen sliced green beans, canned,
    ½ cup...0
Light red kidney beans, canned, ½ cup 1
Pinto beans, canned, ½ cup 1
Pork & beans with tomato sauce,
    canned, ½ cup..2
Red beans, canned, ½ cup 1

Spicy chilli beans, canned, ½ cup 1
Whole green beans, canned, ½ cup 0
Whole green beans, frozen, 1 cup 0

Green Giant Harvest Fresh
Baby lima beans, frozen, ½ cup 1
Green beans & almonds, frozen, ⅔ cup 1

Hain Pure Foods
Black turtle, ½ cup 1
Blue lake cut green beans, ½ cup..............0
French cut green beans, ½ cup..................0
Pinto, ½ cup 1

Hanover
Baby lima beans, ½ cup 1
Blue lake cut green beans, ¾ cup 0
Blue lake French style green beans,
   1 cup 0
Blue lake whole green beans, 1 cup 0
Cut Romano Italian green beans, ¾ cup....0
Fordhook lima beans, ½ cup 2
Premium select whole yellow beans,
   1 cup 0

Hanover The Gold Line Petite whole
   green beans, ¾ cup 0

Heinz Vegetarian beans, 1 cup..................4

Joan of Arc
Black beans, canned, ½ cup......................1
Butter beans, canned, ½ cup.....................1
Dark red kidney beans, canned, ½ cup 1
Garbanzo beans, canned, ½ cup 2
Great northern beans, canned, ½ cup........1
Light red kidney beans, canned, ½ cup 1
Light red kidney beans, canned, ½ cup 1
Pinto beans, canned, ½ cup 1
Pork & beans with tomato sauce,
   canned, ½ cup.......................................2
Red beans, canned, ½ cup 1
Spicy chili beans, ½ cup 1
Spicy chilli beans, canned, ½ cup 1

Old El Paso
Black beans, ½ cup 1
Garbanzos, ½ cup 1
Mexe beans, ½ cup 1
Pinto beans, ½ cup 1

Progresso
Black beans, ½ cup 1
Cannellini beans, ½ cup 1
Chick peas, ½ cup....................................2
Dark red kidney beans, ½ cup...................1
Fava beans, ½ cup 1
Garbanzo beans, ½ cup............................2
Pinto beans, ½ cup 1
Red kidney beans, ½ cup..........................1

Schwan's Cut green beans, ⅔ cup 0

Stouffer's Green bean mushroom
   casserole, ½ cup 3

Sunsun Mayocoba-canar, uncooked,
   ¼ cup 2

Beans, refried
Chi-Chi's
Fat free refried beans, ½ cup 2
Refried beans, ½ cup................................2

Faraon Refried black beans, ½ cup 1

Hain Pure Foods Fat free vegetarian
   refried black beans, ½ cup......................1

Old El Paso
Refried beans, ½ cup................................1
Refried beans with cheese, ½ cup 2
Refried beans with green chillies, ½ cup....1
Refried beans with sausage, ½ cup 4
Refried beans, fat free, ½ cup 1
Refried beans, spicy, fat free, ½ cup...........1
Refried beans, vegetarian, ½ cup 1

Taco Bell Home Originals
Fat free refried beans, ½ cup 1
Fat free refried beans with mild chilies,
   ½ cup 1
Refried beans, ½ cup................................2

Béchamel (white) sauce
Durkee
White sauce, dry mix, 1 Tbsp 1
White sauce, prepared, ¼ cup...................1

Beef
Hormel
Corned beef, 2 oz.....................................3
Roast beef w/ gravy, ½ cup 3

Hormel Pillow Pack Dried beef,
  10 slices (28 g) 1
Tyson Seasoned beef strips, 3 oz 3
Schwan's
  Beef sirloin steak tips, 4 oz 3
  Beef tips and gravy, 1 cup 5
  Big Sam beef steak, 1 (168 g) 5
  Burgundy peppercorn roast, 4 oz 3
  Chopped BBQ beef, ½ cup 3
  Cracked peppercorn beef burger, 1
    (112 g) 5
  Filet mignon, 1 steak (140 g) 3
  Quarter pound beef burger, 1 (112 g) 5
  "E-Z Fix" burgers, 1 (85 g).......................6

Beef jerky or stick
Lance
  Beef & cheese, 1 package (42 g) 4
  Beef jerky, 1 piece (7 g)...........................1
  Beef snack, 1 piece (18 g) 3
  Jumbo beef jerky, 1 piece (16 g)................2
  Jumbo beef snack, 1 piece (28 g) 4
  Kippered beef steak, original,
    1 package (25 g) 1
  Kippered beef steak, peppered,
    1 package (25 g) 1
  Kippered beef steak, teriyaki,
    1 package (25 g) 1
  Supersize beef snack, 1 piece (13 g)..........2
  Supersize beef snack, 1 piece (14 g)..........2
Rustlers Roundup
  Beef jerky, 9 g 1
  Flamin' hot meat stick, 7.4 g 1
  Flamin' hot meat stick, 7.9 g 1
  Smoky steak strip, 22.7 g 1
  Spicy stick, 18 g.....................................2

Beef, dried
Hormel Sliced dried beef, 10 slices
  (28 g) 1

Beef, roast, deli
Alpine Lace Roast beef, extra lean
  97% fat-free, 2 oz...................................2

Boar's Head
  1st cut cooked corned brisket – USDA
    choice, 2 oz......................................2
  1st cut corned beef brisket – uncooked
    USDA choice, 2½ oz...............................3
  1st cut pastrami brisket – USDA choice,
    2 oz...2
  Cajun style seasoned eye rd oven
    roasted beef, 2 oz 2
  Choice cap off top round – whole, no
    salt added, 2 oz..................................2
  Cooked corned beef brisket – USDA
    choice, 2 oz......................................3
  Custom cut beef round, no salt added,
    2 oz...2
  Custom cut cooked corned beef round,
    2 oz...2
  Deluxe low sodium – cap-off top round,
    2 oz...2
  Deluxe low sodium choice top round,
    2 oz...2
  Italian style OR seasoned beef with
    classic bracole seasoning, 2 oz 2
  Natural flat cooked corned beef, 2 oz 2
  No salt added choice cap off top round,
    2 oz...2
  Our deluxe oven roasted eye round,
    low sodium, 2 oz 2
  Oven roasted choice top round, no salt
    added, 2 oz 2
  Pepper seasoned eye round, 2 oz 2
  Red pastrami round, 2 oz 2
  Seasoned filet of roast beef – cap off
    top round, 2 oz...................................2
  USDA choice cooked corned beef top
    round – cap off, 2 oz..............................2

Beer
Budweiser
  Bud dry, 1 can or bottle (12 fl oz).............3
  Bud ice, 1 can or bottle (12 fl oz) 3
  Bud ice light, 1 can or bottle (12 fl oz) 2
  Bud light, 1 can or bottle (12 fl oz) 2
  Budweiser, 1 can or bottle (12 fl oz).........3

Busch
Busch, 1 can or bottle (12 fl oz) 3
Busch ice, 1 can or bottle (12 fl oz) 3
Busch light, 1 can or bottle (12 fl oz) 2

Hurricane, 1 can or bottle (12 fl oz) 3

Lowenbrau
Dark, 1 can or bottle (12 fl oz) 3
Special, 1 can or bottle (12 fl oz) 3
Magnum, 1 can or bottle (12 fl oz) 3

Meister Brau
Meister brau, 1 can or bottle (12 fl oz) 3
Meister brau light, 1 can or bottle,
    (12 fl oz) 2

Michelob
Michelob, 1 can or bottle, (12 fl oz) 3
Michelob amber bock, 1 can or bottle
    (12 fl oz) 3
Michelob black & tan, 1 can or bottle
    (12 fl oz) 3
Michelob classic dark, 1 can or bottle
    (12 fl oz) 3
Michelob dry, 1 can or bottle (12 fl oz) 3
Michelob golden draft, 1 can or bottle
    (12 fl oz) 3
Michelob golden draft light, 1 can or
    bottle (12 fl oz) 2
Michelob hefeweizen, 1 can or bottle
    (12 fl oz) 4
Michelob honey lager, 1 can or bottle
    (12 fl oz) 4
Michelob light, 1 can or bottle (12 fl oz) 3

Miller
Genuine draft light, 1 can or bottle
    (12 fl oz) 2
Genuine draft, 1 can or bottle,
    (12 fl oz) 3
High life ice, 1 can or bottle, (12 fl oz) 3
High life light, 1 can or bottle (12 fl oz) 2
Icehouse 5.0, 1 can or bottle(12 fl oz) 3
Icehouse 5.5, 1 can or bottle (12 fl oz) 3
Lite, 1 can or bottle (12 fl oz) 2
Lite ice 5.0, 1 can or bottle (12 fl oz) 2
Lite ice 5.5, 1 can or bottle, (12 fl oz) 2

Milwaukee's Best
Milwaukee's best, 1 can or bottle
    (12 fl oz) 3
Milwaukee's best ice (12 fl oz) 3
Milwaukee's best light, 1 can or bottle
    (12 fl oz) 2

Natural Light
Natural ice, 1 can or bottle (12 fl oz) 3
Natural light, 1 can or bottle (12 fl oz) 2
Red Wolf, 1 can or bottle (12 fl oz) 3

Southpaw light, 1 can or bottle
    (12 fl oz) 2

Tequiza, 1 can or bottle (12 ml) 3

Beer, non-alcoholic
Busch non-alcoholic beer, 1 can or
    bottle (12 fl oz) 1

O'Doul's
O'Doul's amber non-alcoholic beer,
    1 can or bottle (12 fl oz) 2
O'Doul's non-alcoholic beer, 1 can or
    bottle (12 fl oz) 1

Sharp's, 1 can or bottle (12 fl oz) 1

Beets
Del Monte
Crinkle style sliced, pickled beets,
    ½ cup 1
Sliced beets, ½ cup 0

Green Giant
Harvard beets, ⅓ cup 1
Sliced beets, canned, ½ cup 0
Sliced beets, canned, ½ cup 0
Sliced beets, no salt added, canned,
    ½ cup 0
Whole beets, canned, ½ cup 0

LeSueur Baby whole beets, canned,
    ½ cup 0

Biscuits
Martha White Buttermilk biscuit mix,
    prepared, 1 serving (¼ recipe) 4

Pillsbury
Buttermilk, 3 biscuits (64 g) 3
Country, 3 biscuits (64 g) 3
Tender layer buttermilk, 3 biscuits (64 g) ...3

Pillsbury 1869 Brand Buttermilk,
   1 biscuit (31 g) 2
Pillsbury Big Country
   Butter tastin', 1 biscuit (34 g) 2
   Buttermilk, 1 biscuit (34 g) 2
   Southern style, 1 biscuit (34 g)..................2
Pillsbury Grands!
   Blueberry, 1 biscuit (61 g)..........................5
   Butter tastin', 1 biscuit (58 g) 4
   Buttermilk, 1 biscuit (58 g) 4
   Buttermilk, reduced fat, 1 biscuit (58 g).....4
   Extra rich, 1 biscuit (61 g) 5
   Flaky, 1 biscuit (61 g) 5
   Golden corn, 1 biscuit (61 g) 4
   Homestyle, 1 biscuit (58 g) 4
   Southern style, 1 biscuit (58 g)..................4
   Wheat, reduced fat, 1 biscuit (61 g) 4
Pillsbury Hungry Jack
   Butter tastin, flaky, 1 biscuit (34 g)............2
   Buttermilk, 1 biscuit (34 g) 2
   Cinnamon & sugar, 1 biscuit (35 g) 2
   Flaky, 1 biscuit (34 g) 2
   Honey butter, 1 biscuit (35 g)....................3
   Southern style flaky, 1 biscuit (34 g)..........2
Schwan's
   Cheese and herb biscuits, 1 (34 g) 3
   Southern style biscuits, 1 (62 g) 5

Blueberries
Traverse Bay Fruit Co. Sweetened
   dried blueberries, ¼ cup 2
Tropical Nut & Fruit Dried blueberries,
   40 g 2

Bologna
Boar's Head
   Beef bologna, 2 oz....................................4
   Bologna (pork & beef), 2 oz......................4
   Bologna, 28% lower sodium, 2 oz.............4
   Garlic bologna, 2 oz 4
   Ham bologna, 2 oz 2
   Ring bologna, 2 oz....................................4
Louis Rich Turkey bologna, 1 slice
   (28 g) 1

Oscar Mayer
   Bologna, beef, 1 slice (28 g) 2
   Bologna, beef, light, 1 slice (28 g) 2
   Bologna, garlic, 1 slice (41 g)....................4
   Bologna, light, made with pork, chicken
      and beef, 1 slice (28 g).......................2
   Bologna, made with chicken, pork and
      beef, 1 slice (28 g) 2
   Bologna, Wisconsin made ring, 2 oz 5
Oscar Mayer Free Bologna, made
   with turkey, beef and pork, 1 slice
   (28 g) 0
Perdue Turkey bologna, deli, 2 oz 3

Bouillon
Herb-Ox
   Beef bouillon cubes, 1 cube (3.5 g) 0
   Beef instant bouillon powder, 1 tsp 0
   Beef instant broth & seasoning,
      1 packet (4 g)......................................0
   Beef instant broth & seasoning low
      sodium, 1 packet (4 g) 0
   Beef liquid, 2 tsp 0
   Chicken bouillon cubes, 1 cube (4 g) 0
   Chicken instant bouillon powder, 1 tsp 0
   Chicken instant broth & seasoning,
      1 packet (4 g) 0
   Chicken instant broth & seasoning low
      sodium, 1 packet (4 g) 0
   Chicken liquid, 2 tsp.................................0
   Vegetable bouillon cubes, 1 cube (4 g) 0
Preciosa Chicken bouillon, 1 tsp...............0

Bran, uncooked
Quaker Oats Unprocessed bran, ⅓ cup ...0
Kretschmer Toasted wheat bran, ¼ cup...0

Bratwurst
Boar's Head Natural casing cooked
   bratwurst, 1 (113 g) 8

Brazil nuts
Tropical Nut & Fruit Brazil nuts,
   6 pieces 6

Bread

Beefsteak
Hearty rye bread, 1 slice (28 g) 1
Light soft rye bread, 2 slices (45 g) 1
Soft rye bread, 1 slice (28 g).....................1

Betty Crocker
Banana mix, prepared, 1 slice (1/12 loaf)......4
Cinnamon streusel mix, prepared,
  1 slice (1/14 loaf) 4
Cranberry orange mix, prepared, 1 slice
  (1/12 loaf)...4
Lemon poppyseed mix, prepared, 1 slice,
  (1/12 loaf)...4

Butternut
Honey wheat bread, 1 slice (26 g).............1
White bread, 1 slice (26 g) 1

Cobblestone Mill
100% whole wheat, 1 slice (35 g).............1
Honey wheat berry, 1 slice (35 g).............2

Food for Life
7-sprouted grains, 1 slice (34 g) 1
Cinnamon raisin 7-sprouted grains,
  1 slice (34 g) 1
Ezekiel 4:9 sprouted grains, 1 slice
  (34 g) 1
Organic Ezekiel 4:9 cinnamon raisin,
  1 slice (34 g) 1
Organic Ezekiel 4:9 sprouted with
  sesame, 1 slice (34 g)..............................1
Sprouted wheat, 1 slice (34 g) 1

Home Pride Butter Top
Wheat bread, 1 slice (28 g)......................1
White bread, 1 slice (28 g) 2

Merita
Autumn grain bread, 1 slice (26 g) 1
Old fashioned white bread, 1 slice (26 g) ...1

Millbrook
Cracked wheat bread, 1 slice (31 g) 1
Honey wheat bread, 2 slices (41 g) 2

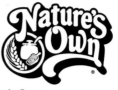

Nature's Own
100% wheat bread, 2 slices (52 g)............1
9-grain, 1 slice (35 g) 1
Butterbread, 1 slice (26 g) 1
Honey wheat, 1 slice (28 g) 1
Light honeywheat, 2 slices (45 g)..............1
Stone ground wheat, 1 slice (26 g).............1
Sugar free bread, 1 slice (25 g) 1
Sugar free bun, 1 bun (53 g)....................2
Whitewheat, 1 slice (28 g).......................1

Otis Spunkmeyer
Apple spice mini loaf, 1 mini loaf
  (3.75 oz) 8
Banana walnut mini loaf, 1 mini loaf
  (3.75 oz) 11
Chocolate fudge pecan mini loaf, mini
  loaf (3.75 oz) 10

Pepperidge Farm
Wheat, 3 slices (45 g) 2
White, 3 slices (45 g)................................2

Pepperidge Farm Light Style
7 grain, 3 slices (57 g) 2
Italian, 3 slices (57 g)...............................2
Oatmeal, 3 slices (57 g)............................2
Wheat, 3 slices (57 g) 2

Pepperidge Farm Natural Whole Grain
9 grain, 1 slice (34 g) 1
Crunchy grain, 1 slice (34 g) 1
Honey oat, 1 slice (34 g) 2
Multi-grain, 1 slice (34 g) 1
Whole wheat, 1 slice (34 g) 2

Pillsbury
French loaf, crusty, 1 slice (62 g) 3
Homestyle loaf, wheat, 1 slice (55 g).........3
Pillsbury Homestyle loaf, white, 1 slice
  (55 g) 3

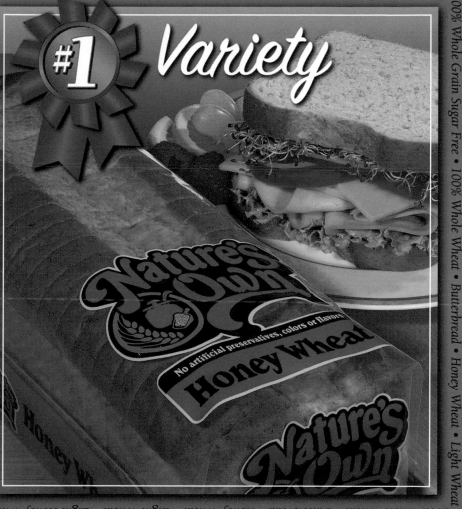

Schwan's
Cheese stuffed bread with sauce, 2 oz.......4
French baguette bread, ¼ loaf (49 g) 2
Honey wheat frozen bread dough, 2 oz 3
White frozen bread dough, 2 oz (56 g) 3
Wonder White bread, 1 slice (26 g)...........1

Wonder Light
Italian bread, 2 slices (45 g) 1
Sourdough bread, 2 slices (45 g)................1
Wheat bread, 2 slices (45 g) 1
White bread, 2 slices (45 g) 1

Bread mixes
Dromedary
Corn bread and muffin mix, prepared,
   2 oz...3
Date bread mix, prepared, 2 oz 4
Gingerbread cake & cookie mix,
   prepared, 2 oz.......................................4
Hot roll mix, prepared, 1 roll (48 g) 2

Harry & David
Autumn harvest bread mix, ⅓ cup 3
Italian bread mix, 1⅓ slices (38 g) 3
Sourdough bread mix, ⅓ cup 3

Pillsbury
Apple cinnamon mix, baked, 1 slice 4
Banana mix, baked, 1 slice 4
Carrot mix, baked, 1 slice 3
Chocolate chip mix, baked, 1 slice.............4
Cinnamon swirl mix, baked, 1 slice 5
Cranberry mix, baked, 1 slice 4
Date mix, baked, 1 slice 4
Lemon poppy seed mix, baked, 1 slice.......4
Nut mix, baked, 1 slice 4
Pecan swirl mix, baked, 1 slice 6
Pumpkin mix, baked, 1 slice.......................4

Pillsbury Ballard
Corn bread, baked, 1 serving
   (⅛₁₈ prepared recipe) 3
Cracked wheat, 1 slice (¹⁄₁₂ loaf) 2
Crusty white, 1 slice (¹⁄₁₂ loaf)....................3
Gingerbread, 1 slice (⅛ loaf)......................5

Bread crumbs
Contadina Seasoned authentic Italian
   style, ¼ cup...2

Progresso
Garlic & herb, ¼ cup 2
Italian style, ¼ cup....................................2
Parmesan, ¼ cup 2
Plain, ¼ cup 2

Breadsticks
Pillsbury
Breadsticks, 2 (52 g) 3
Breadsticks, garlic & herb, 2 (60 g)............4
Breadsticks, Parmesan, garlic & herb,
   2 (60 g) 4

Stella D'oro
Breadsticks, 1 (9 g) 1
Garlic breadsticks, 1 (10 g) 1
Onion breadsticks, 1 (9 g).........................1
Original breadsticks, 1 (9 g).......................1
Potato 'n onion breadsticks, 1 (11 g) 1
Roasted garlic breadsticks, 1 (11 g)...........1
Sesame breadsticks, 1 (11 g) 1
Sesame breadsticks, 1 (11 g) 1
Snack stix, cracked pepper breadsticks,
   1 (10 g) 1
Snack stix, cracked pepper breadsticks,
   4 (16 g) 2
Snack stix, potato onion breadsticks,
   4 (16 g) 2
Snack stix, salted breadsticks, 4 (16 g) 2
Sodium free breadsticks, 1 (10 g) 1
Wheat breadsticks, 1 (9 g).........................1

Breakfast bars
Hain Pure Foods
Country apple, 1 (40 g) 3
Red raspberry, 1 (40 g) 3
Wild blueberry, 1 (40 g).............................3

Breath mints
Breath Savers
Cinnamon, 1 (2.8 g)..................................0
Peppermint, 1 (1.8 g) 0
Spearmint, 1 (1.8 g) 0
Vanilla mint, 1 (1.8 g)...............................0
Wintergreen, 1 (1.8 g)...............................0

Ferrero

Cinnamon, 1 (0.38 g) 0
Fresh mints, 1 (0.38 g) 0
Orange mints, 1 (0.38 g) 0
Spearmints, 1 (0.38 g)............................0
Wintergreen, 1 (0.38 g) 0
Ice Breakers Cool mint, 1 (0.8 g) 0

Broccoli

Boston Markets Broccoli, 1 serving
   (283 g) 5
Freezer Queen Family Side Dish
   Broccoli in cheese sauce, ⅔ cup..............1
Green Giant
   Broccoli cuts, frozen, 1 cup 0
   Broccoli florets, frozen, 1⅓ cups...............0
   Broccoli in cheese flavored sauce,
      frozen, ⅔ cup 1
   Broccoli spears, frozen, 3 oz 0
   Broccoli spears, frozen, 4 oz 1
   Chopped broccoli, frozen, ¾ cup...............0
Green Giant Harvest Fresh
   Broccoli spears, frozen, 3½ oz...................0
   Cut broccoli, frozen, ⅔ cup.......................0
Hanover
   Broccoli florets, 4 florets (85 g) 0
   Cut broccoli, 1 cup.....................................0
Hanover The Gold Line Petite
   broccoli florets, 1¼ cups............................0
Schwan's Broccoli florets, 1 cup...............0
Stouffer's Broccoli au gratin, ½ cup
   (4 oz)..2

Broth

Campbell's Healthy Request
   Chicken broth, 1 cup 0
College Inn
   Beef broth, 99% fat free, 1 cup 0
   Chicken broth with roasted garlic, 1 cup....0
   Chicken broth with roasted vegetables,
      1 cup 0
   Chicken broth, 99% fat free, 1 cup.............0
   Fat free lower sodium beef broth, 1 cup 0
   French onion beef broth, 1 cup 1
   Lemon chicken broth, 1 cup......................0

No fat, lower sodium chicken broth,
   1 cup..0
Turkey broth, 1 cup 0
Vegetable broth, 1 cup..............................0
Hain Pure Foods
   Chicken, 1 cup..1
   Chicken broth, no salt added, 1 cup 1
   Vegetable, 1 cup.......................................0
   Vegetable broth, no salt added, 1 cup 0
Health Valley Chicken, 1 cup 1
Health Valley Fat Free
   Beef, 1 cup 0
   Beef broth, no salt, 1 cup 0
   Beef broth – 1 quart, 1 cup 0
   Chicken, 1 cup...1
   Chicken broth, no salt, 1 cup 1
   Chicken broth - 1 quart, 1 cup 1
   Mushroom, 1 cup.......................................0
   Vegetable, 1 cup..0
   Vegetable broth – 1 quart, 1 cup 0
Swanson's
   Beef broth with onion, 1 serving (245 g) ...0
   Chicken broth, 1 serving (235 g) 0
   Chicken broth w/ Italian herbs, 1 serving
      (240 g) 0
   Chicken broth with roasted garlic,
      1 serving (240 g) 0
   Clear beef broth, 1 serving (235 g)............0
   Clear chicken broth (resealable box),
      1 serving (235 g) 0
   Clear vegetable broth, 1 serving (235 g)....0
   Fat free natural goodness chicken broth,
      1 serving (235 g) 0

Brownies

Betty Crocker
   Chocolate chunk supreme, prepared,
      1 piece (⅟₂₀ pan).....................................4
   Dark chocolate fudge, prepared,
      1 piece (⅟₂₀ pan).....................................4
   Dark chocolate w/ Hershey's syrup,
      prepared, 1 piece (⅟₂₀ pan) 4
   Fall frosted brownie, prepared, 1 piece
      (⅟₂₀ pan) 5

Frosted supreme, prepared, 1 piece
(1/20 pan) 5
Fudge (family size), no-cholesterol/
reduced fat recipe, prepared, 1 piece
(1/20 pan) 3
Fudge (family size), prepared, 1 piece
(1/20 pan) 4
Fudge (megapack – 4 pouches),
prepared, 1 piece (1/20 pan) 4
Fudge (regular size), prepared, 1 piece,
(1/12 pan) 4
German chocolate supreme, prepared,
1 piece (1/20 pan)....................................4
Hot fudge supreme, prepared, 1 piece
(1/20 pan) 4
Original fudge supreme, prepared,
1 piece (1/20 pan)....................................4
Peanut butter chunk w/ Reese's Pieces,
1 piece (1/20 pan) 4
Turtle, prepared, 1 piece (1/20 pan) 4
Walnut supreme, prepared, 1 piece
(1/20 pan) 4

Betty Crocker Pouch Dessert Mix
Dark chocolate brownie mix, prepared,
1 piece (1/9 pan) 4
Fudge brownie mix, prepared, 1 piece
(1/9 pan)..4

Betty Crocker Sweet Rewards
Low fat fudge, mix, 1 serving
(1/18 package) 3
Reduced fat fudge brownie,
no-cholesterol recipe, prepared,
1 piece (1/20 pan) 3
Reduced fat fudge brownie, prepared,
1 piece (1/20 pan) 3

Hostess
Plain brownie bites, 3 (37 g).....................4
Walnut brownie bites, 3 (37 g)..................4
Lance Fudge nut brownie, 1 (78 g)............7

Martha White
Chewy fudge 8" x 8" pan size,
prepared, 1 piece (1/20 pan) 4
Chewy fudge 9" x 13" pan size,
prepared, 1 piece (1/20 pan) 4

Moist 'n fudgy 9" x 13" pan size,
prepared, 1 piece (1/20 pan) 4
Walnut 9" x 13" pan size, prepared,
1 piece (1/20 pan) 4
Otis Spunkmeyer Double chocolate,
1 brownie (2 oz) 6
Pillsbury
Fudge mix (15 oz), baked, 1 piece
(1/16 recipe) 3
Fudge mix (19½ oz), baked, 1 piece
(1/18 recipe) 4
Thick 'n fudgy caramel swirl mix, baked,
1 piece (1/14 recipe) 4
Thick 'n fudgy cheesecake swirl, baked,
1 piece (1/18 recipe) 4
Thick 'n fudgy chocolate chunk, baked,
1 piece (1/16 recipe) 4
Thick 'n fudgy double chocolate mix,
baked, 1 piece (1/16 recipe) 4
Thick 'n fudgy hot fudge swirl mix,
baked, 1 piece (1/14 recipe) 4
Thick 'n fudgy walnut mix, baked,
1 piece (1/12 recipe) 4
Pillsbury One Step Fudge brownie,
1/12 recipe (44 g) 4
Weight Watchers
Brownie a la mode, 1 serving (89 g)..........4
Double fudge brownie parfait,
1 serving (109 g) 4

Brussel sprouts
Hanover The Gold Line Petite
brussel sprouts, ½ cup 0
Green Giant Baby brussels sprouts,
frozen, ⅔ cup..1

Burritos
Amy's
Bean & cheese burrito, 1 package
(6 oz)..5
Bean & rice burrito – non dairy,
1 package (6 oz).......................................5
Black bean vegetable burrito,
1 package (6 oz)..6
Breakfast burrito, 1 package (6 oz) 8

Patio

Bean & cheese burrito, 1 (5 oz)..............6
Beef & bean burrito, hot, 1 (5 oz)............7
Beef & bean burrito, medium, 1 (5 oz)......6
Beef & bean burrito, mild, 1 (5 oz)..........7
Beef & bean burrito, red hot red chili
    peppers, 1 (5 oz)..............................7
Chicken burrito, 1 (5 oz)........................6

Butter
Land O Lakes

Butter, salted sticks, 1 Tbsp....................3
Butter, stick, 1 Tbsp.............................3
Light butter, stick, 1 Tbsp.....................3
Light butter, whipped, 1 Tbsp..................1
Whipped butter, 1 Tbsp.........................2

Butter blends
Land O Lakes

Country morning blend light, stick,
    1 Tbsp..2
Country morning blend light, tub,
    1 Tbsp..2
Country morning blend, stick, 1 Tbsp........3
Country morning blend, tub, 1 Tbsp..........3
Spread with sweet cream, stick, 1 Tbsp.....3
Spread with sweet cream, tub, 1 Tbsp.......2

Butter substitutes
Butter Buds

Powdered mix, 1 tsp 0
Sprinkles, 1 tsp 0

Cabbage
Dole Shredded red cabbage, 3 oz............0

Cactus
Faraon, Tender cactus, ½ cup..................0

Cakes
Betty Crocker

Gingerbread cake and cookie mix,
    no-cholesterol recipe, prepared,
    1 slice (⅛ cake) 5
Gingerbread cake and cookie mix,
    prepared, 1 slice (⅛ cake)..................5

Pineapple upside down cake,
    no-cholesterol recipe, prepared,
    1 slice (⅙ cake) 9
Pineapple upside down cake, prepared,
    1 slice (⅙ cake) 9
Pound cake, no-cholesterol recipe,
    prepared, 1 slice (⅛ cake)..................6
Pound cake, prepared, 1 slice (⅛ cake) 6

Betty Crocker Stir 'n Bake

Brownie w/ mini kisses mix, prepared,
    1 piece (⅙ pan) 5
Carrot cake w/ cream cheese mix,
    prepared, 1 slice (⅙ cake) 6
Cinnamon streusel coffee cake mix,
    prepared, 1 slice (⅙ cake)..................5
Devils food cake w/ chocolate frosting
    mix, prepared, 1 slice (⅙ cake) 5
Yellow cake w/ chocolate frosting mix,
    prepared, 1 slice (⅙ cake)..................5

Boar's Head New York cheese cake,
    4 oz..10

Dolly Madison

Cinnamon buttercrumb cakes, 1 (46 g) 4
Crème cake zingers, 2 (53 g)....................5
Devil's food zingers, 2 (73 g) 6
Frosty angel cake, 1 (99 g)......................7
Raspberry zingers, 1 (40 g) 4
Vanilla zingers, 2 (71 g)..........................6

Drake's

Coffee cakes, 1 (33 g) 3
Devil dogs, 1 (45 g)..............................4
Funny bones, 2 (71 g) 6
Ring dings, 2 (77 g)..............................8
Sunny doodles, 2 (57 g)........................5
Yankee doodles, 2 (57 g) 5
Yodels, 2 (62 g)....................................7

Dromedary Pound cake mix, prepared,
    ⅛ cake (80 g) 5

Hostess

Chocolate cup cakes, 1 (50 g)..................4
Ding dongs, 2 (78 g) 8
Ho hos, 2 (57 g)..................................6
Sno balls, 1 (50 g)................................4

C

Suzy Q's, 1 (58 g)......................................5
Twinkies, 1 (43 g) 3

Hostess Lights
Chocolate cup cakes, 1 (46 g) 3
Cinnamon crumb cakes, 1 (28 g)...............2
Twinkies, 1 (43 g) 3

Jell-O Cheesecake Snacks
Original, 1 (93 g) 4
Strawberry, 1 (99 g) 3

Lance
Dunking sticks, 1 piece (39 g) 4
Fat free fig cake, ½ piece (30 g) 2
Fig cake, ½ piece (30 g)...........................2
Pound cake, 1 slice (71 g) 6

Little Debbie
Golden cremes, 1 (43 g) 3
Swiss cake rolls, 2 (61 g) 6

Martha White Pound cake mix,
prepared, 1 serving (¼ package,
prepared)...7

Oregon Farms Carrot cake, ⅙ cake
(83 g) 6

Otis Spunkmeyer
Apple crumb cake, 1 cake (4 oz)...............9
Blueberry crumb cake, 1 cake (4 oz) 9
Cheese crumb cake, 1 cake (4 oz)...........10
Pound cake, 1 cake (3.5 g)......................9

Pet-Ritz Pound homestyle cake, ¼ cake
(85 g) 7

Pillsbury Moist Supreme
Angel food mix, baked, 1 slice
(1/12 cake)...3
Banana mix, baked, 1 slice (1/12 cake).........6
Butter recipe chocolate mix, baked,
1 slice (1/12 cake) 6
Butter recipe yellow mix, baked,
1 slice (1/12 cake) 6
Chocolate chip streusel coffee cake
mix, baked, 1 slice (1/16 recipe).................6
Chocolate mix, baked, 1 slice (1/12 cake) 6
Cinnamon streusel coffee cake mix,
baked, 1 slice (1/16 recipe)........................6
Dark chocolate mix, baked, 1 slice
(1/12 cake)...6

Devil's food mix, baked, 1 slice
(1/12 cake)...6
Easter funfetti mix, baked, 1 slice
(1/12 cake)...6
French vanilla mix, baked, 1 slice
(1/12 cake)...6
Funfetti mix, baked, 1 slice (1/12 cake).........6
German chocolate mix, baked, 1 slice
(1/12 cake)...6
Halloween funfetti mix, baked, 1 slice
(1/12 cake)...6
Holiday funfetti mix, baked, 1 slice
(1/12 cake)...6
Lemon mix, baked, 1 slice (1/12 cake) 6
Strawberry mix, baked, 1 slice (1/12 cake) 6
Valentine's funfetti mix, baked, 1 slice
(1/12 cake)...6
White mix, baked, 1 slice (1/12 cake) 5
Yellow mix, baked, 1 slice (1/12 cake) 6

Sara Lee
Banana cake dessert cake, ⅕ cake.............6
Butter streusel coffee cake, ⅙ cake 5
Carrot cake bites, 5 pieces.......................9
Carrot cake dessert cake, ⅙ cake..............7
Cheese coffee cake, ⅙ cake 4
Cheesecake bites – chocolate dipped
praline bites, 5 pieces 11
Cheesecake bites – toasted almond
crunch bites, 5 pieces...........................12
Cherry cream cheesecake, ¼ cake 8
Chocolate dipped caramel fudge
brownie bites, 2 pieces..........................4
Chocolate dipped original bites,
5 pieces 12
Chocolate swirl pound cake, ¼ cake..........8
Crumb coffee cake, ⅛ cake 5
Double chocolate iced layer cake,
⅛ cake...6
Flaky coconut iced layer cake, ⅛ cake 6
Free & light pound cake, ¼ cake 5
Fudge golden iced layer cake, ⅛ cake........6
German chocolate iced layer cake,
⅛ cake...7

New York style chocolate chip cookie
  cheesecake, ⅙ cake...............................12
New York style classic cheesecake,
  ⅙ cake..13
New York style mixed berry swirl
  cheesecake, ⅙ cake..............................12
Original cream cheesecake, ¼ cake 8
Pecan coffee cake, ⅙ cake 6
Pound cake, ¼ cake 8
Raspberry coffee cake, ⅙ cake 5
Reduced fat pound cake, ¼ cake..............7
Strawberry cream cheesecake, ¼ cake 7
Strawberry shortcake, ⅛ cake 4
Strawberry swirl pound cake, ¼ cake.........7
Vanilla iced layer cake, ⅛ cake..................6

SuperMoist

Butter pecan mix, no-cholesterol recipe,
  prepared, 1 slice (1/12 cake).....................5
Butter pecan mix, prepared, 1 slice
  (1/12 cake)..6
Butter recipe chocolate mix,
  no-cholesterol recipe, prepared,
  1 slice (1/12 cake) 6
Butter recipe chocolate mix, prepared,
  1 slice (1/12 cake) 6
Butter recipe yellow mix, no-cholesterol
  recipe, prepared, 1 slice (1/12 cake) 6
Butter recipe yellow mix, prepared,
  1 slice (1/12 cake) 6
Carrot cake mix, no-cholesterol recipe,
  prepared, 1 slice (1/10 cake).....................6
Carrot cake mix, prepared, 1 slice
  (1/10 cake)..8
Cherry chip mix, egg white recipe,
  prepared, 1 slice (1/10 cake).....................7
Cherry chip mix, prepared, 1 slice
  (1/10 cake)..7
Chocolate chip mix, no-cholesterol
  recipe, prepared, 1 slice (1/12 cake) 6
Chocolate chip mix, prepared, 1 slice
  (1/12 cake)..6
Chocolate fudge mix, prepared, 1 slice
  (1/12 cake)..6

Chocolate swirl angel food cake,
  prepared, 1 slice (1/12 cake).....................3
Chocolate with creamy swirls of fudge
  mix, no-cholesterol recipe, prepared,
  1 slice (⅑ cake) 5
Chocolate with creamy swirls of fudge
  mix, prepared, 1 slice (⅑ cake) 5
Confetti angel food cake mix, prepared,
  1 slice (1/12 cake) 3
Devils food mix, no-cholesterol recipe,
  prepared, 1 slice (1/12 cake).....................6
Devils food mix, prepared, 1 slice
  (1/12 cake)..6
Double chocolate swirl mix,
  no-cholesterol recipe, prepared,
  1 slice (1/12 cake) 6
Double chocolate swirl mix, prepared,
  1 slice (1/12 cake) 6
Easy angel food mix (pouch), prepared,
  1 slice (¼ cake) 3
French vanilla mix, no-cholesterol
  recipe, prepared, 1 slice (1/12 cake) 5
French vanilla mix, prepared, 1 slice
  (1/12 cake)..6
Fudge marble mix, no-cholesterol
  recipe, prepared, 1 slice (1/10 cake) 7
Fudge marble mix, prepared, 1 slice
  (1/10 cake)..7
German chocolate mix, no-cholesterol
  recipe, prepared, 1 slice (1/12 cake) 6
German chocolate mix, prepared,
  1 slice (1/12 cake) 6
Golden vanilla mix, no-cholesterol
  recipe, prepared, 1 slice (1/12 cake) 5
Golden vanilla mix, prepared, 1 slice
  (1/12 cake)..6
Lemon mix, no-cholesterol recipe,
  prepared, 1 slice (1/12 cake).....................5
Lemon mix, prepared, 1 slice (1/12 cake)......6
Milk chocolate mix, no-cholesterol
  recipe, prepared, 1 slice (1/12 cake) 5
Milk chocolate mix, prepared, 1 slice
  (1/12 cake)..5

One-step white mix, prepared, 1 slice
($\frac{1}{12}$ cake)......................................3

Party swirl mix, no-cholesterol recipe,
prepared, 1 slice ($\frac{1}{12}$ cake)..................5

Party swirl mix, prepared, 1 slice
($\frac{1}{12}$ cake)......................................6

Pineapple mix, no-cholesterol recipe,
prepared, 1 slice ($\frac{1}{12}$ cake)..................5

Pineapple mix, prepared, 1 slice
($\frac{1}{12}$ cake)......................................6

Rainbow chip mix, egg white recipe,
prepared, 1 slice ($\frac{1}{10}$ cake)..................7

Rainbow chip mix, prepared, 1 slice
($\frac{1}{10}$ cake)......................................7

Sour cream white mix, prepared,
1 slice ($\frac{1}{10}$ cake) 7

Sour cream white mix, whole egg
recipe, prepared, 1 slice ($\frac{1}{10}$ cake) 7

Spice mix, no-cholesterol recipe,
prepared, 1 slice ($\frac{1}{12}$ cake)..................5

Spice mix, prepared, 1 slice ($\frac{1}{12}$ cake) 6

Strawberry mix, no-cholesterol recipe,
prepared, 1 slice ($\frac{1}{12}$ cake)..................5

Strawberry mix, prepared, 1 slice
($\frac{1}{12}$ cake)......................................6

Strawberry swirl mix, egg white recipe,
prepared, 1 slice ($\frac{1}{10}$ cake)..................7

Strawberry swirl mix, prepared, 1 slice
($\frac{1}{10}$ cake)......................................7

Traditional white mix, prepared,
1 slice ($\frac{1}{12}$ cake) 3

White chocolate mix, egg white recipe,
prepared, 1 slice ($\frac{1}{12}$ cake)..................5

White chocolate mix, prepared, 1 slice
($\frac{1}{12}$ cake)......................................6

White mix, prepared, 1 slice ($\frac{1}{12}$ cake) 5

White mix, richer recipe, prepared,
1 slice ($\frac{1}{12}$ cake) 6

Yellow mix, no-cholesterol recipe,
prepared, 1 slice ($\frac{1}{12}$ cake)..................5

Yellow mix, prepared, 1 slice ($\frac{1}{12}$ cake) 6

Yellow with creamy swirls of fudge
mix, no-cholesterol recipe, prepared,
1 slice ($\frac{1}{9}$ cake) 5

Yellow with creamy swirls of fudge
mix, prepared, 1 slice ($\frac{1}{9}$ cake) 5

Sweet 'N Low

Banana cake mix, $\frac{1}{5}$ package (45 g)..........3

Chocolate cake mix, $\frac{1}{5}$ package (45 g) 3

Gingerbread cake mix, $\frac{1}{5}$ package
(45 g) 3

Lemon cake mix, $\frac{1}{5}$ package (45 g) 3

White cake mix, $\frac{1}{5}$ package (45 g) 3

Sweet Rewards

Devils food mix, no-cholesterol recipe,
prepared, 1 slice ($\frac{1}{12}$ cake)..................4

Devils food mix, prepared, 1 slice
($\frac{1}{12}$ cake)......................................4

White mix, prepared, 1 slice ($\frac{1}{12}$ cake) 4

White mix, whole egg recipe, prepared,
1 slice ($\frac{1}{12}$ cake) 4

Yellow mix, no-cholesterol recipe,
prepared, 1 slice ($\frac{1}{12}$ cake)..................4

Yellow mix, prepared, 1 slice ($\frac{1}{12}$ cake) 4

Weight Watchers

Double fudge cake, 1 serving (77 g) 4

French style cheesecake, 1 serving
(110 g) 3

New York style cheesecake, 1 serving
(70 g) 3

Calzone
Sara Lee

Classic Italian calzone, 1 8

Santa fe black bean calzone, 1................7

Smoked ham & Cheddar calzone, 1 9

Thai peanut chicken calzone, 1 8

Zesty Italian sausage calzone, 1 11

Candy

3 Musketeers, 1 bar (60.4 g) 6

Amazin' Fruit Gummy bears, 1 bag
(53 g) 4

Andes Creme de menthe thins,
8 pieces (38 g) 5

Cadbury's

Caramello, 1 bar (35 g) 4

Dairy milk, 9 pieces (40 g) 5

Dairy milk (5 oz bar), 9 pieces (40 g).........5

Fruit & nut, 9 pieces (40 g) 5
Krisp, 9 pieces (40 g)................................5
Mini-eggs, 1 bag (42 g) 5
Roast almond, 9 pieces (40 g)...................5
Candy Cane Pops, 1 (17 g) 1
Caramel Apple Pops, 1 (18 g)..............1
Caramel-Lot, 1 (20 g) 2
Cella's
Dark, 2 chocolate covered cherries
   (28 g) 2
Milk, 2 chocolate covered cherries
   (28 g) 2
Charleston Chew
Chocolate, 1 (53 g) 5
Mini, vanilla, 13 pieces (40 g) 4
Strawberry, 1 (53 g) 5
Vanilla, 1 (53 g) 5
Charm's
Blow pop, junior, 1 (15 g) 1
Blow pop, regular, 1 (18 g) 1
Blow pop, super, 1 (38 g)..........................3
Charm's way 2 sour blow pop, junior,
   1 (15 g) 1
Charm's way 2 sour blow pop, regular,
   1 (18 g) 1
Charm's way 2 sour blow pop, super,
   1 (38 g) 3
S'moresels, 1 pouch (43 g) 4
Sour balls, 1 (5 g) 0
Sour pop, 1 junior flat pop (15 g) 1
Sour pop, 1 regular flat pop (18 g) 1
Squares, 2 pieces (6 g) 1
Sweet pop, 1 junior flat pop (15 g)............1
Sweet pop, 1 regular flat pop (18 g)..........1
Sweet/sour pop, 1 junior flat pop (15 g) 1
Sweet/sour pop, 1 regular flat pop
   (18 g) 1
Zip-a-dee-doo-da pop, 3 (15 g) 1
Dots
Crows, 12 pieces (43 g) 3
Dots, 12 pieces (43 g) 3
Tropical dots, 12 pieces (43 g) 3

Dove
Dove dark chocolate, 1 bar (36.9 g) 5
Dove milk chocolate, 1 bar (36.9 g)...........5
Estee
No sugar added caramels, 5 pieces
   (38 g) 3
Sugar free assorted fruit hard candies,
   5 pieces (16 g) 1
Sugar free assorted fruit lollipops,
   2 (16 g) 1
Sugar free gummy bears, 16 pieces
   (40 g) 3
Sugar free hard butterscotch candies,
   2 pieces (12 g) 1
Sugar free hard peppermint swirls
   candies, 3 pieces (14 g) 1
Sugar free toffee hard candies,
   5 pieces (16 g) 1
Sugar free tropical fruit hard candies,
   5 pieces (16 g) 1
Estee Smart Treats
Sugar free chocolate fudge candy bar,
   1 (28 g) 2
Sugar free citrus slices, 9 pieces (39 g) 1
Sugar free cookie dough candy bar, 1
   (28 g) 1
Sugar free gummy apple rings, 5 pieces
   (41 g) 1
Sugar free gummy bears, 17 pieces
   (42 g) 1
Sugar free jelly beans, 26 pieces (40 g)......1
Sugar free licorice gum drops, 11 pieces
   (42 g) 2
Ferrero Rocher
Confetterie, 1 package 4
Hazelnut chocolate, 3 pieces (38 g)...........6
Fluffy Stuff, 1 small bag (1.06 oz) 2
Fruitfield's
Adult fruit shapes, cherry, 10 pieces
   (30 g) 2
Adult fruit shapes, orange, 10 pieces
   (30 g) 2
Adult fruit shapes, strawberry, 10 pieces
   (30 g) 2

C

Harmony

Bold beans, totally tropical, 27 pieces
(40 g) 3

Gourmet jelly beans, 24 pieces (41 g).........3

Gourmet orange slices, 9 pieces (42 g) 3

Gum drops, 5 pieces (45 g) 3

Gummy bears, 17 pieces (42 g) 3

Gummy worms, 4 pieces (40 g) 3

Milk chocolate caramel patties,
3 pieces (39 g) 4

Milk chocolate double dipped peanuts,
12 pieces (41 g)....................................5

Milk chocolate maltballs, 7 pieces
(42 g) 5

Red fish, 5 pieces (43 g) 3

Sour bears, 19 pieces (40 g).......................3

Sour worms, 5 pieces (42 g) 3

Sugarfree gummy worms, 4 pieces
(40 g) 3

Yogurt peanut caramel clusters,
2 pieces (46 g) 6

Harry & David

Australian black licorice, 4 pieces (40 g) 3

Black licorice sticks, 6 pieces (39 g)...........3

Chocolate licorice, 3 pieces (42 g) 3

Fruit licorice twists, 12 pieces (42 g)..........3

Gel berries, 20 pieces (45 g) 3

Green apples candy, 7 pieces (39 g) 3

Gummi bears, 22 pieces (42 g) 3

Gummi frogs, 6 pieces (42 g) 3

Gummi fruit salad, 6 pieces (42 g) 3

Gummi grapefruit, 6 pieces (42 g)..............3

Gummi peach o's, 6 pieces (42 g) 3

Gummi squiggles, 5-6 pieces (42 g)...........3

Orange 'n cream nibbles, 7 pieces (42 g).....3

Red licorice sticks, 6 pieces (38 g) 3

Sour sour fruit gummis, 16 pieces
(42 g) 3

Hershey's

5th avenue, 1 bar (57 g)............................6

Almond joy coconut & almond bits,
1 Tbsp...1

Assorted miniatures, 5 pieces (42 g)..........5

Candy coated milk chocolate eggs,
1 package (4 g) 5

Cherry nibs, 27 pieces (40 g).....................3

Chocolate covered almonds (chocolate
world), 11 pieces (38 g) 5

Chocolate covered marshmallow novelty
shape – pumpkin, 2 pieces (34 g) 3

Chuckles (individually wrapped),
4 pieces (45 g) 3

Coconut & almond bits, 1 Tbsp 1

Cookies 'n' crème, 1 bar (43 g) 5

Cookies n' mint, 1 bar (43 g) 5

Creamy milk chocolate nuggets with
raisins & almonds, 4 pieces (39 g)..........4

Creamy milk chocolate nuggets with
toffee and almonds, 4 pieces (38 g) 5

Crispy rice snacks peanut butter,
2 bars (32 g) 3

Dark chocolate nuggets with almonds,
4 pieces (38 g) 5

Good & fruity, 1 box (50 g)........................4

Good & plenty, 1 box (50 g) 3

Gummi bears, 1 package (40 g) 2

Heath bits, 1 Tbsp 2

Heath bits 'o brickle, 1 Tbsp......................2

Heath milk chocolate english toffee
bar, 1 package (39 g) 5

Hershey-els (pastel), 1 package (62 g) 7

Hugs, 9 pieces (39 g).................................5

Hugs with almonds, 9 pieces (41 g)...........5

Jujubes, 1 box (42 g) 3

Kisses, 9 pieces (42 g) 5

Kisses with almonds, 9 pieces (40 g) 6

Kit kat, three 2-piece bars 6

Krackel, 1 bar (34 g) 4

Milk chocolate, 1 bar (34 g).......................5

Milk chocolate nuggets, 4 pieces (40 g).....5

Milk chocolate with almond nuggets,
4 pieces (38 g) 5

Milk chocolate with almonds, 1 bar
(41 g) 6

Milk chocolate with almonds bites,
17 pieces (39 g)....................................5

Milk duds, 1 box (52 g) 6
Mini robin eggs, 1 package (25 g).............2
Mini whopper eggs, 1 envelope (49 g) 5
Mr. Goodbar, 1 bar (49 g) 6
Payday, 1 bar (52 g) 6
Robin eggs, 8 pieces (40 g).......................4
Rolo, 1 package (53 g) 6
Shell topping, heath, 2 Tbsp 6
Sixlets, 1 package (49 g) 5
Skor, 1 bar (39 g) 5
Special dark, 1 bar (41 g) 5
Whatchamacallit, 1 bar (48 g) 5
Wunderbeans, 1 box (42 g).........................3
Zagnut, 1 bar (49 g)..................................5
Zero, 1 bar (52 g).....................................5

Hershey's Classic
Caramel, 6 pieces (37 g)............................4
Chocolate filled caramels, 6 pieces
   (37 g) 4

Hershey's Sweet Escapes
Caramel & peanut butter crispy bar,
   1 bar (20 g)..2
Chocolate toffee crisp bar, 1 bar (39 g)......4
Chocolate toffee crisp bar, 1 bar (18 g).....2
Crispy caramel fudge bar, 1 bar (20 g).......2
Crunchy peanut butter bar, 1 bar (20 g).....2

Hershey's Symphony
Milk chocolate, 1 bar (42 g).......................5
Milk chocolate with almond toffee,
   1 bar (42 g) 6

Hershey's TasteTations
Butterscotch hard candy, 3 pieces
   (16 g) 1
Caramel hard candy, 3 pieces (16 g)..........1
Chocolate hard candy, 3 pieces (16 g) 1
Chocolate mint hard candy, 3 pieces
   (16 g) 1
Peppermint hard candy, 3 pieces (17 g) 1

Jolly Rancher
Gummis, 10 pieces (39 g) 2
Jolly beans, 25 pieces (40 g) 3
Lollipops (apple, cherry, watermelon),
   1 piece (17 g).......................................1
Junior Mints, 16 pieces (40 g) 3

Lance
Assorted suckers, 3 pieces (14 g) 1
Cinnamon chews, 11 pieces (30 g) 2
Crispy marshmallow treats, 1 piece
   (45 g) 4
Fruit chews, 11 pieces (30 g) 2
Mint chews, 11 pieces (30 g) 2
Peanut bar, 1 (50 g) 6
Pop-a-lance, 1 piece (12 g) 1
Soft mints, 2 pieces (12 g) 1
Starlight mints, 3 pieces (15 g) 1
Strawberry chews, 11 pieces (30 g) 2
Whistle pop, 1 piece (19 g).......................1

Life Savers
Butter rum, 4 (6 g)....................................1
Chill-o-mints, 2 (5 g) 0
Cryst-o-mint, 2 (5 g).................................0
Five flavor, 4 (16 g) 1
Gummi savers, 1 package (42 g) 3
Hot cinnamon, 2 (5 g)...............................0
Pep-o mint, 4 (16 g) 1
Tangy fruits, 4 (16 g) 1
Tropical fruits, 4 (16 g) 1
Wild berries, 4 (16 g) 1
Wild cherry, 4 (16 g)..................................1
Wint-o-green, 4 (16 g)...............................1

M&M's
M&M's almond, 1 bag (37.1 g) 5
M&M's peanut, 1 bag (49.3 g) 5
M&M's peanut butter, 1 bag (46.2 g) 5
M&M's plain, 1 bag (47.9 g) 5

Mars Almond bar, 1 (49.9 g) 6

Milky Way
Milky way bar, 1 (58.1 g)...........................6
Milky way dark bar, 1 (49.9 g) 5
Milky way lite bar, 1 (44.5 g) 4

Mon Cheri Hazelnut chocolate,
4 pieces (43 g) 6

Mutant Fruitants Pops, 1 (17 g)..........1

Nestle
100 Grand, 1 package (42.5 g) 4
Baby Ruth, 1 (59.5 g) 5
Baby Ruth – fun size, 1 (28 g)...................3
Bit-o-honey, 1 (48.1 g) 4

Bittyfinger, 2 (38 g) 4
Buncha crunch, 1 bag (39.6 g) 4
Butterfinger, 1 (59.5 g) 5
Butterfinger – fun size, 1 (21 g) 2
Butterfinger BB's, 1 bag (48.1 g) 5
Chunky bar, 1 (39.6 g) 4
Crunch, 1 (43.9 g) 5
Crunch – fun size, 4 (40 g) 4
Flipz – peanut butter, 8 pieces (28 g) 3
Flipz – white chocolate, 8 pieces (28 g) 3
Flipz – white fudge, 7 pieces (28 g)...........3
Goobers, 1 bag (39.1 g) 4
Graham flipz – milk chocolate, 9 pieces
   (28 g) 3
Graham flipz – white fudge, 8 pieces
   (28 g) 3
Milk chocolate, 1 (41.1 g) 5
Mocha crunch, 1 (36.8 g) 4
Oh Henry!, 1 (26 g) 3
Raisinets, 1 bag (44.7 g) 4
Sno caps, 1 box (65.2 g) 6
Spree – mini chewy, 19 pieces (15 g) 1
Spree – regular, 8 pieces (15 g).................1
SweeTarts – mini chewy, 23 pieces
   (15 g) 1
SweeTarts – regular, 8 pieces (15 g) 1
Treasures – peanut butter, 4 pieces
   (43 g) 5
Treasures – w/ butterfinger, 3 pieces
   (35 g) 4
Treasures – w/ caramel, 3 pieces (35 g) 4
Turtles, 2 pieces (33 g) 4
White crunch, 1 (39.6 g)...........................5
Wonderball, 1 (28 g) 3

Nips

Butter rum, 2 pieces (14 g) 1
Caramel, 2 pieces (14 g)............................1
Chocolate parfait, 2 pieces (14 g) 1
Coffee, 2 pieces (14 g) 1
Peanut butter parfait, 2 pieces (14 g) 1
Vanilla almond cafe, 2 pieces (14 g)..........1
Orange Cream Pops, 1 (18 g) 1

Peter Paul

Almond joy, 1 package (49 g) 5
Almond joy bites, 18 pieces (40 g) 5
Mounds, 1 package (53 g) 5

Planet Harmony

Natural fruit bears, 18 pieces (40 g) 2
Natural gummy bears, 17 pieces (40 g) 2

Planters Original peanut bar,
   1 package (45 g) 5

Pull 'N' Peel

Cherry (individually wrapped), 3 pieces
   (37 g)..2
Paradise punch, 1 piece (34 g) 2
Pink lemonade, 1 piece (34 g)...................2
Red razz, 1 piece (34 g)..............................2

Reese's

Bites, 16 pieces (39 g) 5
Crunchy cookie cups, 1 package (17 g)......2
Ground peanut butter cup, 2 Tbsp.............3
Nutrageous, 1 bar (54 g)...........................7
Peanut butter cup, 2 pieces (34 g).............4
Peanut butter cup, 1 package (79 g).......10
Pieces, 1 package (46 g)............................5
Reesesticks, 1 piece (17 g)........................2

Snickers

Snickers bar, 1 (58.7 g)...............................7
Snickers munch bar, 1 (40.3 g) 5

Starburst

Starburst fruit twists, 1 bag (56.7 g)..........4
Starburst, California fruit, 1 package
   (58.7 g)...5
Starburst, original fruits, 1 package
   (58.7 g)...5
Starburst, tropical fruits, 1 package
   (58.7 g)...5

Sugar Babies, 30 pieces (44 g)..............4

Sugar Daddy

Sugar daddy, 3 junior pops (38 g) 3
Sugar daddy, 1 large pop (48 g)................4

Switzer Cherry bites, 18 pieces (40 g) 3

Tootsie Roll

Tootsie flavor rolls, 6 pieces (40 g) 4
Tootsie frooties, 12 pieces (36 g)...............3

Tootsie pops, 1 regular pop (17 g).............1
Tootsie pops, 1 small pop (13 g) 1
Tootsie roll, ½ bar (32 g) 3
Tootsie roll, ½ bar (43 g) 4
Tootsie roll, 6 regular midgees (36 g) 4
Tootsie roll, 12 small midgees (36 g) 3
Tootsie roll, 2 snack bars (36 g) 3
Twix caramel bar, 2 bars (56.7 g) 7
Twizzlers
Chocolate twists, 3 pieces (42 g)...............3
Licorice bites, 16 pieces (40 g) 3
Licorice twists, 1 package (70 g) 5
Strawberry twists, 1 package (49 g) 3
Twist-n-fill red raspberry/tropical,
  1 piece (28 g).......................................2
Twist-n-fill watermelon/cherry, 1 piece
  (28 g) 2
Weight Watchers
Candy bars, chocolate fudge, 1 (33 g)........2
Candy bars, chocolate peanut butter, 1
  (33 g) 2
Candy bars, chocolate raspberry, 1
  (33 g) 2
Whopper
Eggs, 6 pieces (37 g) 4
Whoppers, 1 pouch (21 g) 2
York
Bites, 15 pieces (39 g) 3
Peppermint pattie, 1 package (40 g)..........3

Cantaloupe
Chiquita Cantaloupe, ¼ medium
  (134 g) 1
Dole Cantaloupe, ¼ 1

Caponata
Progresso Eggplant (caponata), 2 Tbsp 0

Cappuccino
Maxwell House Cappuccino, prepared
  with 2% reduced fat milk, 8 fl oz............4
Maxwell House Cafe
Amaretto, 8 fl oz.....................................2
Irish cream, prepared, 8 fl oz 2
Mocha decaffeinated, prepared, 8 fl oz 2

Mocha, prepared, 8 fl oz 2
Mocha, prepared, sugar free, 8 fl oz 1
Vanilla decaffeinated, prepared, 8 fl oz......2
Vanilla, prepared, 8 fl oz 2
Vanilla, prepared, sugar free, 8 fl oz 1

Carrot chips
Hain Pure Foods Carrot chips, 22
  (31 g) 4

Carrot juice
Hain Pure Foods Carrot juice, 1 can
  (354 ml)..2

Carrots
Del Monte Sliced carrots, ½ cup 0
Dole
Peeled mini carrots, 3 oz 0
Shredded carrots, 3 oz..............................0
Green Giant
Honey glazed carrots, frozen, 1 cup...........2
Sliced carrots, canned, ½ cup....................0
Hanover
Crinkle sliced carrots, ½ cup 0
Whole baby carrots, ⅔ cup.......................0
LeSueur Baby whole carrots, canned,
  ½ cup 0

Cashews
EXPRESSnacks
Cashews, salted, 1½ oz 7
Cashews, unsalted, 1½ oz 7
Frito-Lay Salted cashews, 3 Tbsp 4
Lance
Cashews, 1 package (43 g).........................7
Cashews, ¼ cup.......................................4
Planters
Cashew halves with pieces, 1 oz 4
Fancy cashews, 1 oz.................................4
Fancy cashews, 1 package (57 g) 9
Honey roasted cashews, 1 oz....................4
Honey roasted cashews, 1 package
  (42 g) 6
Honey roasted cashews, 1 package
  (57 g) 8

Honey roasted cashews dry roasted,
1 package (42 g) 6
Honey roasted cashews dry roasted,
1 package (57 g) 8
Whole cashews, 1 oz................................4
Whole cashews, 1 package (57 g) 9

Tropical Nut & Fruit
Cashew butts, 1 oz 5
Cashew pieces, roasted, salted, 1 oz 5
Cashew splits, 1 oz 5
Honey roasted cashews, ¼ cup 5
Large whole cashews, 1 oz 5
Raw cashew butts, ¼ cup...........................4
Raw cashew splits, ¼ cup...........................4
Super large cashews, raw, ¼ cup...............4
Whole cashews, 1 oz................................5
Whole, raw cashews, ¼ cup.......................4

Cauliflower
Green Giant
Cauliflower florets, frozen, 1 cup...............0
Cauliflower in cheese flavored sauce,
frozen, ½ cup 1
Hanover Cauliflower florets, 5 florets
(78 g) 0

Cereal bars
Health Valley
Fat-free apple fruit bar, 1 (42 g) 2
Fat-free apricot fruit bar, 1 (42 g) 2
Fat-free bakes, apple, 1 (27 g)...................1
Fat-free bakes, date, 1 (27 g) 1
Fat-free bakes, raisin, 1 (27 g)....................1
Fat-free breakfast bakes, apple, 1 (38 g) 2
Fat-free breakfast bakes, blueberry, 1
(38 g) 2
Fat-free breakfast bakes, raspberry, 1
(38 g) 2
Fat-free breakfast bakes, strawberry, 1
(38 g) 2
Fat-free date fruit bar, 1 (42 g)...................2
Fat-free raisin fruit bar, 1 (42 g) 2

Health Valley Low fat
Apple cobbler cereal bar, 1 (37 g) 3
Blueberry cobbler cereal bar, 1 (37 g) 3
Strawberry cobbler cereal bar, 1 (37 g) 3

Hostess
Apple fruit & grain cereal bars, 1 (37 g).....2
Banana nut fruit & grain cereal bars,
1 (37 g) 2
Blueberry fruit & grain cereal bars,............1
(37 g) 2
Raspberry fruit & grain cereal bars, 1
(37 g) 2
Strawberry fruit & grain cereal bars, 1
(37 g) 2

Kellogg's Nutri-grain
Apple cinnamon, 1 bar (37 g) 3
Blueberry, 1 bar (37 g) 3
Cherry, 1 bar (37 g) 3
Mixed berry, 1 bar (37 g) 3
Peach, 1 bar (37 g) 3
Raspberry, 1 bar (37 g) 3
Strawberry, 1 bar (37 g) 3

Kellogg's Nutri-grain Fruit-full Squares
Apple, 1 bar (49 g)...................................4
Banana, 1 bar (49 g) 4
Cinnamon raisin, 1 bar (49 g) 4

Kellogg's Nutri-grain Twists
Apple cinnamon & brown sugar, 1 bar
(37 g) 3
Banana & strawberry, 1 bar (37 g) 3
Strawberry & blueberry, 1 bar (37 g) 3
Strawberry & crème, 1 bar (37 g) 3

Kellogg's Rice Krispies Treats
Squares cocoa, 1 bar (22 g) 2
Squares original, 1 bar (22 g) 2
Squares peanut butter chocolate, 1 bar
(23 g) 3

Kudos
Chocolate chip, 1 bar (27.8 g)...................3
Chocolate fudge, 1 bar (27.8 g) 3
M&M's milk chocolate mini's, 1 bar
(23.2 g)..2
Peanut butter, 1 bar (27.8 g).....................3
Snickers bar, 1 bar (23.2 g) 2

Nabisco
Fruit & grain bars – apple cinnamon, 1
(37 g) 3

Fruit & grain bars – blueberry, 1 (37 g)......3
Fruit & grain bars – mixed berry, 1
  (37 g) 3
Fruit & grain bars – raspberry, 1 (37 g)......3
Fruit & grain bars – strawberry, 1 (37 g).....3

Quaker Oats
Fruit & oatmeal bar with calcium –
  apple cinnamon, 1 (37 g) 3
Fruit & oatmeal bar with calcium –
  blueberry, 1 (37 g) 3
Fruit & oatmeal bar with calcium –
  cherry cobbler, 1 (37 g) 3
Fruit & oatmeal bar with calcium –
  strawberry, 1 (37 g) 3
Fruit & oatmeal bar with calcium –
  strawberry banana, 1 (37 g) 3
Fruit & oatmeal bar with calcium –
  strawberry cheesecake, 1 (37 g)..............3
Fruit & oatmeal bar with calcium –
  very berry, 1 (37 g) 3

Sunbelt Snacks & Cereals
Blueberry fruit filled cereal bar, 1 (37 g).....3
Raspberry fruit filled cereal bars, 1
  (37 g) 3
Strawberry fruit filled cereal bars, 1
  (37 g) 3

Weight Watchers
Breakfast bars, apple cinnamon,
  1 serving (28 g) 2
Breakfast bars, blueberry, 1 serving
  (28 g) 2
Breakfast bars, raspberry, 1 serving
  (28 g) 2

Cereals, hot
General Mills Wheat hearts, ¼ cup 2
Health Valley
Apple cinnamon flavor cereal cup,
  1 package (57 g) 4
Banana nut flavor cereal cup,
  1 package (63 g) 4
Maple madness cereal cup, 1 package
  (66 g) 4
Terrific 10 grain cereal cup, 1 package
  (59 g) 4

Jim Dandy
Grits, quick, ¼ cup 3
Grits, quick, iron fortified, ¼ cup 3
Grits, regular, ¼ cup.................................3
Martha White
Grits, instant, original, 1 pouch (28 g) 2
Grits, yellow, ¼ cup..................................3
Nabisco
Cream of wheat instant multigrain –
  banana nut bread, 1 packet (40 g)..........3
Cream of wheat instant multigrain –
  blueberry muffin, 1 packet (38 g)............2
Cream of wheat instant multigrain –
  raspberry danish, 1 packet (40 g)............2
Cream of wheat, 1 minute, 1 cup 2
Cream of wheat, 10 minute, 1 cup 2
Cream of wheat, 2½ minute, 1 cup 2
Instant cream of wheat – baked apple
  cinnamon, 1 packet (35 g)....................2
Instant cream of wheat – cinnamon
  brown sugar, 1 packet (35 g).................2
Instant cream of wheat – maple brown
  sugar, 1 packet (35 g) 2
Instant cream of wheat - original,
  1 packet (28 g) 2
Quaker Oats
Cinnamon-spice instant oatmeal,
  1 packet (46 g) 3
Creamy wheat – enriched farina,
  ¼ cup 3
Fruit & cream instant oatmeal, artificial
  blueberry flavor, 1 packet (35 g) 2
Instant oatmeal – baked apple flavor,
  1 packet (40 g) 3
Instant oatmeal – French vanilla flavor,
  1 packet (43 g) 3
Instant oatmeal – low sodium,
  1 packet (28 g) 2
Instant oatmeal – maple/brown sugar,
  1 packet (43 g) 3
Instant oatmeal with apples and
  cinnamon, 1 packet (35 g)....................2
Mother's instant oatmeal, ½ cup...............2

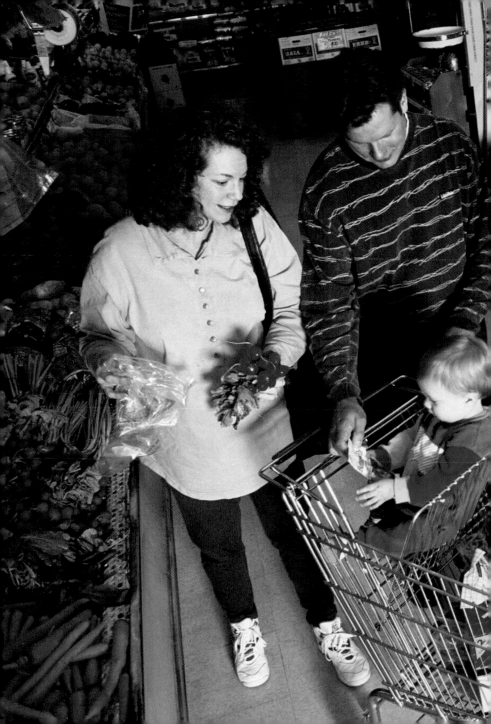

Cereals, hot, Quaker Oats (con't)   POINTS

Multigrain hot cereal, ½ cup 2
Oat bran, ½ cup 2
Old fashioned oats, ½ cup 2
Peaches & cream instant oatmeal,
   1 packet (35 g) 2
Quick oats, ½ cup 2
Raisin, date, walnut instant oatmeal,
   1 packet (37 g) 3
Raisin-spice instant oatmeal, 1 packet
   (43 g) 3
Strawberries & cream instant oatmeal,
   1 packet (35 g) 2
Whole wheat natural cereal, ½ cup 2

Cereals, ready-to-eat
Country Inn Specialities

Green Gables Inn blend, ½ cup 4
Inn at Hormsby Hill blend, 1 cup 4
Greyfield Inn blend, ¾ cup 4

General Mills

Apple cinnamon cheerios, ¾ cup 2
Basic 4, 1 cup 4
Berry berry kix, ¾ cup 3
Boo berry, 1 cup 2
Cheerios, 1 cup 2
Cinnamon grahams, ¾ cup......................2
Cinnamon toast crunch, ¾ cup 3
Cocoa puffs, 1 cup 2
Cookie crisps, 1 cup 2
Corn chex, 1 cup.....................................2
Count chocula, 1 cup 2
Country corn flakes, 1 cup 2
Fiber One, 1 cup 2
Frankenberry, 1 cup 2
French toast crunch, ¾ cup 2
Frosted cheerios, 1 cup...........................2
Frosted wheaties, ¾ cup 2
Golden grahams, ¾ cup 2
Honey nut cheerios, 1 cup 2
Honey nut chex, 1 cup 2
Honey nut clusters, 1 cup 4
Kaboom, 1 ¼ cups 2
Kix, 1 ⅓ cups..2
Lucky charms, 1 cup................................2

POINTS

Millenios, 1 cup 2
Multi-bran chex, 1 cup 3
Multi-grain cheerios plus, 1 cup 2
Nesquik chocolate, ¾ cup 3
Oatmeal crisp almond, 1 cup 4
Oatmeal crisp apple cinnamon, 1 cup........4
Oatmeal crisp raisin, 1 cup 4
Raisin nut bran, ¾ cup............................4
Reese's peanut butter puffs, ¾ cup 3
Rice chex, 1¼ cups 2
Sunrise, ¾ cup..2
Team cheerios, 1 cup 2
Total brown sugar & oat, ¾ cup 2
Total corn flakes, ¾ cup 2
Total raisin bran, 1 cup...........................3
Total whole grain, ¾ cup 2
Trix, 1 cup 2
Wheat chex, 1 cup 3
Wheaties, 1 cup 2
Wheaties raisin bran, 1 cup 3

Health Valley

Apple crunch o's, ¾ cup 2
Banana gone nuts crunches & flakes,
   ¾ cup 3
Corn crunch-em's!, 1 cup 2
Cranberry crunch, ¾ cup 3
Fat-free healthy crunches and flakes,
   ¾ cup 2
Fat-free honey crunch o's, ¾ cup 2
Lowfat granola date almond flavor,
   ⅔ cup 3
Lowfat granola, raisin cinnamon,
   ⅔ cup 3
Lowfat granola, tropical fruit, ⅔ cup 3
Organic amaranth flakes, ¾ cup 1
Organic apple crunch bran cereal,
   ¾ cup 2
Organic blue corn flakes, ¾ cup...............1
Organic fiber 7 flakes, ¾ cup 1
Organic golden flax cereal, ½ cup 3
Organic healthy fiber flakes, ¾ cup 1
Organic honey fiber 7 multigrain flakes,
   ¾ cup...1

Cereals, ready-to-eat, Health Valley (con't)

POINTS

Organic honey nut o's, ¾ cup 2
Organic oat bran flakes with raisins,
  ¾ cup..1
Organic oat bran o's, ¾ cup 1
Organic oat brand flakes, ¾ cup 1
Organic raisin bran flakes, 1¼ cups 3
Organic raisin crunch bran cereal,
  ¾ cup..2
Puffed corn cereal, 1 cup...........................2
Raspberry rhapsody cereal, ¾ cup 3
Real oat bran, cereal – almond crunch,
  ½ cup..3
Rice crunch-ems!, 1¼ cups 2

Health Valley Soyo's

Apple cinnamon, 1 cup 3
Honey nut, 1 cup 3
Original, 1 cup 3

Healthy Choice from Kellogg's

Almond crunch with raisins, 1 cup 4
Low fat granola, ½ cup 3
Low fat granola with raisins, ⅔ cup 4
Mueslix raisin & almond crunch with
  dates, ⅔ cup 3
Toasted brown sugar squares, 1 cup..........3

Kellogg's

All-bran, bran buds, ⅓ cup 1
All-bran, extra fiber, 1 cup 1
All-bran, original, ½ cup 1
Apple jacks, 1 cup.....................................2
Cocoa frosted flakes, ¾ cup 2
Cocoa krispies, ¾ cup 2
Complete oat bran flakes, ¾ cup 1
Complete wheat bran flakes, ¾ cup 1
Corn flakes, 1 cup.....................................2
Corn pops, 1 cup.......................................2
Cracklin' oat bran, ¾ cup 4
Crispix, 1 cup 2
Froot loops, 1 cup 2
Frosted flakes, ¾ cup 2
Honey crunch corn flakes, ¾ cup 2
Just right fruit & nut, 1 cup 4
Marshmallow blasted froot loops,
  1 cup..2

POINTS

Mini-wheats apple cinnamon, ¾ cup 3
Mini-wheats blueberry, ¾ cup 3
Mini-wheats frosted bite size,
  24 pieces (59 g).......................................3
Mini-wheats frosted original, 5 pieces
  (51 g) 3
Mini-wheats raisin, ¾ cup.........................3
Mini-wheats strawberry, ¾ cup 3
Product 19, 1 cup 2
Raisin bran, 1 cup 3
Raisin bran crunch, 1 cup 3
Razzle dazzle rice krispies, ¾ cup 2
Rice krispies, 1 ¼ cups 2
Rice krispies treats, ¾ cup.........................3
Smacks, ¾ cup 2
Smart start, 1 cup 3

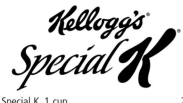

Special K, 1 cup 2
Special K plus, 1 cup 4

Morning Traditions

Banana nut crunch, 1 cup..........................5
Blueberry morning, 1¼ cups 4
Cranberry almond crunch, 1 cup 4
Great grains crunch pecan, ⅔ cup.............4
Great grains raisins, dates & pecans,
  ⅔ cup..4

Nabisco

100% bran, ⅓ cup 1
Frosted shredded wheat bite size, 1 cup 3
Honey nut shredded wheat bite size,
  1 cup..3
The original shredded wheat, 2 biscuits
  (46 g) 2
The original shredded wheat 'n bran,
  1¼ cups..3
The original shredded wheat spoon size,
  1 cup..3

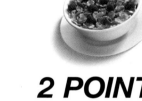

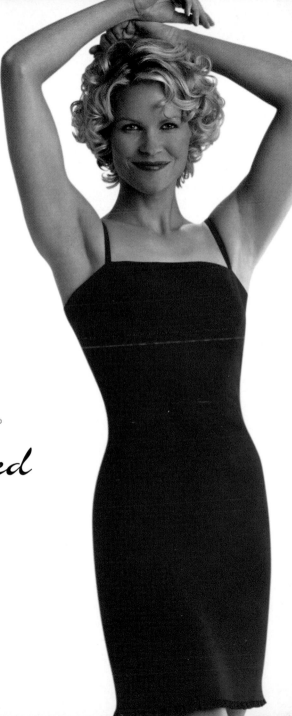

2 POINTS®
never tasted
so great.

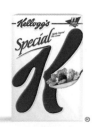

Cereals, ready-to-eat (con't)

Nature Valley Low fat fruit granola,
⅔ cup 4

Nature's Choice
Low fat granola cereal, ⅔ cup 4
Muesli, ⅔ cup 3
Oats, raisins & almonds, 1 cup 4

Post
Alpha-bits, 1 cup 3
Bran flakes, ¾ cup 1
Cocoa pebbles, ¾ cup 2
Fruit & fibre peaches, raisins & almonds,
1 cup 4
Fruity pebbles, ¾ cup 2
Golden crisp, ¾ cup 2
Grape-nuts, ½ cup 3
Grape-nuts flakes, ¾ cup 1
Honey bunches of oats honey roasted,
¾ cup...2
Honey bunches of oats with almonds,
¾ cup...3
Honeycomb, 1⅓ cups 2
Marshmallow alpha-bits, 1 cup 2
Post toasties, 1 cup 2
Raisin bran, 1 cup 3
Waffle crisp, 1 cup 3

Quaker Oats
100% natural granola oats & honey,
½ cup...5
100% natural granola oats, honey &
raisins, ½ cup 5
Cap'n crunch, ¾ cup 2
Cinnamon life, ¾ cup 2
Cinnamon oatmeal squares, 1 cup 4
Life, ¾ cup 2
Low fat 100% natural granola with
raisins, ⅔ cup.......................................4
Oat bran cereal, 1¼ cups 4
Oatmeal squares, 1 cup............................4
Puffed rice, 1 cup.....................................1
Puffed wheat, 1¼ cups.............................1
Toasted oatmeal cereal – honey nut,
1 cup..3
Toasted oatmeal cereal – original,
1 cup..3

Sunbelt Snacks & Cereals
Berry basic whole grain flakes with
real fruit pieces, ½ cup 4
Granola cereal with cinnamon & raisins,
½ cup 3

Chai
Pacific
Spice, 3 Tbsp 2
Vanilla, 3 Tbsp...2
Vanilla decaf, 3 Tbsp 2

Cheese

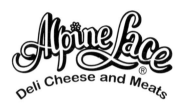

Alpine Lace
American flavor pasteurized process
cheese product, 1 oz.............................2
American flavor pasteurized process
cheese product with jalapeno peppers,
1 oz..2
Cheddar cheese, 1 oz 2
Colby cheese, 1 oz 2
Feta, 1 oz 1
Feta cheese, sun dried tomato & basil,
1 oz..1
Lightly smoked provolone cheese, 1 oz......2
Mozzarella cheese, 1 oz 2
Muenster cheese, reduced sodium, 1 oz 3
Swiss cheese, 1 oz 2

Boars's Head
American cheese, 2 slices (28 g) 3
American cheese (loaf), 1 oz.....................3
Baby Swiss cheese, 1 oz 3
Butterkase cheese, 1 oz............................3
Canadian Cheddar cheese 3 yr. old,
1 oz..3
Cream havarti cheese, 1 oz.......................3
Cream havarti cheese w/ jalapeño, 1 oz.....3

Cream havarti cheese with dill, 1 oz..........3
Creamy blue cheese, 1 oz 2
Double Gloucester Cheddar cheese –
  white & yellow, 1 oz 3
Edam cheese, 1 oz 2
Feta cheese, 1 oz 2
Fontina cheese, 1 oz...................................3
Gold label prem. imp. Swiss – low
  sodium, 1 oz 3
Gouda cheese – wheel, 1 oz.....................3
Hickory smoked pasteurized process
  gruyere cheese, 1 oz 3
Lacey Swiss cheese, 1 oz 2
Longhorn colby cheese, 1 oz.....................3
Low sodium muenster cheese, 1 oz 3
Monterey Jack cheese, 1 oz 3
Monterey Jack cheese with jalapeño,
  1 oz..3
Mozzarella cheese – low moisture,
  1 oz..2
Muenster cheese, 1 oz...............................3
Natural Swiss cheese, 1 oz 3
Neufchatel cheese, 2 Tbsp 2
No salt added natural Swiss cheese,
  1 oz..3
Picante/sharp provolone cheese, 1 oz 3
Pre-cut 3 yr. old Canadian Cheddar,
  1 oz..3
Pre-cut edam cheese, 1 oz........................2
Pre-cut extra aged Cheddar cheese
  (white & yellow), 1 oz...........................3
Pre-cut gouda cheese, 1 oz.......................3
Pre-cut gruyere, 1 oz.................................3
Pre-cut longhorn colby cheese, 1 oz 3
Pre-cut picante/sharp provolone, 1 oz........3
Provolone cheese, ½ lower sodium,
  1 oz..3
Sharp slicing Cheddar cheese
  (white & yellow), 1 oz............................3
Sliced pasteurized process American
  cheese, 1 slice (19 g)..............................2
Smoked butterkase cheese, 1 oz 3

Di Giorno
100% grated Parmesan, 2 tsp...................1
100% grated Romano cheese, 2 tsp 1
100% shredded Parmesan cheese,
  2 tsp..1
100% shredded Romano cheese, 2 tsp 1
Parmesan cheese, 2 tsp 0
Romano cheese, 2 tsp 1

Finlandia
Heavenly light imported Swiss cheese,
  1 oz..2
Imported Swiss cheese, 1 oz 3
Healthy Choice
Balls, 1 serving (30 g)...............................1
Shreds, 1 serving (28 g).............................1
Singles, 1 serving (21 g) 1
String, 1 serving (28 g)..............................1
Kraft
100% grated Parmesan cheese, 2 tsp 1
100% Parmesan, 2 tsp 1
Bacon, spread, 2 Tbsp 2
Cheddar & Monterey Jack (shredded),
  ¼ cup..3
Cheddar medium (shredded), ¼ cup..........3
Cheddar, extra sharp, 1 oz 3
Cheddar, medium, 1 oz..............................3
Cheddar, mild, 1 oz 3
Cheddar, mild (finely shredded), ⅓ cup 3
Cheddar, mild (shredded), ¼ cup...............3
Cheddar, sharp, 1 oz...................................3
Cheddar, sharp (finely shredded), ⅓ cup 3
Cheddar, sharp (shredded), ¼ cup 3
Cheddary melts pasteurized process
  medium Cheddar cheese food, 1 oz 3
Cheddary melts pasteurized process
  medium Cheddar cheese food shreds,
  ¼ cup 3

c

Cheddary melts pasteurized process
mild Cheddar cheese food, 1 oz..............3

Cheddary melts pasteurized process
mild Cheddar cheese food shreds,
¼ cup....................3

Colby, 1 oz..............3

Colby & Monterey Jack (finely shredded),
⅓ cup....................3

Colby & Monterey Jack (shredded),
¼ cup....................3

Colby Monterey Jack, 1 oz........................3

Deluxe American pasteurized process
American cheese, 1 oz...........................3

Deluxe American pasteurized process
American cheese (white), 1 oz................3

Low-moisture part-skim mozzarella,
1 oz.....................2

Low-moisture part-skim mozzarella
(finely shredded), ⅓ cup.........................2

Low-moisture part-skim mozzarella
(shredded), ⅓ cup..................................2

Monterey Jack, 1 oz..................................3

Monterey Jack (shredded), ¼ cup..............3

Monterey Jack with jalapeño peppers,
1 oz.....................3

Olive and pimento, spread, 2 Tbsp............2

Pasteurized process cheese food with
garlic, 1 oz...................2

Pasteurized process cheese food with
jalapeño peppers, 1 oz.....................2

Pimento, spread, 2 Tbsp...........................2

Pineapple, spread, 2 Tbsp........................2

Roka brand blue, spread, 2 Tbsp...............2

Swiss, 1 oz..............3

Swiss (finely shredded), ⅓ cup..................3

Swiss (shredded), ⅓ cup...........................3

Whole milk low-moisture mozzarella
(shredded), ⅓ cup..................................3

Kraft 2%

Cheddar, mild, 1 oz..................................2

Cheddar, mild (finely shredded), ⅓ cup......3

Cheddar, mild (shredded), ¼ cup...............2

Cheddar, sharp, 1 oz.................................2

Cheddar, sharp (finely shredded), ⅓ cup....3

Cheddar, sharp (shredded), ¼ cup.............2

Colby, 1 oz..............2

Colby & Monterey Jack (shredded),
¼ cup....................2

Monterey Jack, 1 oz..................................2

Mozzarella (shredded), ⅓ cup...................2

Pizza cheese (Cheddar & mozzarella),
shredded, ⅓ cup..................................2

Reduced fat Swiss cheese slices, 1 slice
(38 g)....................3

Kraft 2% Singles

American reduced fat pasteurized
cheese food, ¾ oz.................................1

American reduced fat pasteurized
process cheese food (white), ¾ oz..........1

Kraft Cracker Barrel

Baby Swiss, 1 oz.......................................3

Cheddar, extra sharp, 1 oz.......................3

Cheddar, marbled sharp, 1 oz...................3

Cheddar, New York aged reserve, 1 oz.......3

Cheddar, sharp, 1 oz.................................3

Cheddar, Vermont sharp, 1 oz...................3

Extra sharp Cheddar spread, 2 Tbsp..........2

Sharp Cheddar spread, 2 Tbsp (25 g).........2

Sharp Cheddar with herbs spread,
2 Tbsp....................2

Kraft Cracker Barrel 2%

Cheddar, extra sharp, 1 oz.......................2

Cheddar, sharp, 1 oz.................................2

Cheddar, Vermont sharp, 1 oz...................2

Kraft Deli-Thin

Low-moisture part-skim mozzarella,
1 slice (28 g)...2

Swiss, 1 slice (23 g)..................................2

Swiss aged, 1 slice (23 g).........................2

**Kraft Deluxe Singles Pasteurized
Process Cheese**

American, ⅔ oz...2

American, ¾ oz...2

American, 1 oz..3

American (white), ⅔ oz.............................2

American (white), ¾ oz.............................2

American (white), 1 oz 3

Pimento, 1 oz 3

Swiss, ¾ oz 2

Kraft Free

Cheddar cheese (shredded), ¼ cup............1

Mozzarella cheese (shredded), ¼ cup 1

Nonfat grated topping, 2 tsp 0

Kraft Free Singles

American, ⅔ oz 1

American, ¾ oz 1

American (white), ⅔ oz...........................1

American (white), ¾ oz 1

Sharp Cheddar, ⅔ oz...............................1

Swiss artificially flavored, ¾ oz.................1

Kraft Handi-Snacks Low-moisture
part-skim mozzarella string cheese,
1 piece (28 g)......................................2

Kraft Italian Style

Classic garlic (shredded), ⅓ cup 3

Hearty Italian (shredded), ⅓ cup 3

Mozzarella & Parmesan (shredded),
⅓ cup...3

Kraft Light N' Lively American
flavor pasteurized process cheese
product singles, ¾ oz.............................1

Kraft Marbled

Cheddar and Monterey Jack, 1 oz 3

Cheddar and whole milk mozzarella,
1 oz..3

Cheddar, mild, 1 oz 3

Colby Monterey Jack, 1 oz.......................3

Kraft Mexican Style

Cheddar and Monterey Jack, ⅓ cup 3

Cheddar and Monterey Jack with
jalapeño peppers (shredded), ⅓ cup........3

Four cheese (shredded), ⅓ cup.................3

Taco cheese (shredded), ⅓ cup 3

Kraft Natural Cheese Slices

Cheddar, mild, 1 slice (28 g) 3

Colby, 1 slice (45 g)................................5

Low-moisture part-skim mozzarella,
1 slice (43 g) 3

Low-moisture part-skim mozzarella,
1 slice (45 g) 3

Provolone with smoked flavor added,
1 slice (43 g) 4

Swiss, 1 slice (23 g)................................2

Swiss, 1 slice (38 g)................................4

Swiss, 1 slice (43 g)................................4

Swiss, 1 slice (45 g)................................5

Swiss aged, 1 slice (43 g) 4

Kraft Off the Block

Cheddar, extra sharp, 1 oz 3

Cheddar, medium, 1 oz............................3

Cheddar, mild, 1 oz 3

Cheddar, sharp, 1 oz...............................3

Colby Monterey Jack, 1 oz.......................3

Low-moisture part-skim mozzarella, 1 oz ...2

Monterey Jack, 1 oz................................3

Kraft Old English

American cheese slice, 1 oz 3

Sharp pasteurized process American
cheese, 1 oz 3

Sharp pasteurized process cheese
spread, 2 Tbsp 2

Kraft Parm Plus!

Seasoning blend garlic herb, 2 tsp.............0

Seasoning blend zesty red pepper, 2 tsp 0

Kraft Pizza

Four cheese (shredded), ¼ cup..................2

Low-moisture mozzarella and Cheddar
(shredded), ⅓ cup................................3

Low-moisture mozzarella and provolone
with smoke flavor (shredded), ¼ cup.......2

**Kraft Singles Pasteurized Process
Cheese Food**

American, ⅔ oz 2

American, ¾ oz 2

American, 1.2 oz.....................................3

American (white), ⅔ oz...........................2

American (white), ¾ oz 2

Mild Mexican style, ¾ oz 2

Monterey, ¾ oz 2

Pimento, ⅔ oz 2

Pimento, ¾ oz 2

Pimento, 1 oz 3

Sharp, ¾ oz...2

Swiss, ¾ oz 2

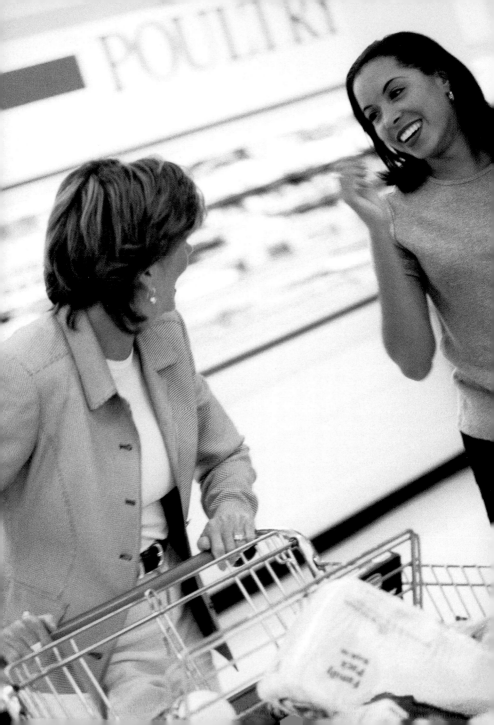

Kraft Velveeta

Hot Mexican, 1 oz.....................................2
Mild Mexican, 1 oz 2
Plain, 1 oz 2
Shredded mild Mexican pasteurized
    process cheese food with jalapeno
    pepper, ¼ cup 3
Shredded pasteurized process cheese
    food, ¼ cup...3

Kraft Velveeta Light Reduced fat

pasteurized process cheese product,
    1 oz...1

Land O' Lakes

American cheese, slice, yellow or white,
    1 slice..2
American cheese, slice, yellow or white,
    2 slices (1 oz) 3
Chedarella cheese, 1 oz...........................3
Cheddar cheese, mild, medium, sharp,
    extra sharp, 1 oz 3
Co-Jack cheese, 1 oz 3
Colby cheese, 1 oz 3
Hot pepper Monterey Jack cheese, 1 oz.....3
Monterey Jack cheese, 1 oz 3
Mozzarella cheese, 1 oz 2
Pasteurized process cheese food,
    individually wrapped slices, 1 slice..........2
Pasteurized process cheese spread,
    golden velvet loaf, 1 oz 2
Swiss cheese, 1 oz 3

Land O' Lakes Deli

American cheese loaf, sharp, yellow
    or white, 1 oz 3
American cheese, less salt, 1 oz 3
Brick cheese, 1 oz 3
Cheddar cheese prints, medium & sharp,
    1 oz...3
Co-Jack cheese, 1 oz 3
Extra sharp flavor process Cheddar
    cheese, 1 oz 3
Italian mozzarella cheese, 1 oz 2
Italian provolone cheese, 1 oz...................3
Jalapeno flavor process Jack cheese,
    1 oz...3

Jalapeno flavor process cheese food,
    1 oz...2
Longhorn colby cheese, 1 oz 3
Monterey Jack cheese prints, 1 oz.............3
Muenster cheese naturals, 1 oz.................3
Process American cheese loaf yellow
    or white, 1 oz 3
Process light jalapeno cheese loaf, 1 oz.....2
Process pasteurized American cheese
    loaf, yellow or white, 1 oz 3
Swiss & American cheese, 1 oz 3
Swiss cheese, 1 oz 3

Polly-O

Light mozzarella cheese, 1 oz 1
Lite string cheese, 1 oz..............................1
Part skim mozzarella, 1 oz 2

Schwan's

American process cheese, 1 slice (19 g).....2
Breaded mozzarella sticks, 2 (29 g)...........2

Shedd's Country Crock Easy squeeze

Cheddar, 2 Tbsp.....................................1

Cheese nuggets

Banquet Mozzarella cheese nuggets,

6 pieces (3 oz).......................................7

Cheese sauce

Di Giorno

Four cheese sauce, ¼ cup 4
Garlic pesto sauce, ¼ cup........................10

Five Brothers

Five cheese, ½ cup 1
Quattro formaggio, ¼ cup 3

Kraft Sqeezable, 2 Tbsp........................3

Kraft Cheez Whiz

Jalapeño pepper, 2 Tbsp 2
Mild salsa, 2 Tbsp....................................3
Plain, 2 Tbsp..2

Kraft Cheez Whiz Light Pasteurized

process cheese product, 2 Tbsp...............2

Ragu Cheese Creations

Creamy tomato Romano, ¼ cup.................1
Double Cheddar, ¼ cup 3
Four cheese, ¼ cup 3
Roasted garlic Parmesan, ¼ cup.................3

Ragu Robusto Six cheese, ½ cup............1

Cheese snacks

Boston's Cheez bopps, 1 oz 3

Cheetos

Crunchy, 21 pieces (1 oz)...........................4

Curls, 15 pieces (1 oz)................................4

Flamin' hot, 31 pieces (1 oz).....................4

Hot puff rods, 13 pieces (1 oz) 4

Jumbo puffs, 13 pieces (1 oz)....................4

Puffed balls, 38 pieces (1 oz) 4

Puffs, 29 pieces (1 oz) 4

X's & O's, 23 pieces (1 oz) 4

Zig zags, 17 pieces (1 oz) 4

Jax Cheddar cheese curls, 25 pieces

(30 g) 3

Lance

Cheese balls, 32 (28 g).............................4

Cheese balls, 56 (50 g).............................6

Crunchy cheese twist, 30 pieces (32 g) 5

Weight Watchers Cheese curls,

1 serving (14 g) 2

Cheese, breaded, frozen

Giorgio Italian breaded pizza cheese

sticks, 2 (37 g).......................................3

Cheese, cottage

Breakstone's®

Breakstone

Cottage cheese – 4% milkfat, large

curd, ½ cup 3

Cottage cheese – 4% milkfat, small

curd, ½ cup 3

Cottage cheese – 4% milkfat, small

curd (snack size), 4 oz...........................3

Dry curd cottage cheese less than ½%

milkfat with added skim milk, ¼ cup 1

Lowfat cottage cheese – 2% milkfat,

large curd, ½ cup....................................2

Lowfat cottage cheese – 2% milkfat,

small curd, ½ cup 2

Lowfat cottage cheese – 2% milkfat,

small curd (snack size), 4 oz 2

Breakstone Cottage Doubles

Lowfat cottage cheese and peach

topping, 6 oz..3

Lowfat cottage cheese and pineapple

topping, 6 oz..3

Lowfat cottage cheese and strawberry

topping, 6 oz..3

Breakstone Free

Fat free cottage cheese, ½ cup.................2

Fat free cottage cheese (snack size),

4 oz...1

Foremost

Cottage cheese, 4%, ½ cup 3

Reduced fat cottage cheese, ½ cup 2

Golden Guernsey

Cottage cheese, 4%, ½ cup 3

Reduced fat cottage cheese, ½ cup 2

Knudsen®

Knudsen

Cottage cheese – 4% milkfat, large

curd, ½ cup 3

Cottage cheese – 4% milkfat, small

curd, ½ cup 3

Lowfat cottage cheese – 2% milkfat,

small curd, ½ cup 2

Lowfat cottage cheese with pineapple –

1.5% milkfat, small curd, ½ cup 3

Knudsen Free Fat free cottage cheese,

½ cup 2

Knudsen On The Go

Lowfat cottage cheese – 2% milkfat,

small curd, 4 oz......................................2

Peach lowfat cottage cheese & fruit –

1.5% milkfat, 4 oz 2

Pineapple lowfat cottage cheese &

fruit – 1.5% milkfat, 4 oz 2

Strawberry lowfat cottage cheese &

fruit – 1.5% milkfat, 4 oz 2

Tropical fruit lowfat cottage cheese

& fruit – 1.5% milkfat, 4 oz....................2

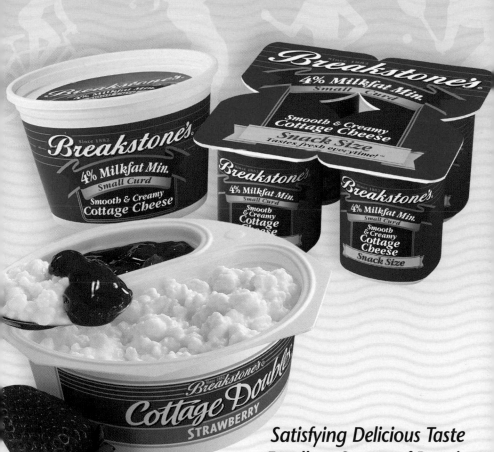

Add Variety to your Healthy Lifestyle.

**Satisfying Delicious Taste
Excellent Source of Protein**

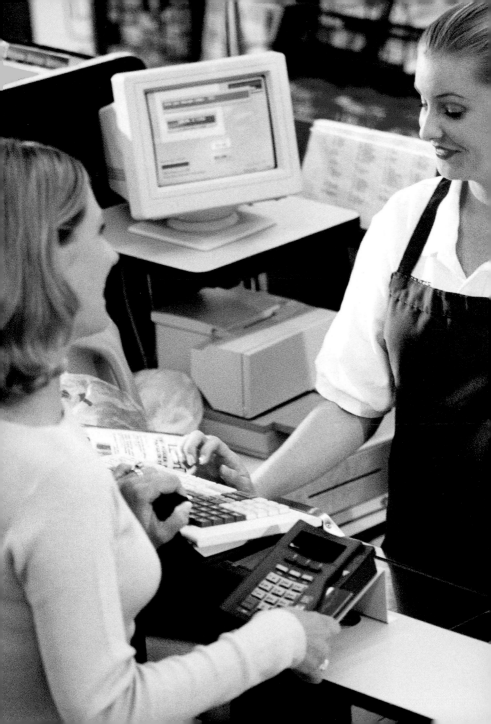

Cheese, cottage (con't) POINTS

Knudsen On The Go Free Fat free
cottage cheese, 4 oz 1

Light N' Lively
Garden salad, ½ cup 2
Peach & pineapple, ½ cup 2
Plain, ½ cup 2

Light N' Lively Free
Fat free cottage cheese with added
    calcium, ½ cup 2

Morning Glory
Cottage cheese, 4%, ½ cup 3
Reduced fat cottage cheese, ½ cup 2

Cheese, cream

Alpine Lace Sun dried tomato & basil
    cream cheese, reduced-fat, 2 Tbsp 2

Boar's Head Cream cheese, 2 Tbsp..........3

Kraft Breakstone's Temp-Tee
    Pasteurized whipped cream cheese,
    2 Tbsp...................................2

Kraft Philadelphia Brand
Cream cheese, 2 Tbsp................3
Cream cheese, 1 oz 3
Cream cheese with chives, 1 oz 3
Neufchatel cheese – ⅓ less fat than
    cream cheese, 1 oz 2
Plain, whipped, 2 Tbsp 2
With chives, whipped, 2 Tbsp......2
With smoked salmon, whipped, 2 Tbsp......2

Kraft Philadelphia Brand Free
Fat free cream cheese, 1 oz 1
Plain, 2 Tbsp..............................1
With garden vegetables, 2 Tbsp 1
With strawberries, 2 Tbsp 1

Kraft Philadelphia Brand Light
    Light Cream Cheese, 2 Tbsp.........2

Kraft Philly Flavors
Apple cinnamon, 2 Tbsp 3
Cheesecake, 2 Tbsp 3
Chive & onion, 2 Tbsp 3
Garden vegetable, 2 Tbsp 3
Honey nut flavor, 2 Tbsp 3
Jalapeño, light, 2 Tbsp...............2
Pineapple, 2 Tbsp......................3

POINTS

Raspberry, light, 2 Tbsp 2
Roasted garlic, light 2 Tbsp..........2
Salmon, 2 Tbsp 3
Strawberry, 2 Tbsp 3

Rite
Cream cheese & lox spread, 2 Tbsp..........2
Cream cheese & scallion spread, 2 Tbsp 2
Whipped cream cheese spread, 2 Tbsp 3

Cheese, ricotta

Breakstone Ricotta cheese, ¼ cup..........3

Polly-O
Part skim ricotta, ¼ cup 2
Reduced fat ricotta cheese, ¼ cup.............2

Cherries

Del Monte Dark, pitted cherries in
    heavy syrup, ½ cup 2

Dole Cherries, 1 cup....................1

Futuro Nance yellow cherries, 1 oz...........0

Traverse Bay Fruit Co. Sweetened
    dried cherries, ⅓ cup...............2

Tropical Nut & Fruit
Bing cherries, ¼ cup..................2
Dried cherries, ¼ cup 2

Chicken

Banquet
Breast nuggets, 7 pieces (3 oz) 7
Country fried chicken, 3 oz 7
Fat free baked breast patties, 1 (3 oz) 2
Fat free baked breast tenders, 3 pieces
    (3 oz).....................................2
Firehouse big wings, 4 oz 5
Grilled honey BBQ chicken breast
    patties, 1 (2.6 oz) 3
Grilled honey mustard chicken breast
    patties, 1 (2.6 oz) 3
Honey BBQ skinless fried chicken, 3.2 oz.....5
Honey BBQ wings, 4½ oz 10
Hot 'n spicy fried chicken, 3 oz..........7
Hot 'n spicy wings, 4 pieces (4 oz)..........7
Our original breast tenders, 3 pieces
    (3.1 g) 6
Our original chicken nuggets, 6 (3 oz) 7

C

Chicken, Banquet (con't)   POINTS

Our original chicken patties, 1 (2¼ oz) 5
Our original fried chicken, 3 oz 7
Our original fried chicken, jumbo pack,
   3 oz..7
Skinless fried chicken, 3 oz 5
Smokehouse big wings, 2 pieces (4 oz)......5
Southern breast tenders, 3 (3.1 oz) 6
Southern chicken nuggets, 5 pieces
   (3 oz)..7
Southern chicken patties, 1 (2.1 oz)...........5
Southern fried chicken, 3 oz......................7

Butterball

Baked breast tenders, 3 pieces (3.1 oz)......4
Crispy baked breasts, Italian style herb,
   1 piece (3½ oz) 4
Crispy baked breasts, original, 1 piece
   (3½ oz) 4
Crispy baked breasts, Parmesan, 1 piece
   (3½ oz) 4
Crispy baked breasts, southwestern,
   1 piece (3½ oz) 4
Crispy baked breats, lemon pepper,
   1 piece (3½ oz) 4
Hickory smoked grilled tenders,
   1 serving (4.3 oz)....................................3
Oriental grilled tenders, 1 serving
   (4.3 oz)...3

Country Skillet

Chicken bites, value pack, 5 pieces
   (3.2 oz)..7
Chicken breast tenders, value pack, 3
   (3.3 oz)..6
Chicken chunks, 5 pieces (3.3 oz)..............7
Chicken nuggets, 10 (3.3 oz)....................7
Chicken patties, 1 (2½ oz) 5
Chicken patties, value pack, 1 (2½ oz).......5
Fried chicken, 3 oz 7
Southern fried chicken chunks, 5 (3.3 oz) 7
Southern fried chicken patties, 1
   (2½ oz)..5

Foster Farms Fast Favorites

Diced chicken breasts, ⅔ cup...................3
Grilled chicken breasts, 1 fillet (112 g).......3
Grilled chicken breast strips, ⅔ cup...........3

                                POINTS

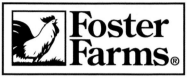

Foster Farms Savory Servings

Honey dijon chicken, 1 fillet (112 g) 3
Lemon herb chicken, 1 fillet (112 g) 3
Mesquite barbecue chicken, 1 fillet
   (112 g) 3
Roasted garlic & herb chicken, 1 fillet
   (112 g) 2
Sun-dried tomato & basil chicken,
   1 fillet, (112 g) 2

Foster Farms Select Servings

Chicken breast strips, refrigerated,
   1 serving (112 g) 2
Chicken breast tenders, refrigerated,
   1 serving (112 g) 2
Chicken nuggets, refrigerated, 1 serving
   (112 g) 2

Hormel

Chunk breast of chicken, 2 oz 1
Chunk breast of chicken – no salt, 2 oz 1
Chunk chicken, 2 oz 2

Kid Cuisine Muchers

Dino mite chicken nuggets, 4 pieces
   (3 oz)..8
Radical racin' chicken nuggets with
   cheese, 4 pieces (3 oz) 8

Perdue

Breaded breast cutlets, 1 (98 g) 6
Breaded breast nuggets, 5 (95 g) 6
Breaded breast tenderloins, 3 oz 4
Chicken and cheese nuggets, 5 (95 g) 7
Fajita marinated thighs, 1 (68 g) 3
Fun shapers chicken nuggets –
   dinosaurs, 3 (84 g)..................................5
Fun shapes chicken nuggets – stars
   & drumsticks, 4 (92 g)............................6
Garlic herb seasoned boneless skinless
   breasts, cooked, 3 oz..............................2

Healthy cooking has never been easier

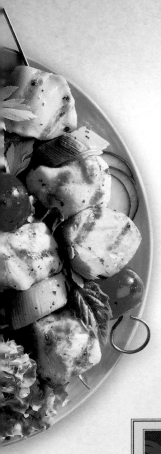

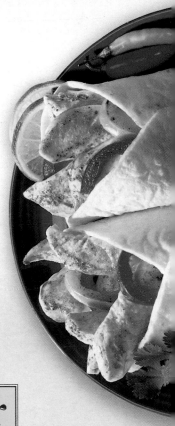

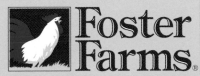

Select Servings™ • Savory Servings™ • Fresh & Easy • Fast Favorites™

 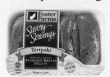

Fresh Foster Farms Chicken has always been a great choice for lean, healthy cooking.
Now with premium Select Servings cuts, already-marinated Savory Servings, quick Fresh & Easy and
fully cooked Fast Favorites entrées, our chicken is as easy to prepare as it is low in fat and calories.

For more information on our product line
call the Foster Farms Helpline at 1-800-255-7227 or visit our website at www.fosterfarms.com

Ground breast meat, cooked, 3 oz.............2
Ground, cooked, 3 oz 4
Honey mustard marinated chicken
thighs, 1 (68 g) 3
Honey roasted short cuts, ½ cup 2
Hot 'n spicy chicken wings, 1 serving
(84 g) 5
Italian seasoned boneless skinless
breasts, cooked, 3 oz............................2
Italian short cuts, ½ cup 2
Lemon pepper seasoned boneless
skinless breasts, cooked, 3 oz 2
Lemon pepper short cuts, ½ cup 2
Low fat breaded breast cutlets,
homestyle, 1 (84 g) 3
Low fat breaded breast cutlets, Italian
style, 1 (84 g) 3
Roasted short cuts, ½ cup 2
Rotisserie chicken, barbecue flavor,
roasted dark, 1 serving (3 oz) 5
Rotisserie chicken, barbecue flavor,
roasted white, 1 serving (3 oz)................3
Rotisserie chicken, Italian flavor, roasted
dark, 1 serving (3 oz) 5
Rotisserie chicken, Italian flavor, roasted
white, 1 serving (3 oz) 3
Rotisserie chicken, lemon pepper flavor,
roasted dark, 1 serving (3 oz) 5
Rotisserie chicken, lemon pepper flavor,
roasted white, 1 serving (3 oz)................3
Rotisserie chicken, oven roasted, dark,
1 serving (3 oz) 5
Rotisserie chicken, oven roasted, white,
1 serving (3 oz) 3
Seasoned roasting, dark, cooked, 3 oz.......5
Seasoned roasting, white, cooked, 3 oz 4
Southwestern short cuts, ½ cup 2
Toasted garlic rotisserie, dark, cooked,
3 oz...6
Toasted garlic rotisserie, light, cooked,
3 oz (84 g) 4

***Stouffer's Lean Cuisine Skillet
Sensations*** Chicken oriental, 1 serving
(10 oz)...5

Swanson's
Premium chunk chicken breast in water,
1 serving (56 g) 1
Premium chunk mixin' chicken in broth,
1 serving (56 g) 2
Premium white & dark chunk chicken in
water, 1 serving (56 g) 1

Tyson
Basted boneless skinless chicken
breasts, 4 oz...2
Basted chicken drumstick, 4 oz 3
Basted chicken tenders, 4 oz.....................2
Basted chicken thigh, 4 oz 7
Basted chicken wings, 4 oz 6
Basted skinless split breast, 4 oz...............3
Basted split breast, 4 oz 5
BBQ chicken drumsticks, 1 piece (88 g) 4
BBQ chicken wings, 3 pieces (91 g) 5
Boneless skinless breasts, 1 piece
(133 g) 3
Boneless skinless chicken breast,
1 piece (106 g) 3
Boneless skinless chicken breast strips,
4 oz...3
Boneless skinless chicken breasts with
rib meat, 4 oz...3
Boneless skinless chicken thigh cutlets,
4 oz...4
Boneless skinless tenderloins, 4 pieces
(130 g) 2
Boneless skinless teriyaki breast, 4 oz 2
Boneless skinless thighs, 1 piece (112 g) 4
Breaded chicken breast fillet, 2 pieces
(81 g) 4
Breaded chicken breast fillets, 1 piece
(80 g) 3
Breaded chicken breast pattie, 1 (73 g) 5
Breaded chicken breast tenders,
5 pieces (85 g) 5
Breaded chicken southern fried breast
pattie, 1 piece (73 g)..............................5
Breast chunks, 6 pieces (85 g) 6
Breast pattie, 1 piece (84 g)......................5

Buffalo chicken breast strips, 2 pieces
(85 g) 4
Chicken breast strips, 3 oz 3
Chicken breast tenderloins, 4 oz................2
Chicken breast tenders, 2 pieces (92 g)......4
Chicken drumsticks, 4 oz 4
Chicken grill pack, 4 oz 7
Chicken nuggets, 4 pieces (90 g)...............5
Chicken nuggets, 6 pieces (85 g)...............6
Chicken nuggets, 6 pieces (108 g) 6
Chicken patties, 1 piece (74 g) 5
Chicken tenders, 5 pieces (85 g)................4
Chicken thigh, 4 oz 7
Chicken thigh, 1 piece (139 g) 10
Chicken wing drummettes, 4 oz 7
Chicken wings, 4 oz 7
Chick'n chunks, 6 pieces (84 g) 6
Chick'n w/ Cheddar patties, 1 (74 g) 6
Chile-lime boneless skinless chicken
breasts, 4 oz..2
Crispy chicken strips, 2 pieces (72 g) 4
Diced chicken breast, 3 oz 2
Drumsticks, 2 pieces (115 g) 3
Fresh young chicken, 4 oz.........................7
Ground chicken, 4 oz 4
Half bird with skin, 3 oz 4
Half bird without skin, 3 oz 3
Half breast, 1 piece (147 g) 6
Honey battered tenders, 5 pieces (84 g) 6
Honey battered tenders, 5 pieces (85 g) 5
Hot & spicy wings, 3 pieces (97 g) 6
Hot BBQ Style chicken drumsticks,
2 pieces (100 g)......................................4
Italian boneless skinless chicken breasts,
4 oz..2
Italian style chicken meatballs,
6 pieces (84 g) 4
Jumbo split griller, 4 oz 7
Lemon herb boneless skinless chicken
breasts, 4 oz..2
Lemon pepper chicken breasts, 1 fillet
(78 g) 2
Low fat breast patties, 1 (74 g).................2

Low fat breast tenders, 3 pieces (92 g) 3
Mesquite chicken breasts, 1 pattie
(78 g) 3
Mixed fryer chicken parts, 4 oz 6
Pick of the chick, 4 oz 5
Plain ground chicken pattie, 1 piece
(112 g) 4
Roasted leg quarter with skin, 1 piece
(160 g) 10
Roasted leg quarter without skin,
1 piece (133 g) 6
Seasoned ground chicken pattie,
1 piece (112 g) 4
Single serve breasts with skin, 1 piece
(145 g) 6
Single serve breasts without skin,
1 piece (122 g) 3
Single serve drumstick with skin,
3 pieces (164 g)......................................8
Single serve drumstick without skin,
3 pieces (143 g)......................................5
Single serve thighs with skin, 1 piece
(103 g) 7
Single serve thighs without skin, 1 piece
(82 g) 4
Skinless chicken thighs, 4 oz 5
Skinless drumstick, 4 oz 3
Skinless pick of the chix, 4 oz 4
Skinless split breast, 4 oz 3
Southern fried breast fillets, 2 pieces
(98 g) 5
Southern fried chicken chunks, 6 pieces
(84 g) 7
Southwestern chicken breast strips, 3 oz
(84 g) 2
Split chicken breasts with ribs, 4 oz...........5
Sunday best roaster, 4 oz..........................6
Tabasco wings, 3 pieces (77 g)..................4
Teriyaki style chicken wings, 4 pieces
(96 g) 4
Thick'n crispy chicken pattie, 1 piece
(73 g) 5
Thin & fancy chicken breast fillets, 4 oz 3

Chicken, Tyson (con't)   POINTS

Tray BBQ wings, 4 pieces (88 g) 5
Tray hot & spicy wings, 4 pieces (91 g) 5
Whole bird with skin, 3 oz 4
Whole bird without skin, 3 oz 3
Whole chicken cut up, 4 oz 7
Whole chicken leg, 4 oz 8
Wings, 4 pieces (120 g) 6
Young roaster, 4 oz 6

Chicken, deli
Boar's Head
Bar B Q sauce basted breast of chicken,
  2 oz 1
Golden oven roast chicken breast, 2 oz 1
Hickory smoked chicken breast, 2 oz 1

Chili
Austex
Chili, no beans, 1 cup 13
Chili, with beans, 1 cup 8
Castleberry's
Chili, no beans, 1 cup 13
Chili, with beans, 1 cup 8
Health Valley
Mild vegetarian chili, 1 cup 2
Mild vegetarian chili, no salt, 1 cup...........2
Mild vegetarian lentil chili, 1 cup 2
Mild vegetarian lentil chili, no salt,
  1 cup 2
Spicy vegetarian chili, 1 cup 2
Spicy vegetarian chili, no salt, 1 cup..........2
Health Valley 99% Fat Free
Burrito flavored, 1 cup 2
Enchilada flavored, 1 cup 2
Fajita flavored, 1 cup 2
Mild 3 bean, 1 cup..................................2
Mild black bean, 1 cup.............................2
Spicy black bean, 1 cup 2
Turkey chili, 1 cup 4
Health Valley Chili in a Cup
Healthy mild black bean, ¾ cup.................2
Healthy spicy Texas style, ¾ cup 2
Hormel
Chili no beans, canned, 1 cup 4
Chili with beans, canned, 1 cup 5

POINTS

Chunky chili with beans, canned, 1 cup 5
Hot chili no beans, canned, 1 cup..............4
Hot chili with beans, canned, 1 cup...........5
Turkey chili no beans, canned, 1 cup..........3
Turkey chili with beans, canned, 1 cup.......4
Vegetarian chili, canned, 1 cup 3
Hormel Microcup Meals
Chili no beans, 1 cup................................4
Chili with beans, 1 cup.............................4
Hot chili with beans, 1 cup 4
Old El Paso Chili with beans, 1 cup 5
Stagg
Chicken grande chili, 1 cup 6
Chili laredo, 1 cup 7
Classic chili, 1 cup 7
Country brand chili, 1 cup 7
Double barrel beef chili, 1 cup 8
Dynamite hot chili, 1 cup..........................7
Ranch house chicken chili, 1 cup...............6
Silverado beef chili, 1 cup.........................4
Steak house chili, 1 cup............................8
Turkey ranchero chili, 1 cup 4
Vegetable garden chili, 1 cup....................3

Chili sauce
Del Monte Sauce, chili, 1 Tbsp 0
Heinz Chili sauce, 1 Tbsp.........................0

Chips, vegetable
Harry's
Beet garlic, 1 oz 3
Bell pepper, 1 oz 3
Garlic blue, 1 oz.......................................3
Jalapeno bean, 1 oz 3
Veggie mix, 1 oz 3

Chocolate drinks
Hershey's Chocolate shake,
  1 container (210 ml) 5
Yoo-hoo
Yoo-hoo, 8 fl oz (240 ml) 3
Yoo-hoo, 1 bottle (9 fl oz)........................3
Yoo-hoo light, 8 fl oz (240 ml) 1
Yoo-hoo light, 1 bottle (9 fl oz) 1

Chocolate, baking
Baker's
Bittersweet chocolate bar, ½ square
(14 g) 2
German's sweet chocolate bar,
2 squares (13 g) 1
Real milk chocolate chips, ½ oz (14 g).......2
Real semi-sweet chocolate chips, ½ oz
(14 g) 1
Semi-sweet chocolate bar, ½ square
(14 g) 2
Semi-sweet chocolate flavored chips,
½ oz (14 g) 2
Unsweetened bar, ½ square (14 g)............2
White chocolate bar, ½ square (14 g) 2

Chow mein noodles
Tropical Nut & Fruit Chow mein
noodles, 1 oz..........................3

Churros
Tio Pepe's Cinnamon churros, 1 (28 g).....2

Chutney
Harry & David Fall harvest chutney,
¼ cup 2

Cinnamon rolls
Lance Cinnamon roll, 1 (113 g).................8
Otis Spunkmeyer
Cinnamon roll, 4- pack, 1 roll (35 g)..........4
Cinnamon roll, 8-pack, 1 roll (32 g)..........3
Giant cinnamon roll, ½ roll (57 g) 6
Sara Lee Deluxe cinnamon rolls with
icing, 1 roll/1 packet of icing 8

Clam juice
Chincoteague
Ocean clam juice, 8 fl oz 0
Eastern sea clam juice, ½ cup 0
Doxsee All natural clam juice, 1 Tbsp 0
Snow's All natural clam juice, 1 Tbsp........0

Clam sauce
Chincoteague Premium white clam
sauce, ½ cup 3

Progresso
Creamy clam, ½ cup 3
Red clam, ½ cup.....................................1
White clam, ½ cup..................................4
White clam (authentic), ½ cup 4
Snow's
Red clam sauce, ½ cup............................2
White clam sauce, ½ cup..........................2

Clams
Chincoteague
Chopped ocean clams, ½ cup 1
Eastern chopped sea clams, ½ cup...........1
Fried clams, 3 oz.....................................6
Stuffed clams, frozen, 1 piece (57 g).........3
Doxsee
Chopped clams in clam juice, ¼ cup..........1
Minced clams in clam juice, ¼ cup 1
Progresso Minced clams, ¼ cup 1
Snow's
Chopped clams in clam juice, ¼ cup..........1
Minced clams, ¼ cup 1

Cobblers
Marie Callender's
Apple, ¼ cobbler (4¼ oz) 9
Berry, ¼ cobbler (4¼ oz) 9
Cherry, ¼ cobbler (4¼ oz)........................9
Peach, ¼ cobbler (4¼ oz) 9
Mrs. Smith's
Apple cobbler, ⅛ cobbler (113 g) 5
Blackberry cobbler, ⅛ cobbler (113 g)........5
Cherry cobbler, ⅛ cobbler (113 g) 5
Peach cobbler, ⅛ cobbler (113 g) 5
Pet-Ritz
Apple cinnamon homestyle cobbler,
⅙ cobbler (123 g) 7
Blackberry homestyle cobbler,
⅙ cobbler (123 g) 6
Cherry homestyle cobbler, ⅙ cobbler
(123 g) 7
Peach homestyle cobbler, ⅙ cobbler
(123 g) 5

C

C

Cocktail sauce
Captain Huey's
Hot, ¼ cup 2
Regular, ¼ cup...........................2
Sweet 'n smokey, ¼ cup 2
Del Monte Sauce, seafood cocktail,
¼ cup 2
Heinz Seafood cocktail sauce, ¼ cup........1
Kraft Cocktail sauce, ¼ cup 1
Naturally Fresh Seafood cocktail
sauce, 2 Tbsp...........................0

Cocoa
Harmony Swiss mix, ¼ cup 4
Hershey's
Goodnight hug hot cocoa mix,
1 envelope (35 g) 3
Goodnight kiss milk chocolate hot
cocoa mix, 1 envelope (35 g)...................3
Hershey's Classic
Hot cocoa mix, 1 envelope (28 g)..............2
Hot cocoa mix with marshamallows,
1 envelope (28 g) 2
Hershey's Hot Cocoa Collection
Chocolate amaretto, 1 envelope (35 g)......3
Chocolate mint, 1 envelope (35 g) 3
Chocolate raspberry, 1 envelope (35 g)......3
Dutch chocolate, 1 envelope (35 g) 3
Fat free chocolate irish cream,
1 envelope (25 g) 2
Fat free dutch chocolate, 1 envelope
(15 g) 1
Fat free French vanilla, 1 envelope
(15 g) 1
French vanilla, 1 envelope (35 g) 3
Irish crème, 1 envelope (35 g)...............3
Swiss mocha, 1 envelope (35 g)...............3
Nestle
Double chocolate meltdown,
1 envelope (35 g) 3
Fat free w/ marshmallows, 1 envelope
(12 g) 1
French vanilla, 1 envelope (28 g) 3
Homemade classics dark chocolate,
1⅓ Tbsp................................1

Homemade classics milk chocolate,
1⅓ Tbsp................................2
Marshmallow madness, 1 envelope
(44 g) 4
Milk chocolate, 3 Tbsp............................3
Rich chocolate, 3 Tbsp...........................3
Rich chocolate fat free, 1 envelope (8 g) 1
Rich chocolate no sugar added, 3 Tbsp......1
Rich w/ mini marshmallows, 3 Tbsp...........3
Weight Watchers Hot cocoa mix,
1 serving (19 g) 1

Coconut
Baker's Angel Flake
Coconut (bag), 2 Tbsp 2
Coconut (can), 2 Tbsp 2
Premium shred coconut, 2 Tbsp 2
Dole Coconut, 1 cup 7
Tropical Nut & Fruit Angel flake
coconut, 2 Tbsp 2

Coffee drinks
General Foods
Café Francais, prepared, 8 fl oz 1
Cafe Vienna, prepared, 8 fl oz 2
French vanilla cafe decaffeinated,
prepared, 8 fl oz 1
French vanilla cafe decaffeinated (sugar
free, fat free), prepared, 8 fl oz 1
French vanilla cafe, prepared, 8 fl oz 1
French vanilla cafe (sugar free, fat free),
prepared, 8 fl oz 1
Hazelnut Belgian cafe, prepared, 8 fl oz.....2
Irish cream cafe, prepared, 8 fl oz 1
Italian cappuccino, prepared, 8 fl oz..........1
Kahlua cafe, prepared, 8 fl oz 1
Orange cappuccino, prepared, 8 fl oz 2
Suisse mocha decaffeinated, prepared,
8 fl oz...................................1
Suisse mocha decaffeinated (sugar
free, fat free), prepared, 8 fl oz 1
Suisse mocha, prepared, 8 fl oz................1
Suisse mocha (sugar free, fat free),
prepared, 8 fl oz 1
Viennese chocolate cafe, prepared,
8 fl oz...................................1

Nestle

Amaretto cappuccino mix, 3 Tbsp 2
Caramel cappuccino mix, 3 Tbsp 2
Chocolate hazelnut mocha mix, 3 Tbsp......2
Chocolate mint mocha mix, 3 Tbsp............2
Chocolate mocha mix, 3 Tbsp 2
Chocolate raspberry mocha mix, 3 Tbsp.....2
French vanilla cappuccino mix, 3 Tbsp 2
Latte cappuccino mix, 3 Tbsp....................2

Starbucks Coffee

Coffee frappucino, 1 bottle 4
Mocha amaretto frappucino, 1 bottle 4
Mocha frappucino, 1 bottle 4
Mocha frappucino, light, 1 bottle 2
Vanilla frappucino, 1 bottle.......................4

Coffee substitute

Postum

Coffee flavor instant hot beverage,
    prepared, 8 fl oz 0
Instant hot beverage, prepared, 8 fl oz 0

Cookie mixes

Betty Crocker

Chocolate peanut butter bars,
    prepared, 1 piece (1/12 pan) 5
Date bar mix, 1 serving (1/12 package) 3
Easy layer dessert bar, prepared,
    1 piece (1/16 pan) 3
Hershey cookie bars, prepared,
    1 piece (1/16 pan) 4
Sunkist lemon bar, prepared, 1 piece
    (1/16 pan)..3

Betty Crocker Pouch Dessert Mix

Chocolate chip cookie mix, prepared, 2 4
Chocolate peanut butter cookie mix,
    prepared, 2 4
Double chocolate chunk cookie mix,
    prepared, 2 4
Oatmeal chocolate chip cookie mix,
    prepared, 2 4
Peanut butter cookie mix, prepared, 2 4
Sugar cookie mix, prepared, 2...................4

Pillsbury

Chocolate chip mix, 3 Tbsp......................3

Chocolate chunk mix, 3 Tbsp 3
White chunk, 3 Tbsp 4

Sweet 'N Low Chocolate chip cookie
    mix, 4 (28 g) 2

Cookies

Dunkaroos

Chocolate chip w/ chocolate frosting,
    1 (28 g) 3
Cinnamon graham w/ vanilla frosting,
    1 (28 g) 3
Cookies 'n creme chocolate cookies w/
    vanilla frosting, 1 (28 g) 3

Dutch Twins

Artificially flavored lemon sugar/crème
    wafers (10 oz tray), 5 pieces (30 g) 3
Artificially flavored lemon sugar/crème
    wafers (14 oz tray), 4 pieces (33 g) 4
Artificially flavored vanilla ice cream
    sandwich wafers, 2 pieces (32 g) 4
Artificially flavored vanilla sugar/crème
    wafers (10 oz tray), 5 pieces (30 g) 3
Artificially flavored vanilla sugar/crème
    wafers (14 oz tray), 4 pieces (33 g) 4
Assorted sugar/crème wafers, 4 pieces
    (33 g) 4
Assorted sugar/crème wafers, 5 pieces
    (28 g) 3
Assorted sugar/crème wafers, 5 pieces
    (30 g) 3
Caramel ice cream sandwich wafers,
    2 pieces (32 g) 4
Crème wafers – neapolitan, 2 pieces
    (25 g) 3
Crème wafers – vanilla, 2 pieces (25 g) 3
Dutch twins party sticks, 2 pieces
    (32 g) 3
Fudge covered crème wafers, 3 pieces
    (27 g) 3
Mini crème wafers, 5 pieces (30 g)............4
Mini fudge covered crème wafers,
    5 pieces (28 g) 3
Striped peanut butter wafers, 2 pieces
    (25 g) 3

Waffle cremes, 4 pieces (32 g) 4

Yes yes, 1 piece (23 g)..............................3

Estee Smart Treats

Sugar free raspberry candy bar, 1 (28 g) 2

Sugar free, reduced fat chocolate chip,
3 (30 g) 2

Sugar free, reduced fat chocolate
walnut, 3 (30 g).....................................2

Sugar free, reduced fat coconut, 3
(30 g)..2

Sugar free, reduced fat lemon, 3 (30 g) 2

Famous Amos

Chocolate chip, 4 (29 g) 3

Chocolate chip & pecan, 4 (29 g) 3

Chocolate chip Belgian-style, 4 (29 g) 3

Chocolate chip toffee, 4 (29 g)..................3

Oatmeal Chocolate chip & walnut, 4
(29 g) 3

Frito-Lay

Combinado suplex sandwich cookie, 3
(30 g) 3

Emperador cookies chocolate, 2 (25 g) 3

Emperador cookies vanilla, 2 (25 g) 3

Merengue sandwich cookies, 3 (28 g) 2

Piruetas cookies lemon, 3 (30 g) 3

Piruetas cookies strawberry, 3 (30 g).........3

Golden Graham Treats

Marshmallow graham w/ mini
marshmallows, 1 (22 g)..........................2

Peanut butter chocolate, 1 (22 g) 2

S'Mores chocolate chunk, 1 (22 g) 2

S'Mores chocolate chunk – king size, 1
(45 g) 4

Grandma's

Fudge sandwich, 3 4

Fudge vanilla sandwich, 3 3

Mini cookies – fudge, 9..............................3

Mini cookies – peanut butter, 9 3

Mini cookies – vanilla, 9.............................3

Peanut butter sandwich, 5..........................5

Rich n' chewy, 1 package 6

Sugar wafers strawberry, 3 4

Sugar wafers vanilla, 3...............................4

Tiny bites animal crackers, 11 6

Tiny bites chocolate chip, 12.....................6

Tiny bites oatmeal raisin, 12 6

Tiny bites sugar, 12 6

Vanilla sandwich, 3....................................4

Vanilla sandwich, 5....................................5

Grandma's Homestyle Big Cookies

Chocolate chip, 1 (39 g) 4

Fudge chocolate chip, 1 (39 g) 4

Molasses, 1 (39 g) 3

Oatmeal raisin, 1 (39 g) 4

Peanut butter, 1 (39 g) 4

Peanut butter chocolate chip, 1 (39 g).......4

Hain Pure Foods

Animal crackers, 9 (28 g)...........................2

Peanut butter flavor cookie jar bits,
17 bits (15 g) 1

Health Valley

Biscotti cookies, amaretto, 2 cookies
(30 g) 2

Biscotti cookies, chocolate, 2 cookies
(30 g) 2

Fat free cookies, apple raisin jumbo,
1 cookie (25 g).......................................1

Fat free cookies, apple spice, 3 cookies
(33 g) 1

Fat free cookies, apricot delight,
3 cookies (33 g)......................................1

Fat free cookies, date delight,
3 cookies (33 g)......................................1

Fat free cookies, Hawaiian fruit,
3 cookies (33 g)......................................1

Fat free cookies, raisin oatmeal,
3 cookies (33 g)......................................1

Fat free healthy chips cookies, double
chocolate, 3 cookies (33 g)......................1

Fat free old fashioned healthy chips
cookies, 3 cookies (33 g).........................1

Fat free original healthy chips cookies,
3 cookies (33 g)......................................1

Fat free raspberry jumbo cookies,
1 cookie (25 g).......................................1

Fat-free marshmallow bars, chocolate
chip, 1 bar (30 g) 2

Fat-free marshmallow bars, old
 fashioned, 1 bar (30 g)..........................2
Low fat sandwich bars, Bavarian
 creme, 1 (40 g) 3
Low fat sandwich bars, vanilla creme,
 1 (40 g) 3
Wheat free, dairy free cookies, chocolate
 chip, 1 cookie (23 g) 2
Wheat free, dairy free cookies, peanut,
 1 cookie (23 g) 2

Health Valley Cobbler Bites
Blueberry, 2 cookies (25 g) 2
Fig, 2 cookies (25 g)....................................2
Strawberry, 2 cookies (25 g) 2

Kraft Handi-Snacks Cookies & fruit
 spread, 1 (37 g) 3

Lance
Chocolate crème filled sugar wafers,
 4 (31 g) 4
Choc-o-lunch, 6 (43 g) 4
Choc-o-lunch, 7 (48 g) 5
Double big town, all flavors, ½ cookie
 (39 g) 4
Lem-o-lunch, 7 (48 g)................................6
Low fat apple bar, 1 (50 g) 3
Low fat strawberry bar, 1 (50 g)................4
Mini chocolate chip cookies, 4 (28 g) 3
Nut-o-lunch, 7 (48 g) 5
Oatmeal crème, 1 (57 g)............................5
Peanut butter crème wafer, ½ piece
 (28 g) 4
Regular big town, all flavors, 1 (57 g)........4
Strawberry crème, 7 (48 g) 5
Strawberry crème filled cookies, 6 (43 g).....4
Strawberry crème filled sugar wafers,
 4 (31 g) 4
Vanilla crème filled sugar wafers, 4
 (31 g) 4
Van-o-lunch, 6 (43 g) 5
Van-o-lunch, 7 (48 g) 5

Little Debbie
Apple flips, 1 (35 g) 3
Chocolate flavored marshmallow pies,
 1 (43 g) 4

Fig bars, 2 (43 g)..3
Fudge rounds, 1 (34 g) 3
Ginger cookies, 1 (21 g)..............................2
Marshmallow supremes, 1 (32 g) 3
Raisin crème pies, 1 (34 g) 3
Star crunch, 1 (31 g) 3

Little Debbie Snack Smart Oatmeal
 lights, 1 (38 g)..3
Mi-Del Ginger snaps, 5 (30 g) 3
Nabisco
Caramel delights, 1 cookie (18 g) 2
Chips ahoy, 3 cookies (32 g) 4
Chips ahoy, reduced-fat, 3 cookies
 (31 g) 3
Mint crème, 2 cookies (25 g) 2
Oatmeal raisin, 2 cookies (27 g)................2
Oreo, 3 cookies (33 g) 4
Oreo, reduced-fat, 3 cookies (32 g) 3

Nabisco SnackWell's
Chocolate chip, 13 cookies (29 g) 3
Chocolate chip crisps, 18 crisps (34 g) 3
Chocolate crisps, 18 crisps (31 g) 3
Chocolate sandwich, 2 cookies (26 g) 2
Coconut crème, 2 cookies (25 g) 3
Crème sandwich, 2 cookies (26 g)............2
Devil's food, 1 cookie (16 g) 1
Double chocolate chip, 13 cookies
 (30 g) 3
Golden devil's food, 1 cookie (16 g) 1
Peanut butter chip, 13 cookies (29 g) 3

Otis Spunkmeyer Otis Express
Chocolate chunk, frozen, 1 cookie
 (2 oz)..6
Double chocolate chip, frozen, 1 cookie
 (2 oz)..6
Oatmeal raisin, frozen, 1 cookie (2 oz) 5
Peanut butter, frozen, 1 cookie (2 oz) 7

Payaso
Animal cookies, 15 (30 g) 2
Cookie rolls, 8 (31 g) 3

Peek Freans
Arrowroot, 4 (34 g)....................................3
Assorted creme, 2 (28 g) 3

Assorted tea, arrowroot, 4 pieces
(34 g) 3
Assorted tea, fruit shortcake, 3 pieces
(35 g) 4
Assorted tea, nice, 4 pieces (4 g)...............4
Assorted tea, petit beurre, 4 pieces
(28 g) 3
Assorted tea, rich tea, 4 pieces (34 g)........4
Assorted tea, shortcake, 2 pieces (27 g).....3
Coffee crème, 2 (30 g)................................3
Dream puffs, 2 (26 g)..................................3
Dream puffs, cappuccino, 2 (26 g) 3
Fruit crème biscuits, 2 (27 g).....................3
Ginger crisp, 4 (34 g) 3
Nice, 4 (34 g)..4
Petit beurre, 4 (28 g) 3
Rich tea, 4 (34 g) 4
Shortcake, 2 (27 g)......................................3
Sweetmeal, 3 (34 g)....................................4
Traditional oatmeal, 1 (20 g) 2

Peek Freans Petit Beret
Black forest, 2 (24 g)...................................2
Crème caramel, 2 (24 g)..............................3
Fudge truffle, 2 (24 g) 3

Peek Freans Tropical Cremes
Calypso lime, 2 (27 g) 3
Lemon sunrise, 2 (27 g)...............................3
South sea mango, 2 (27 g) 3

Stella D'oro
Anisette toast, 1 (30 g) 2
Anisette toast, 3 (35 g) 3
Breakfast treats, 2 (43 g)............................4
Chinese dessert cookies, 1 (33 g) 4
Chocolate breakfast treats, 1 (23 g) 2
Chocolate castelets, 2 (28 g).......................3
Chocolate margherite cookies, 2 (31 g) 3
Cinnamon raisin breakfast cake, 1 piece
(28 g) 2
Como delight, 1 (32 g) 3
Egg jumbo, 2 (24 g) 2
Fat free fruit slices, 1 (17 g) 1
Golden bars, 1 (25 g) 2
Kichel, 21 (29 g) 4

Lady Stella cookie assortment, 3 (28 g) 3
Margherite, 2 (32 g).....................................3
Margherite combination, 2 (32 g) 3
Margherite, low sodium, 2 (32 g) 3
Roman egg biscuits, 1 (34 g) 3
Sesame (Regina), 3 (32 g) 3
Swiss fudge, 3 (35 g)...................................4
Swiss fudge, low sodium, 2 (26 g).............3
Viennese cinnamon breakfast treats,
1 (23 g) 2

Stella D'oro Holiday
Chocolate powder puffs, 3 (30 g) 3
Fruit slices, 2 (33 g) 3
Pfeffernusse spice drops, 3 (27 g)..............3
Rings and stars, 3 (33 g)..............................4
Trinkets, 4 (32 g) 4

Tropical Nut & Fruit
Fat free blueberry, 1 bar (50 g)...................3
Fig bars, fat free, 1 bar (50 g) 3
Wheat honey apple bars, 1 bar (30 g) 2
Wheat honey fig bar, 1 bar (30 g) 1
Wheat honey peach apricot, 1 bar
(30 g) 2

Walkers
Pure butter chocolate chip shortbread,
2 pieces (28 g) 3
Pure butter shortbread, 1 piece (19 g) 3
Pure butter shortbread highlanders,
1 piece (22 g) 3
Pure butter shortbread triangles,
2 pieces (20 g) 3

Weight Watchers
Apple raisin bar, 1 serving (21 g) 1
Chocolate chip cookies, 1 serving
(30 g) 3
Chocolate sandwich cookies, 1 serving
(31 g) 3
Fig fruit filled cookies, 1 serving (20 g) 1
Oatmeal raisin cookies, 1 serving (30 g) 2
Raspberry fruit filled cookies, 1 serving
(20 g) 1
Vanilla sandwich cookies, 1 serving
(31 g) 3

C

Cookies, from dough
Otis Spunkmeyer
Butter sugar, 1 bite size cookie (¾ oz).......2
Butter sugar, 1 cookie (2 oz) 6
Butter sugar, 1 large cookie (4 oz)...........11
Carnival, 1 cookie (2 oz)............................6
Carnival, 1 large cookie (4 oz) 11
Chocolate chip, 1 bite size cookie
  (¾ oz) 2
Chocolate chip, 1 cookie (2 oz) 6
Chocolate chip, 1 cookie (3 oz) 8
Chocolate chip, 1 large cookie (4 oz).......11
Double chocolate chip, 1 bite size
  cookie (¾ oz) 2
Double chocolate chip, 1 cookie (2 oz) 6
Double chocolate chip, 1 large cookie
  (4 oz)..11
Milk chocolate chunk, 1 cookie (2 oz) 6
Oatmeal raisin, 1 bite size cookie (1 oz) 2
Oatmeal raisin, 1 cookie (2 oz) 5
Oatmeal raisin, 1 large cookie (4 oz) 11
Peanut butter, 1 bite size cookie (¾ oz).....2
Peanut butter, 1 cookie (2 oz) 6
Peanut butter, 1 large cookie (4 oz).........12
Rocky road, 1 cookie (2 oz) 5
Triple chocolate, 1 cookie (2 oz) 6
Turtle, 1 cookie (2 oz)...............................6
White chocolate macadamia nut,
  1 bite size cookie (¾ oz) 2
White chocolate macadamia nut,
  1 cookie (2 oz) 7
White chocolate macadamia nut,
  1 large cookie (4 oz) 12

Otis Spunkmeyer Sweet Discovery
Butter sugar, 1 medium cookie (1.3 oz) 4
Carnival, 1 medium cookie (1.3 oz) 4
Chocolate chip, 1 medium cookie
  (1.3 oz)...4
Chocolate chip pecan, 1 medium
  cookie (1.3 oz) 4
Chocolate chip walnut, 1 medium
  cookie (1.3 oz) 4
Double chocolate chip, 1 medium
  cookie (1.3 oz) 4

Milk chocolate chunk, 1 medium
  cookie (1.3 oz) 4
Oatmeal raisin, 1 medium cookie
  (1.3 oz) 4
Peanut butter, 1 medium cookie (1.3 oz) 4
Peanut butter chocolate chunk,
  1 medium cookie (1.3 oz).....................4
Rocky road, 1 medium cookie (1.3 oz).......4
Triple chocolate, 1 medium cookie
  (1.3 oz) 4
Turtle, 1 medium cookie (1.3 oz) 4
White chocolate macadamia nut,
  1 medium cookie (1.3 oz).....................4

Otis Spunkmeyer Traditional Recipe
Carnival, 1 cookie (1½ oz) 2
Carnival, 1 cookie (2½ oz) 7
Chocolate chip, 1 cookie (1½ oz) 4
Chocolate chip, 1 cookie (2½ oz) 7
Double chocolate chip, 1 cookie (1½ oz)....4
Double chocolate chip, 1 cookie (2½ oz)....7
Oatmeal raisin, 1 cookie (1½ oz)...............4
Oatmeal raisin, 1 cookie (2½ oz)...............7
Peanut butter, 1 cookie (1½ oz) 5
Peanut butter, 1 cookie (2½ oz) 8
Ranger, 1 cookie (1½ oz) 4
Ranger, 1 cookie (2½ oz) 7
Sugar, 1 cookie (1½ oz) 4
Sugar, 1 cookie (2½ oz) 7
White chocolate macadamia nut,
  1 cookie (1½ oz)...................................5
White chocolate macademia nut,
  1 cookie (2½ oz)...................................8

Pillsbury
Chocolate chip, 1 oz..................................3
Chocolate chip with walnuts, 1 oz.............3
Chocolate chip, reduced fat, 1 oz 2
Chocolate chunk, 1 oz 3
Double chocolate, 1 oz 3
Gingerbread, 1 oz 3
Holiday shapes, 2 (28 g) 3
M&M's, 1 oz...3
Oatmeal chocolate chip, 1 oz....................3
Peanut butter, 1 oz...................................3

Cookies, from dough, Pillsbury (con't)   POINTS

Sugar, 2 (32 g)..3
White chocolate chunk, 1 oz.....................3
Pillsbury One Step Chocolate chip,
   1⁄10 recipe (32 g).......................................3

Cooking spray
Butter Buds Non stick cooking spray,
   1⁄3 second spray (0.31 g)..........................0
I Can't Believe It's Not Butter,
   Spray, 5 sprays (1 g)................................0
Mazola
No stick, 1⁄3 second spray (0.3 g) 0
Pro chef, corn oil, 1⁄3 second spray (0.3 g) 0
Pro chef, oilive oil, 1⁄3 second spray
   (0.3 g)...0
Shedd's Country Crock Cooking &
   topping spray, 5 sprays (1 g)...................0

Corn
Boston Markets Sweet corn,
   1 serving (140 g) 4
Del Monte
Fiesta corn, whole kernel supersweet,
   1⁄2 cup 1
Gold & white, whole kernel supersweet,
   1⁄2 cup 1
Golden, cream style, 1⁄2 cup........................1
Golden, cream style supersweet, 1⁄2 cup 1
Golden, cream style, no salt added,
   1⁄2 cup 1
Golden, whole kernel, 1⁄2 cup 1
Golden, whole kernel supersweet,
   1⁄2 cup 1
Golden, whole kernel supersweet/
   no sugar, 1⁄2 cup 1
Golden, whole kernel supersweet/vac
   pack, 1⁄2 cup 1
Golden, whole kernel supersweet/vac
   pack NSA, 1⁄2 cup 1
White, cream style, 1⁄2 cup...........................2
White, whole kernel, 1⁄2 cup 1
Green Giant
Cream style corn, canned, 1⁄2 cup 2
Cream style corn, frozen, 1⁄2 cup 2

POINTS

Extra sweet corn on the cob, frozen,
   1 (125 g)..2
Extra sweet niblets corn, frozen, 2⁄3 cup 1
Gold & white corn, frozen, 3⁄4 cup 1
Mexicorn (corn with peppers), canned,
   1⁄3 cup 1
Nibblers corn on the cob, frozen,
   1 small ear (61 g) 1
Niblets corn on the cob, frozen, 1
   (142 g) 2
Niblets corn, 50% less sodium, canned,
   1⁄3 cup 1
Niblets corn, canned, 1⁄3 cup 1
Niblets corn, extra sweet, canned,
   1⁄3 cup 1
Niblets corn, frozen, 2⁄3 cup (84 g) 1
Niblets corn, frozen, 2⁄3 cup (123 g) 2
Niblets corn, no added salt or sugar,
   canned, 1⁄3 cup..1
Shoepeg white corn, frozen, 3⁄4 cup
   (93 g) 1
Shoepeg white corn, frozen, 3⁄4 cup
   (112 g) 2
Southwestern style corn & roasted
   peppers, frozen, 3⁄4 cup...........................2
White shoepeg corn, canned, 1⁄3 cup..........1
Whole kernel sweet corn, 50% less
   sodium, canned, 1⁄2 cup 1
Whole kernel sweet corn, canned,
   1⁄2 cup 1
Green Giant Harvest Fresh
Niblets corn, frozen, 2⁄3 cup.......................1
Shoepeg white corn, frozen, 1⁄2 cup 1
Hain Pure Foods Whole kernel golden
   corn, 1⁄2 cup 1
Hanover Yellow sweet corn, 2⁄3 cup..........1
Hanover The Gold Line
White shoepeg corn, 2⁄3 cup.......................1
White sweet corn, 2⁄3 cup 1
Schwan's
Corn, 2⁄3 cup 1
Corn on the cob, 1 (162 g) 3
Stouffer's Corn souffle, 1⁄2 cup.................4

Corn bread
Boston Markets Cornbread,
  1 serving (64 g) 4
Gladiola
  Mexican cornbread mix, prepared,
    1 piece (⅙ recipe) 3
  Sweet yellow cornbread mix, prepared,
    1 piece (⅙ recipe) 4
  White cornbread mix, prepared, 1 piece
    (⅙ recipe) 3
  Yellow cornbread mix, prepared, 1 piece
    (⅙ recipe) 3
Marie Callender's Cornbread & honey
    butter, 1 serving (2.28 oz) 3
Martha White
  Buttermilk cornbread mix, prepared,
    1 piece (⅕ recipe) 3
  Cotton pickin' buttermilk cornbread
    mix, prepared, 1 piece (⅕ recipe) 3
  Golden honey cornbread mix, prepared,
    1 piece (⅕ recipe) 4
  Mexican cornbread mix, prepared,
    1 piece (⅕ recipe) 3
  Sweet yellow cornbread mix, prepared,
    1 piece (⅕ recipe) 4
  Yellow cornbread mix, prepared,
    1 piece (⅕ recipe) 4
Pillsbury Cornbread twists, 1 (41 g) 3

Corn chips
Fritos
  B.B.Q., 29 pieces (1 oz) 3
  Chili cheese, 31 pieces (1 oz) 4
  King size, 12 pieces (1 oz) 4
  Original, 32 pieces (1 oz) 4
  Racerz honey BBQ, 12 pieces (1 oz) 4
  Racerz nacho cheese, 12 pieces (1 oz) 4
  Racerz original, 15 pieces (1 oz) 4
  Sabrositas flamin' hot, 28 pieces (1 oz) 4
  Sabrositas lime 'n chile, 28 pieces
    (1 oz) 4
  Scoops, 10 pieces (1 oz) 4
  Texas grill honey BBQ, 15 pieces (1 oz) 4
Jax Corn chips, ⅔ cup, 30 g 3

Lance
  BBQ corn chips, 35 (35 g) 5
  Nacho tortilla chips, triangles, 15 (28 g) 4
  Plain corn chips, 31 (28 g) 4
  Regular corn chips, 39 (35 g) 5

Corn dogs
Kid Cuisine Muchers Mystical mini
    corn dogs, 4 pieces (3 g) 6
State Fair
  Beef corn dogs, 1 (2.67 oz) 5
  Beef mini corn dogs, 4 (2.67 oz) 6
  Low fat corn dogs, 1 (2.67 oz) 3
  Original corn dogs, 1 (2.67 oz) 5
  Original mini corn dogs, 4 (2.67 oz) 6

Corn snacks
Tropical Nut & Fruit
  Corn nuts, ⅓ cup 3
  Hot rancheritos, ½ cup 2
  Spicy rancheritos, ½ cup 2
  Toasted sweet corn, 1 oz 3

Corn starch
Argo Corn starch, 1 Tbsp 1
Kingsford's Corn starch, 1 Tbsp 1

Cornflake crumbs
Kellogg's Corn flake crumbs, 2 Tbsp.........1

Cornish hen
Perdue
  Fresh cornish hen, dark, 1 serving (3 oz) 5
  Fresh cornish hen, white, 1 serving
    (3 oz) 4
Tyson Cornish game hen, 4 oz 5

Cornmeal
Gladiola
  Buttermilk corn meal mix, self rising,
    3 Tbsp 2
  White corn meal mix, self rising, 3 Tbsp.....2
Jim Dandy
  Degerminated, white, 3 Tbsp 2
  Self rising, degerminated, white, 3 Tbsp.....2
  Self rising, white, 3 Tbsp 2

Martha White

Buttermilk corn meal mix, self rising, 3 Tbsp	3
Plain, white, 3 Tbsp	2
Plain, yellow, 3 Tbsp	2
White corn meal mix, self rising, 3 Tbsp	2
Yellow corn meal mix, self rising, 3 Tbsp	2

Couscous
Golden Grain Near East

Broccoli & cheese couscous, 2 oz	3
Couscous, ⅓ cup	4
Garlic and olive oil couscous, 2 oz	4
Herbed chicken couscous, 2 oz	3
Tomato lentil couscous, 2 oz	3

Crab

Lascco Seafood & crab cocktail, 4 oz	2

Crackers
Estee Smart Treats

Sugar free chocolate graham crackers, 2 (30 g)	2
Sugar free cinnamon graham crackers, 2 (30 g)	2
Sugar free cracked pepper, 18 (30 g)	2
Sugar free golden, 10 (30 g)	3
Sugar free old fashioned graham crackers, 2 (30 g)	2
Sugar free wheat, 17 (30 g)	2

Frito-Lay

Cheetos bacon Cheddar, 1 package	4
Cheetos Cheddar cheese, 1 package	5
Cheetos golden toast, 1 package	6
Doritos jalapeno cheese, 1 package	5
Doritos nacho cheesier, 1 package	6
Peter pan cheese peanut butter, 1 package	5
Peter pan toast peanut butter, 1 package	5

Hain Pure Foods

Chocolate flavor animal grahams, 15 (30 g)	2
Chocolate flavor graham crackers, 2 (30 g)	2
Cinnamon flavor graham crackers, 2 (28 g)	2
French vanilla flavor graham crackers, 2 (30 g)	2
Golden Cheddar cheese bites, 22 (30 g)	2
Herb, fat free, 11 (30 g)	2
Honey flavor animal grahams, 15 (28 g)	2
Honey flavor graham crackers, 2 (28 g)	2
Oyster crackers, 36 (15 g)	1
Peanut butter flavor animal grahams, 15 (30 g)	3
Rich, 11 (30 g)	3
Saltine, 5 (15 g)	1
Sesame, 11 (30 g)	3
Vegetable, 11 (30 g)	3
White Cheddar cheese bites, 22 (30 g)	2
Whole wheat, fat free, 11 (30 g)	2

Health Valley

Low fat bruchetta vegetable crackers, 6 (14 g)	1
Low fat bruschetta vegetable-no salt, 6 (14 g)	1
Low fat cracked pepper crackers, 5 (14 g)	1
Low fat French onion crackers, 6 (14 g)	1
Low fat garden herb crackers, 6 (14 g)	1
Low fat roasted garlic crackers, 10 (14 g)	1
Low fat sesame crackers, 5 (14 g)	1
Low fat stoned wheat crackers, 5 (14 g)	1
Low fat whole wheat crackers, 6 (14 g)	1
Original amaranth graham crackers, 6 (28 g)	4
Original oat bran graham crackers, 6 (28 g)	4
Rice bran crackers, 6 (28 g)	4

Keebler

Club reduced fat crackers, 5	2
Grahams low fat cinnamon crackers, 8	2
Grahams low fat honey crackers, 9	2
Munch'ems ranch crackers, 40	3
Snackin' grahams chocolate crackers, 21	2
Snackin' grahams cinnamon crackers, 21	2

Toasteds reduced fat wheat crackers, 5 1
Town house reduced fat crackers, 6...........1
Wheatables reduced fat original crackers, 13 3
Zesta fat free crackers, 5 1
Zesta original crackers, 5 1

Keebler Harvest Bakery
Cornbread, 2 (16 g)...................................2
Country butter, 2 (16 g)............................2
Multigrain, 2 (16 g)...................................1

Lance
Cheddar cheese on capt. Wafer, 6 (37 g) 4
Cheese-on-wheat, 6 (37 g) 4
Cream cheese & chives on capt. Wafer, 6 (37 g) 5
Gold-n-chees, ¾ cup 3
Gold-n-chees, 1 package (28 g) 3
Gold-n-chees, 1 package (35 g) 4
Gold-n-chees, 1 package (39 g) 4
Grilled cheese, 4 (25 g) 3
Honey graham crackers, 1 package (22 g) 2
Lemon nekot, 6 (43 g) 5
Malt, 6 (35 g) 4
Nekot, 6 (43 g) 5
Nip chee, 6 (37 g) 4
Peanut butter & honey on capt. Wafers, 6 (37 g) 5
Peanut butter wheat, 6 (37 g)...................5
Pizza cheese, 4 (23 g)................................2
Reduced fat toastchee, 6 (39 g) 4
Reduced fat toasty, 6 (35 g)......................4
Ryechee, 6 (41 g) 5
Salsa & lanchee, 6 (35 g)..........................4
Smokehouse Cheddar, 6 (39 g)..................4
Snack mix, 1 package (50 g).....................7
Toastchee, 6 (39 g)....................................5
Toastchee – kids pack, 4 (27 g).................3
Toasty, 6 (35 g) 5

Nabisco
Air crisps, original, 24 crisps (29 g)...........3
Air crisps, ranch, 23 crisps (30 g)..............3
Cheese nips air crisps, original, 32 crisps (30 g) 3
Chocolate grahams, 8 crackers (30 g)........3
Cinnamon grahams, 8 crackers (30 g)........3
Honey grahams, 8 crackers (30 g) 3
Low fat honey grahams, 8 crackers (30 g) 3
Oatmeal crunch grahams, 8 crackers (30 g) 3
Ritz air crisps, original, 24 crisps (30 g).....3
Ritz air crisps, sour cream & onion, 23 crisps (30 g) 3

Nabisco SnackWell's
Cracked pepper crackers, 5 (14 g) 1
French onion snack crackers, 38 pieces (30 g) 3
Wheat crackers, 5 pieces (15 g).................2
Zesty cheese snack crackers, 38 (30 g) 3

Red Oval Farms
Mini stoned wheat thins, lemon pepper, 20 (31 g)...3
Mini stoned wheat thins, original, 19 (30 g) 3
Mini stoned wheat thins, roasted garlic & sun dried tomatoes, 20 (31 g) 3
Mini stoned wheat thins, toasted sesame, 19 (31 g) 3
Some of each – assorted crackers, 3 (13 g) 1
Stoned wheat thins, classic, 4 (16 g) 1
Stoned wheat thins, cracked pepper, 4 (16 g) 1
Stoned wheat thins, grilled onion, 4 (16 g) 1
Stoned wheat thins, lower sodium, 2 (14 g) 1
Wheat crackers, 2 (14 g)............................1
Tropical Nut & Fruit Cheddar whales, 53 (30 g)...4

Cranberries
Dole Cranberries, ½ cup 0
Ocean Spray Dried cranberries, 40 g.......2
Sunsweet Cranberry fruitlings, 1½ oz 2
Traverse Bay Fruit Co. Sweetened dried cranberries, ⅓ cup.........................2

Cream, sour
Breakstone
Reduced fat sour cream, 2 Tbsp 1
Sour cream, 2 Tbsp 2
Breakstone Free Fat free sour cream,
2 Tbsp....................1
Foremost
Reduced fat sour cream, naturally
cultured, 2 Tbsp.......................1
Sour cream, naturally cultured, 2 Tbsp.......2
Golden Guernsey
Reduced fat sour cream, 2 Tbsp 1
Sour cream, 2 Tbsp 2
Knudsen Free Fat free sour cream,
2 Tbsp....................1
Knudsen Hampshire Sour cream,
2 Tbsp....................2
Knudsen Light Light sour cream,
2 Tbsp....................1
Morning Glory
Reduced fat sour cream, 2 Tbsp 1
Sour cream, 2 Tbsp 2

Creamers
Carnation Coffee-Mate
Ameretto, liquid, 1 Tbsp 1
Amaretto, powder, 4 tsp 1
Cafe mocha, liquid, 1 Tbsp.......................1
Chocolate raspberry, liquid, 1 Tbsp 1
Cinnamon vanilla creme, liquid, 1 Tbsp......1
Cinnamon, powder, 4 tsp...........................1
Fat free, liquid, 1 Tbsp 0
Fat free, powder, 1 tsp..............................0
Fat free cafe mocha, liquid, 1 Tbsp 1
Fat free French vanilla, liquid, 1 Tbsp.........1
Fat free French vanilla, powder, 4 tsp 1
Fat free hazelnut, liquid, 1 Tbsp 1
Fat free hazelnut, powder, 4 tsp 1
Fat free Irish cream, liquid, 1 Tbsp 1
Fat free Swiss chocolate, powder, 4 tsp......1
French vanilla, liquid, 1 Tbsp.....................1
French vanilla, powder, 4 tsp 1
Hazelnut, liquid, 1 Tbsp 1
Hazelnut, powder, 4 tsp............................1

Irish creme, liquid, 1 Tbsp 1
Irish creme, powder, 4 tsp.........................1
Lite, powder, 1 tsp 0
Low fat, liquid, 1 Tbsp..............................0
Mocha almond, powder, 4 tsp...................1
Regular, liquid, 1 Tbsp 0
Regular, powder, 1 tsp...............................0
Swiss chocolate, powder, 4 tsp..................0
Toasted almond, liquid, 1 Tbsp..................1
Vanilla nut, liquid, 1 Tbsp 1
International Delight
Amaretto, 1 Tbsp 1
Butter pecan, 1 Tbsp 1
Cinnamon hazelnut, 1 Tbsp 1
Classic original, 1 Tbsp..............................0
French vanilla, 1 Tbsp................................1
Irish crème, 1 Tbsp 1
Kahlua, 1 Tbsp..1
Swiss chocolate, 1 Tbsp 1
Vanilla toffee caramel, 1 Tbsp...................1

Croissants
Sara Lee
Original, 1 4
Petite, 2 5

Cucumber
Chiquita Cucumber, ⅓ medium (99 g) 0

Currants
Tropical Nut & Fruit Currants, ¼ cup 2

Dairy shakes
Alba
Chocolate, 8 fl oz.....................................1
Double fudge, 8 fl oz................................1
Strawberry, 8 fl oz....................................1
Vanilla, 8 fl oz 1
Weight Watchers Chocolate fudge
shake mix, 1 serving (21 g).....................1

Danish
Otis Spunkmeyer
Apple danish, 12-pack, 1 pastry (78 g) 8
Bear claw, 4-pack, 1 pastry (57 g) 6

Breakfast claw, 8-pack, 1 pastry (57 g) 6

Buttercrumb danish, 4-pack, 1 pastry
(57 g) 6

Cheese danish, 12-pack, 1 pastry (78 g) 8

Cherry danish, 1 pastry (78 g)...................8

Cinnamon danish, 4-pack, 1 pastry
(57 g) 6

Fruit danish, 8-pack, 1 pastry (57 g) 6

Raisin danish, 8-pack, 1 pastry (57 g)........6

Dates
Dole
Chopped, 1 oz 2

Pitted, 5-6 items, 40 g..............................2

Sunsweet
Chopped dates, ¼ cup...............................2

Pitted dates, 1½ oz 2

Tropical Nut & Fruit
Date pieces, 40 g 2

Deglet noor dates, 40 g............................2

Medjool dates, 40 g 2

Dessert mixes
Hain Pure Foods
Cherry, ¼ package (21 g)...........................1

Orange, ¼ package, (21 g)........................1

Raspberry, 1 package (21 g) 1

Strawberry, ¼ package (21 g) 1

Jell-O No Bake
Cherry cheesecake, prepared as
directed, 1 serving, ⅛ cake (136 g) 8

Chocolate silk pie, prepared as
directed, 1 serving, ⅛ pie (125 g)............8

Double layer chocolate, prepared as
directed, 1 serving, ⅛ dessert (126 g)......6

Double layer cookies and creme,
prepared as directed, 1 serving,
⅛ dessert (129 g) 9

Double layer lemon, prepared as
directed, 1 serving, ⅛ dessert (126 g)......6

Homestyle cheesecake, prepared as
directed, 1 serving, ⅛ cake (132 g) 18

Peanut butter cup, prepared as directed,
1 serving, ⅛ dessert (109 g) 9

Real cheesecake, prepared as directed,
1 serving, ⅛ cake (130 g) 8

Strawberry cheesecake, prepared as
directed, 1 serving, ⅛ cake (136 g) 8

Strawberry swirl cheesecake (reduced
fat), prepared as directed, 1 serving,
⅛ cake (113 g) 6

Desserts, frozen
Weight Watchers Smart Ones
Strawberry parfait royale, 1 serving
(104 g) 4

Dinner in a box
Old El Paso
Burrito dinner, prepared, 1 burrito
(⅛ package) 6

Fajita dinner, prepared, 2 fajitas
(⅕ package) 7

Soft taco dinner, prepared, 2 tacos
(⅕ package) 9

Taco dinner, prepared, 2 tacos
(⅙ package) 7

Taco dinner, prepared, soft, 2 tacos
(⅓ package) 8

Taco dinner, prepared, hard, 2 tacos
(⅓ package) 7

Old El Paso One Skillet Mexican
Rice burrito dinner kit, prepared,
1 burrito 7

Salsa flavored tacos, prepared, 2 tacos 10

Taco flavored, prepared, 2 tacos 10

Pancho Villa Taco dinner, prepared,
2 tacos 9

Taco Bell Home Originals
Chicken fajita dinner, prepared,
2 fajitas (198 g) 7

Soft taco dinner, prepared, 2 tacos
(180 g) 9

Taco dinner, prepared, 2 tacos (124 g) 6

Ultimate bean burrito dinner, prepared,
1 burrito (124 g)..................................4

Ultimate nachos, prepared, about
12 nachos (131 g) 5

D

Dinner mixes

Chicken Helper

Cheddar & broccoli, prepared, 1 cup 7
Chicken & herb rice, prepared, 1 cup 6
Chicken & stuffing, prepared, 1 cup...........6
Chicken fried rice, prepared, 1 cup 6
Chicken potato augratin, prepared,
1 cup 6
Fettuccini alfredo, prepared, 1 cup 6
Roasted garlic, prepared, 1 cup.................6

Hamburger Helper

BBQ beef, prepared, 1 cup 7
Beef pasta, prepared, 1 cup 6
Beef romanoff, prepared, 1 cup.................7
Beef stew, prepared, 1 cup 6
Beef taco, prepared, 1 cup......................6
Beef teriyaki, prepared, 1 cup 6
Cheddar and broccoli, prepared, 1 cup 8
Cheddar melt, prepared, 1 cup..................7
Cheddar 'n bacon, prepared, 1 cup...........7
Cheeseburger macaroni, prepared,
1 cup 8
Cheesy hashbrowns, prepared, 1 cup........9
Cheesy Italian, prepared, 1 cup 7
Cheesy shells, prepared, 1 cup 8
Chili macaroni, prepared, 1 cup 6
Fettuccine alfredo, prepared, 1 cup...........7
Four cheese lasagna, prepared, 1 cup........8
Italian Parmesan w/rigatoni, prepared,
1 cup 7
Lasagne, prepared, 1 cup.........................6
Meat loaf, prepared, 1 serving (⅙ loaf)......7
Meaty spaghetti & cheese, prepared,
1 cup 6
Mushroom & wild rice, prepared, 1 cup 7
Nacho cheese, prepared, 1 cup 7
Pizza pasta w/ cheese topping,
prepared, 1 cup 6
Pizzabake, prepared, 1 serving (⅙ pan)......6
Potato stroganoff, prepared, 1 cup 6
Potatoes augratin, prepared, 1 cup...........6
Ravioli w/ white cheese topping,
prepared, 1 cup 7
Ravioli, prepared, 1 cup...........................6

Rice Oriental, prepared, 1 cup...................6
Salisbury, prepared, 1 cup........................6
Spaghetti, prepared, 1 cup.......................6
Stroganoff, prepared, 1 cup 7
Swedish meatballs, prepared, 1 cup 7
Three cheese, prepared, 1 cup...................8
Zesty Italian, prepared, 1 cup....................6
Zesty Mexican, prepared, 1 cup 6

Hamburger Helper Reduced Sodium

Cheddar spirals, prepared, 1 cup 7
Cheddar spirals, reduced fat chicken
recipe, prepared, 1 cup...........................5
Italian herb, prepared, 1 cup....................6
Italian herb, reduced fat chicken recipe,
prepared, 1 cup 4
Southwestern beef, prepared, 1 cup 6
Southwestern beef, reduced fat chicken
recipe, prepared, 1 cup...........................4

Skillet Chicken Helper Stir-fried
chicken, prepared, 1 cup 6

Tuna Helper

Augratin, 50% less fat recipe, prepared,
1 cup 5
Augratin, prepared, 1 cup.......................7
Cheesy broccoli, 50% less fat recipe,
prepared, 1 cup 5
Cheesy broccoli, prepared, 1 cup..............6
Cheesy pasta, 50% less fat recipe,
prepared, 1 cup 5
Cheesy pasta, prepared, 1 cup 7
Creamy broccoli, 50% less fat recipe,
prepared, 1 cup 5
Creamy broccoli, prepared, 1 cup 7
Creamy pasta, 50% less fat recipe,
prepared, 1 cup 5
Creamy pasta, prepared, 1 cup 7
Fettuccine alfredo, 50% less fat recipe,
prepared, 1 cup 5
Fettuccine alfredo, prepared, 1 cup...........7
Garden Cheddar, 50% less fat recipe,
prepared, 1 cup 5
Garden Cheddar, prepared, 1 cup..............7
Pasta salad, low-fat recipe, prepared,
⅔ cup..3

Pasta salad, prepared, ⅔ cup **10**
Tetrazzini, 50% less fat recipe,
    prepared, 1 cup **5**
Tetrazzini, prepared, 1 cup **7**
Tuna melt, prepared, 1 cup **7**
Tuna melt, reduced fat recipe,
    prepared, 1 cup **5**
Tuna pot pie, prepared, 1 cup **11**
Tuna romanoff, 50% less fat recipe,
    prepared, 1 cup **5**
Tuna romanoff, prepared, 1 cup **6**

Dinners, frozen
Amy's
Asian noodle stir-fry, 1 package (10 oz) **4**
Black bean enchilada whole meal,
    1 package (10 oz) **5**
Black bean vegetable enchilada,
    1 package (4¾ oz) **3**
Cannelloni whole meal, 1 package
    (9 oz) **7**
Cheese enchilada, 1 package (4¾ oz) **5**
Cheese enchilada whole meal,
    1 package (9 oz) **7**
Cheese lasagna, 1 package (10¼ oz) **6**
Chili & cornbread whole meal,
    1 package (10½ oz) **6**
Country dinner, 1 package (11 oz) **8**
Macaroni & cheese, 1 package (9 oz) **9**
Macaroni & soy cheeze, 1 package
    (9 oz) **8**
Pasta primavera, 1 package (9½ oz) **7**
Ravioli with sauce, 1 (8 oz) **7**
Thai stir-fry, 1 package (9½ oz) **6**
Tofu vegetable lasagna, 1 package
    (9½ oz) **6**
Vegetable lasagna, 1 package (9½ oz) **6**
Veggie loaf whole meal, 1 package
    (10 oz) **5**

Banquet
Beef enchilada, 1 package (11 oz) **8**
Beef enchilada & tamale combo,
    1 package (11 oz) **10**
Beef patty with country style
    vegetables, 1 package (9½ oz) **7**

Boneless pork rib, 1 package (10 oz) **9**
Boneless white fried chicken,
    1 package (8¼ oz) **13**
Cheese enchilada, 1 package (11 oz) **7**
Chicken fingers meal, 1 package
    (7.1 oz) **18**
Chicken fried beef steak, 1 package
    (10 oz) **10**
Chicken nuggets, 1 package (6¾ oz) **10**
Chicken Parmigiana, 1 package (9½ oz) **7**
Chicken pasta primavera, 1 (9½ oz) **7**
Chimichanga meal, 1 package (9½ oz) **11**
Fettucini alfredo, 1 package (9½ oz) **8**
Fish sticks, 1 package (6.6 oz) **6**
Fried rice with chicken & egg rolls,
    1 package (6½ oz) **7**
Grilled chicken, 1 package (9.9 oz) **7**
Homestyle noodles and chicken,
    1 package (12 oz) **9**
Honey roast turkey breast, 1 package
    (9 oz) **6**
Lasagna with meat sauce, 1 package
    (9½ oz) **5**
Macaroni and cheese, 1 package
    (12 oz) **9**
Meatloaf, 1 package (9½ oz) **6**
Mexican style enchilada combo, 1
    (11 oz) **7**
Our original fried chicken, 1 package
    (9 oz) **11**
Pepperoni pizza, 1 (6¾ oz) **11**
Pork cutlet meal, 1 package (10¼ oz) **10**
Salisbury steak, 1 package (9½ oz) **9**
Sliced beef, 1 package (9 oz) **5**
Turkey (mostly white meat),
    1 package (9¼ oz) **6**
Veal Parmigiana, 1 package (8¾ oz) **7**
Western style beef patty, 1 package
    (9½ oz) **8**
White meat fried chicken, 1 package
    (8¾ oz) **12**
Yankee pot roast, 1 package (9.4 oz) **5**

D

D

Banquet Extra Helping Dinners/ Hearty Ones

Boneless pork riblet, 1 package (15¼ oz) 17

Boneless white fried chicken, 1 package, 13 oz 17

Chicken fried beef steak, 1 package (16 oz)..20

Fried chicken, 1 package (14.7 oz) 22

Meatloaf, 1 package (16 oz) 15

Salisbury steak, 1 package (16½ oz)........19

Turkey & gravy with dressing, 1 package (17 oz)..................................14

Yankee pot roast, 1 package (14½ oz).......9

Banquet Family Size Entrees/ Meals Made Easy

Brown gravy & 6 salisbury steaks, 1 patty with gravy (5 oz)........................6

Brown Gravy & sliced beef, 2 slices with gravy (5.6 oz) 3

Chicken & broccoli alfredo, 1 cup 6

Country-style chicken & dumplings, 1 cup..7

Creamy broccoli, chicken, cheese & rice, 1 cup 6

Egg noodles with beef & brown gravy, 1 cup..3

Hearty beef stew, 1 cup............................3

Hearty chicken pie, 1 cup.........................11

Homestyle gravy & sliced turkey, 2 slices with gravy (4.3 oz).....................3

Lasagna with meat sauce, 1 cup 6

Macaroni and cheese, 1 cup 5

Mushroom gravy & 6 charbroiled beef patties, 1 patty with gravy (5 oz) 6

Potato, ham & broccoli au gratin, ⅔ cup..5

Savory gravy & meatloaf, 1 patty with gravy (4.7 oz) 5

Banquet Hot Sandwich Toppers

Creamed chip beef, 1 package (4 oz).........3

Gravy and salisbury steak, 1 package (5 oz)..5

Gravy and sliced beef, 1 package (4 oz).....2

Gravy and sliced turkey, 1 package (5 oz)..4

Boston Markets

Beef pot roast, 1 serving (425 g)..............9

Country fried chicken, 1 serving (382 g) 14

Grilled chicken breast fillet, 1 serving (428 g) 9

Macaroni & cheese, 1 serving (220 g)........6

Meatloaf, 1 serving (255 g) 12

Meatloaf, 1 serving, (453 g)....................18

Oven roasted chicken, 1 serving (109 g) 4

Oven roasted chicken, 1 serving (138 g) 7

Oven roasted chicken, 1 serving (370 g) 10

Oven roasted chicken, 1 serving (389 g) 16

Oven roasted turkey medallions, 1 serving (226 g) 5

Oven roasted turkey medallions, 1 serving (440 g) 10

Oven roasted turkey medallions, 1 serving (453 g) 13

Sliced beef sirloin, 1 serving (396 g)..........9

Swedish meatballs, 1 serving (226 g) 10

Budget Gourmet

Angel hair pasta with chunky tomato, 1 serving (226 g) 5

Beef Cheddar melt, 1 serving (241 g) 7

Beef pepper steak with rice, 1 serving (241 g) 5

Beef salisbury steak, 1 serving (241 g) 5

Beef stroganoff, 1 serving (226 g) 5

Broccoli chicken bake, 1 serving (368 g) 6

Cheese manicotti with marinara, 1 serving (241 g) 6

Chicken a la king, 1 serving (397 g) 12

Chicken and egg noodles, 1 serving (241 g) 9

Chicken Oriental & vegetables, 1 serving (241 g) 5

Chicken with fettucini, 1 serving (241 g) 8

Chinese style vegetables, 1 serving
(226 g) 5

Country fried beef steak, 1 serving
(368 g) 10

Escalloped noodles and white turkey in
sauce, 1 serving (226 g) 7

Fettucini alfredo with four cheeses,
1 serving (397 g) 12

Fettucini alfredo with four cheeses,
1 serving (226 g) 7

Fettucini and meatballs in wine,
1 serving (241 g) 6

Fettucini primavera in herb sauce,
1 serving (241 g) 5

French recipe chicken, 1 serving (241 g) 4

Glazed turkey, 1 serving (241 g)................5

Golden fried chicken supreme,
1 serving (368 g) 9

Homestyle macaroni & cheese,
1 serving (226 g) 7

Italian style meatballs and vegetables,
1 serving (241 g) 6

Italian style vegetables & white chicken
in sauce with rice, 1 serving (226 g)........5

Lasagna alfredo with broccoli, 1 serving
(226 g) 7

Lasagna mozzarella, 1 serving (226 g).......6

Lasagna with meat sauce, 1 serving
(226 g) 6

Lasagna with meat sauce, 1 serving
(241 g) 5

Linguini with clams & shrimp,
1 serving (226 g) 6

Linguini with clams and bay shrimp,
1 serving (226 g) 6

Linguini with tomatoes & Italian
sausage in sauce, 1 serving (226 g).........6

Macaroni & cheese, 1 serving (163 g)........6

Macaroni & cheese with Cheddar,
1 serving (226 g) 6

Mandarin chicken, 1 serving (241 g) 5

Orange glazed chicken, 1 serving
(241 g) 6

Oriental beef, 1 serving (226 g).................5

Oriental style rice with vegetables,
1 serving (397 g) 15

Pasta in wine & mushroom sauce,
1 serving (241 g) 5

Pasta primavera Parmesan, 1 serving
(226 g) 5

Penne pasta with chunky tomatoes,
1 serving (226 g) 5

Pennini pasta with chicken, 1 serving
(397 g) 9

Potatoes mozzarella, 1 serving (241 g) 7

Rigatoni in cream sauce, 1 serving
(226 g) 5

Roast beef supreme, 1 serving (226 g).......6

Spaghetti marinara, 1 serving (226 g) 5

Spicy szechuan style vegetables,
1 serving (226 g) 6

Stir fry rice and vegetables, 1 serving
(226 g) 8

Swedish meatballs, 1 serving (283 g) 12

Tex-mex rice & beans, 1 serving (397 g)....10

Three cheese lasagna, 1 serving (241 g) 7

Wild rice pilaf with vegetables,
1 serving (226 g) 7

Ziti Parmesano, 1 serving (226 g) 5

Celentano

Cavatelli, ⅔ cup 7

Eggplant Parmigiana, 1 cup 8

Eggplant Parmigiana, ½ tray (196 g) 7

Lasagne, ½ tray (196 g).............................6

Manicotti, ½ tray (196 g) 7

Manicotti without sauce, 2 (198 g) 9

Mini cheese ravioli, 12 (112 g)..................6

Round cheese ravioli, 4 (123 g)..................6

Stuffed shells, ½ tray (196 g) 6

Stuffed shells without sauce, 4 (177 g) 7

Celentano Great Choice

Broccoli stuffed shells, 3 (284 g) 3

Cheese ravioli, low fat, 1 cup 5

Eggplant rollettes, 1 (280 g) 5

Lasagne primavera, 1 (280 g) 5

Manicotti florentine, 2 (280 g) 4

D

Celentano Non-Dairy
Vegetarian Selects
Eggplant medallions with garbanzo
 bean filling, 1 (10 oz)............................7
Eggplant rollettes, 1 tray (10 oz) 5
Eggplant wraps with three bean filling,
 1 (10 oz)..5
Penne with roasted vegetables, 1
 (10 oz)..6
Porcini risotto with roasted vegetables,
 1 (10 oz)..4
Risotto with eggplant tofu & spinach,
 1 (10 oz)..8
Roasted vegetable lasagne, 1 (10 oz) 5
Spinach & broccoli manicotti, 1 tray
 (10 oz)...4
Spinach & broccoli stuffed shells, 1
 (10 oz)...4
Vegan eggplant Parmigiana, 1 (10 oz) 7

Celentano Vegetarian Selects
Broccoli stuffed shells, 1 tray (10 oz) 6
Lasagne primavera, 1 tray (10 oz) 5
Manicotti florentine, 1 tray (10 oz)............5
Spinach tofu ravioli with tomato sauce,
 1 (284 g)..7

Fishery Products
Fish & chips (chips only), 1 cup 3
Fish & chips (fish only), 2 portions
 (112 g) 7
Fish & chips (tartar sauce only), ¾ oz........1
Linguini & shrimp, 6 oz 3
Shrimp scampi, 4 oz..................................8

Fran's Healthy Helpings
Dino chicken chompers, 1 meal..................4
Lucky ducky chicken, 1 meal......................5
Soccer-oni & cheese, 1 meal 4
Twinkle star fish, 1 meal............................5
Wacky whale pizza, 1 meal........................5

Freezer Queen
Char-broiled beef pattie meal, 1 (269 g) 5
Cheese ravioli & tomato sauce meal, 1
 (220 g) 7
Chicken fingers & BBQ sauce meal, 1
 (255 g) 6

Chicken nuggets meal, 1 (170 g)...............6
Chicken pattie meal, 1 (212 g) 8
Gravy & sliced beef meal, 1 (255 g) 2
Meatloaf meal, 1 (269 g)...........................7
Pot roast meal, 1 (262 g)...........................2
Salisbury steak meal, 1 (269 g) 6
Shells & cheese sauce meal, 1 (241 g).......5
Turkey & gravy with dressing meal,
 mostly wh. turkey, gvy. with dressing,
 mashed potatoes & corn, 1 (262 g).........4
Veal parmagiana meal, 1 (255 g) 7

Freezer Queen Cook-In-Pouch
Breaded veal parmagiana with tomato
 sauce, 1 (142 g)......................................4
Chicken a'la king, 1 (113 g) 1
Creamed chipped beef, 1 (113 g) 2
Gravy & salisbury steak, 1 (142 g).............3
Gravy & sliced beef, 1 (113 g)...................1
Gravy & sliced chicken, 1 (113 g) 1
Gravy & sliced turkey, 1 (142 g) 1

Freezer Queen Deluxe
Family Entrée
Beef & peppers with rice, 1 cup 5
Breaded veal parmagiana, 1 pattie
 (140 g) 3
Cheese ravioli & tomato sauce, 1 cup........5
Chicken & biscuits, 1 cup..........................4
Chicken & vegetables, 1 cup 4
Chicken & vegetables with linguini,
 1 cup 5
Gravy & sliced beef, ⅔ cup 2
Lasagna in meat sauce, 1 cup 5
Pasta & stroganoff sauce with
 meatballs, 1 cup 5
Pot roast, 1 cup 4
Turkey & gravy with dressing, 1 serving
 (199 g) 3

Freezer Queen Family Entrée
Chicken nuggets, 6 (85 g).........................6
Gravy & 6 breaded chicken croquettes,
 1 pattie & gravy (132 g).........................3
Gravy & 6 breaded turkey croquettes,
 1 pattie & gravy 132 g)...........................3

Gravy & 6 salisbury steaks, 1 pattie
& gravy (132 g) 4
Gravy & sliced turkey, 4½ oz....................1
Mushroom gravy & 6 charbroiled beef
patties, 1 pattie & gravy (132 g) 4
Noodles with beef, 1 cup..........................4
Onion gravy & beef patties, 1 pattie
& gravy (199 g) 6
Rigatoni with meat sauce, 1 cup 5
Tomato sauce & meatloaf, 1 pattie
& gravy (132 g) 4

Freezer Queen Family Side Dish
Macaroni & cheese, 1 cup 5

Freezer Queen Homestyle Entrée
Beef & peppers with rice, 1 (241 g) 4
Chicken & vegetables with noodles, 1
(227 g) 3
Fettucini alfredo, 1 (256 g) 8
Imperial chicken with rice, 1 (241 g)..........4
Lasagna in meat sauce, 1 (284 g)..............6
Macaroni & beef, 1 (256 g)......................4
Macaroni & cheese, 1 (227 g) 7
Penne with meat sauce, 1 (256 g) 5
Pot roast, 1 (255 g) 3
Salisbury steak & gravy with whipped
potatoes, 1 (241 g) 6
Sweet & sour chicken with rice, 1
(241 g) 5
Turkey & gravy with dressing &
whipped potatoes, 1 (241 g)..................4

Green Giant Create A Meal!
Barbeque chicken, as packaged,
1½ cups................................3
Barbeque chicken, prepared, 1⅓ cups........7
Beef & broccoli stir fry, as packaged,
2⅓ cups................................2
Beef & broccoli stir fry, prepared,
1⅓ cups................................6
Beefy noodle, as packaged, 1¾ cups........3
Beefy noodle, prepared, 1¼ cups 8
Cheesy pasta & vegetable, as packaged,
1¾ cups 4
Cheesy pasta & vegetable, prepared,
¼ cup 10

Chicken & stuffing, as packaged, 6 oz 4
Chicken & stuffing, prepared, 1⅓ cups 8
Chicken alfredo, as packaged, 2 cups 4
Chicken alfredo, prepared, 1¼ cups..........8
Garlic & ginger stir fry, as packaged,
1⅔ cups 2
Garlic & ginger stir fry, prepared,
1½ cups................................5
Garlic herb chicken (oven roasted),
as packaged, 1¾ cups 2
Garlic herb chicken (oven roasted),
prepared, 1¾ cups.........................7
Garlic herb chicken (with vegetables),
as packaged, 2⅓ cups.....................5
Garlic herb chicken (with vegetables),
prepared, 1¼ cups 8
Homestyle stew, as packaged, 1¼ cups 2
Homestyle stew, prepared, 1 cup...........8
Lemon pepper chicken, as packaged,
1½ cups................................2
Lemon pepper chicken, prepared,
1⅓ cups 6
Lo mein stir fry, as packaged, 2⅓ cups 3
Lo mein stir fry, prepared, 1¼ cups...........6
Mushroom wine chicken, as packaged,
1¾ cups 5
Mushroom wine chicken, prepared,
1¼ cups................................8
Parmesan herb chicken, as packaged,
1¾ cups 3
Parmesan herb chicken, prepared,
1¾ cups 7
Skillet lasagna, as packaged, 1¾ cups 2
Skillet lasagna, prepared, 1¼ cups 7
Sweet & sour stir fry, as packaged,
1½ cups................................3
Sweet & sour stir fry, prepared,
1¼ cups................................7
Szechuan stir fry, as packaged, 1¾ cups....3
Szechuan stir fry, prepared, 1¾ cups 7
Teriyaki stir fry, as packaged, 1¾ cups.......1
Teriyaki stir fry, prepared, 1¼ cups 4

D

Healthy Choice

Beef macaroni, 1 (8½ oz) 4
Beef pepper steak Oriental, 1 (9½ oz) 5
Beef pot roast, 1 (11 oz)............................6
Beef stroganoff, 1 (11 oz) 6
Beef tips francais, 1 (9½ oz) 6
Beef tips portabello, 1 (11¼ oz) 5
Breaded chicken breast strips with
   macaroni and cheese, 1 (8 oz) 6
Charbroiled beef patty, 1 (11 oz)................6
Cheddar broccoli potatoes, 1 (10½ oz) 6
Cheese ravioli Parmigiana, 1 (9 oz) 5
Chicken & vegetables marsala, 1
   (11½ oz) 5
Chicken breast con queso burrito, 1
   (10.55 oz) 7
Chicken broccoli alfredo, 1 (11½ oz)..........6
Chicken cantonese, 1 (10¾ oz) 6
Chicken dijon, 1 (11 oz)..............................5
Chicken enchilada sauce, 1 (10 oz)............5
Chicken enchilada suprema, 1 (11.3 oz) 6
Chicken fettuccini alfredo, 1 (8½ oz) 5
Chicken Parmigiana, 1 (11½ oz)................7
Chicken teriyaki, 1 (11 oz) 5
Country breaded chicken, 1 (10¼ oz) 7
Country glazed chicken breast, 1
   (8½ oz) 5
Country herb chicken, 1 (12.15 oz)............6
Country inn roast turkey, 1 (10 oz) 5
Fettuccini alfredo, 1 (8 oz) 5
Garlic chicken Milano, 1 (9½ oz) 5
Grilled chicken Sonoma, 1 (9 oz)................4
Grilled chicken with mashed potatoes,
   1 (8 oz)..3
Herb baked fish, 1 (10.9 oz)......................7
Herb breaded pork patty, 1 (8 oz)..............5
Homestyle chicken and pasta, 1 (9 oz).......5
Honey glazed chicken, 1 (10 oz)................5
Honey mustard chicken, 1 (9½ oz) 6
Lasagna Roma, 1 (13½ oz) 8
Lemon pepper fish, 1 (10.7 oz) 6
Macaroni and cheese, 1 (9 oz) 5
Macaroni with three cheeses, 1 (11 oz) 6

Mandarin chicken, 1 (10 oz) 5
Mesquite beef with barbecue sauce, 1
   (11 oz)..6
Mesquite chicken BBQ, 1 (10½ oz)............6
Oriental-style chicken & vegetables
   stir-fry, 1 (11.9 oz) 7
Oven roasted beef, 1 (10.15 oz) 5
Roast turkey breast, 1 (8½ oz) 4
Roasted chicken, 1 (11 oz)........................4
Sesame chicken, 1 (9¾ oz) 5
Sesame chicken, 1 (10.8 oz).....................7
Shrimp & vegetables, 1 (11.8 oz) 5
Spaghetti and sauce with seasoned
   beef, 1 (10 oz) 5
Stuffed pasta shells, 1 (10.35 oz) 7
Sweet and sour chicken, 1 (11 oz)..............7
Traditional breast of turkey, 1 (10½ oz) 5
Traditional meatloaf, 1 (12 oz) 6
Traditional salisbury steak, 1 (11½ oz).......6
Tuna casserole, 1 (9 oz) 4

Healthy Choice Bowls

Cheese & chicken tortillini, 1 (8.7 oz) 5
Chicken teriyaki with rice, 1 (9½ oz)..........5
Chili and cornbread, 1 (9½ oz)..................7
Colonial chicken pie, 1 (9½ oz) 6
Country chicken bake, 1 (9½ oz) 4
Fiesta chicken, 1 (9½ oz) 4
Garlic lemon chicken with rice, 1
   (9½ oz) 6
Roasted potatoes with ham, 1 (8½ oz)......4
Southwestern chicken & pasta, 1
   (9½ oz) 6
Turkey divan, 1 (9½ oz) 5

Kid Cuisine

Big league hamburger pizza, 1 (8.3 oz) 8
Buckaroo beef patty sandwich with
   cheese, 1 (8½ oz) 9
Circus show corn dog, 1 (8.8 oz)..............11
Cosmic chicken nuggets, 1 (9.1 oz) 11
Funtastic fish sticks, 1 (8¼ oz) 9
Game time taco roll up, 1 (7.35 oz)..........9
High flying fried chicken, 1 (10.1 oz) 10
Magical macaroni & cheese, 1 (10.6 oz) 9

Parachuting pork ribettes, 1 (7.55 oz) 9
Pirate pizza with cheese, 1 (8 oz) 9
Wave rider waffle sticks, 1 (6.6 oz) 8

Marie Callender's

Beef stroganoff and noodles, 1 (13 oz) 3
Beef tips in mushroom sauce, 1
  (13.6 oz) 9
Breaded chicken Parmigiana, 1 (16 oz) 15
Breaded fish with macaroni & cheese,
  1 (12 oz) 13
Cheese ravioli in marinara sauce with
  spirals & garlic bread, 1 (18 oz) 17
Cheesy rice with chicken & broccoli,
  1 (12 oz) 8
Chicken and dumplings, 1 (14 oz) 9
Chicken and noodles, 1 (13 oz) 12
Chicken cordon bleu, 1 (13 oz) 14
Chicken fried beef steak & gravy, 1
  (15 oz) 15
Chicken teriyaki, 1 (13 oz) 11
Chili & cornbread, 1 (16 oz)....................12
Country fried chicken & gravy, 1 (16 oz) 14
Country fried pork chop, 1 (15 oz)...........12
Escalloped noodles & chicken, 1
  (13 oz) 18
Extra cheese lasagna, 1 (15 oz)...............13
Fettuccine alfredo & garlic bread,
  1 (14 oz) 22
Fettuccine alfredo supreme, 1 (13 oz) 10
Fettuccine primavera with tortellini,
  1 (14 oz) 18
Fettucinne with broccoli & chicken,
  1 (13 oz) 17
Glazed chicken, 1 (13 oz) 12
Grilled chicken & mashed potatoes,
  1 (10 oz) 8
Grilled chicken breast & rice pilaf,
  1 (11¾ oz) 8
Grilled chicken in mushroom sauce,
  1 (14 oz) 10
Grilled southwestern style chicken,
  1 (14 oz) 8
Grilled turkey breast & rice pilaf, 1
  (11¾ oz)...6

Herb roasted chicken & mashed
  potatoes, 1 (14 oz)................................14
Homestyle tuna & noodles, 1 (12 oz).......14
Honey roasted chicken, 1 (14 oz) 9
Honey smoked ham steak with
  macaroni & cheese, 1 (14 oz) 10
Lasagna with meat sauce, 1 (15 oz) 15
Macaroni and cheese, 1 (12 oz) 12
Meatloaf & gravy with mashed
  potatoes, 1 (14 oz)................................13
Old fashioned beef pot roast & gravy,
  1 (15 oz) 11
Roast beef, 1 (14½ oz) 9
Sirloin salisbury steak & gravy, 1 (4 oz) 12
Spaghetti & meat sauce with garlic
  bread, 1 (17 oz) 15
Stuffed pasta trio, 1 (10½ oz) 8
Swedish meatballs, 1 (12½ oz) 12
Sweet & sour chicken, 1 (14 oz) 12
Turkey with gravy & dressing, 1 (14 oz)....11

Marie Callender's Family Serve

Chicken fried beef steak & gravy with
  mashed potatoes, 1 patty with gravy,
  ½ cup potatoes (12 oz) 16
Country fried chicken & gravy with
  mashed potatoes, 1 patty with gravy,
  ½ cup potatoes (12 oz) 13
Escalloped noodles & chicken, 1 cup 7
Lasagna with meat sauce, 1 cup 8
Macaroni & cheese, 1 cup 6
Meatloaf and gravy with mashed
  potatoes, 1 patty with gravy, ½ cup
  potatoes (8.8 oz) 7
Turkey & gravy with mashed potatoes,
  2 pieces turkey with gravy & ½ cup
  potatoes (9¾ oz) 7

Marie Callender's Skillet Meals

Beef pot roast, ½ package (11 oz) 6
Beef stroganoff, ½ package (11 oz)...........6
Beef stroganoff, ¼ package (8.8 oz) 5
Chicken & rice with broccoli & cheese,
  ½ package (12½ oz) 9
Chicken alfredo, ½ package (11½ oz) 11

Dinners, frozen, Marie Callender's Skillet Meals (con't)

POINTS

Chicken alfredo, ¼ package (9¼ oz)..........9
Chicken teriyaki, ½ package (12 oz)..........6
Herb chicken, ½ package (12 oz) 5
Penne pasta & meatballs, ½ package
 (12 oz)..14
Rigatoni with vegetables in cheese
 sauce, 1 cup 6
Roast chicken & vegetables, ½ package
 (12½ oz)..4
Roast chicken & vegetables, ¼ package
 (10 oz)...4
White & wild rice with broccoli in
 cheese sauce, 1 cup 7

Mon Cuisine

Vegetarian breaded chicken nuggets,
 .85 oz..1
Vegetarian breaded chicken patties,
 2½ oz...2
Vegetarian grilled steak in mushroom
 gravy, 10 oz...4
Vegetarian moroccan chicken, 10 oz 5
Vegetarian salisbury steak in gravy,
 10 oz..6
Vegetarian spaghetti & meatballs, 10 oz 7
Vegetarian stuffed cabbage in tomato
 sauce, 10 oz 5
Vegetarian vegan breaded chicken
 style cutlet in mushroom sauce, 10 oz.....6
Vegetarian vegan Italian stuffed shell
 pasta, 10 oz 4
Vegetarian vegan veal style schnitzel
 in sauce, 10 oz 6

Morton

Breaded chicken patty, 1 (6¾ oz)..............6
Chicken nuggets, 1 (7 oz) 8
Chili gravy with beef enchilada and
 tamale, 1 (10 oz) 5
Fried chicken, 1 (9 oz) 11
Gravy and charbroiled beef patty, 1
 (9 oz)...7
Gravy and salisbury steak, 1 (9 oz)...........7
Gravy and turkey with dressing, 1 (9 oz) 5
Macaroni & cheese, 1 (16 oz) 5

POINTS

Spaghetti with meat sauce, 1 (8½ oz) 4
Tomato sauce with meat loaf, 1 (9 oz).......5
Veal Parmigiana with tomato sauce, 1
 (8¾ oz)..6

Oven Poppers

Cod augratin, 1 piece (140 g) 5
Cod stuffed with broccoli & cheese,
 1 piece (140 g)......................................3
Crab stuffed flounder, 1 piece (140 g) 6
Crab stuffed sole, 1 piece (140 g)..............6
Fish with cheese & salsa, 1 piece
 (4½ oz)..3
Fish with shrimp, crab & vegetables,
 1 piece (4½ oz) 5
Fish with spinach & cheese, 1 piece
 (4½ oz)..4
Flounder augratin, 1 piece (140 g) 5
Flounder stuffed with broccoli &
 cheese, 1 piece (140 g) 3
Flounder stuffed with garlic, shrimp
 & almonds, 1 piece (140 g).....................6
Haddock with shrimp, crab and
 vegetables, 1 piece (5 oz)......................5
Sole augratin, 1 piece (140 g).................5
Sole stuffed with broccoli & cheese,
 1 piece (140 g)......................................3
Sole stuffed with garlic, shrimp
 & almonds, 1 piece (140) 6
Sole with shrimp & lobster, 1 piece
 (140 g)..3

Patio

Beef enchilada, 1 (12 oz)..........................8
Cheese enchilada, 1 (12 oz)......................8
Chicken enchilada, 1 (12 oz).....................8
Fiesta, 1 (12 oz) 7
Mexican style, 1 (13¼ oz)........................10
Ranchera, 1 (13 oz).................................10

Patio Extra Large Dinners

2 beef & 2 cheese enchiladas chili 'n
 beans, 1 (15½ oz)................................15
4 beef enchiladas chili 'n beans, 1
 (15½ oz) 12

Schwan's

Beef & broccoli with rice, 1 cup 4
Cheese tortellini, 1 cup..............................5
Chicken bites, 3 oz 4
Chicken breast meat for fajitas, 3 oz 2
Chicken breast stir fry w/ rice, ¼ bag
  (276 g) 5
Chicken breast tenderloin fajita, 2
  (220 g) 6
Chicken egg roll, 2 pieces (113 g) 5
Chicken fried rice stir fry kit, ¼ bag
  (276 g) 6
Chicken quesadilla, 1 (98 g).......................5
Diced chicken meat, 3 oz...........................3
Gourmet turkey breast, 3 oz 2
Lasagna w/ beef in sauce, 1 cup 7
Lemon pepper chicken, 1 (128 g) 4
Pork egg rolls, 2 pieces (113 g) 5
Roasted chicken breast halves, 1 piece
  with skin (145 g) 5
Roasted chicken breast halves, 1 piece
  without skin (122 g) 3
Roasted chicken drumstick, 2 with skin
  (98 g) 3
Roasted chicken drumsticks, 2 without
  skin (84 g) 2
Single serve vegetable lasagna, 1
  (340 g) 9
Sliced beef pot roast w/ noodles, 1 cup 4
Sweet & sour chicken with rice, 1 cup 5
Teriyaki chicken breast filet, 1 (112 g) 3
Teriyaki chicken express, 1 bowl (280 g) 7
Teriyaki chicken w/ rice & vegetables,
  ⅓ tray (302 g) 8
Unbrd. chicken breast filet, 1 (112 g).........2
Unbrd. turkey breast filet, 1 (85 g) 1
Vegetable egg roll, 2 pieces (113 g) 3
Vegetable lasagna, 1 cup 6

Sea Cuisine

Baked cod fillets, 1 serving (112 g).............3
Linguini & shrimp, 6 oz 3
Shrimp marinara, 4 oz...............................4
Shrimp scampi, 4 oz..................................8

Stuffed fillet of flounder, 1 serving
  (140 g) 6

Stouffer's

Beef pie, 1 (10 oz)....................................10
Cheddar cheese and chicken bake, 1
  (11½ oz) 10
Cheddar pasta, 1 (11 oz) 12
Cheese manicotti, 1 (9 oz)..........................8
Cheese ravioli, 1 9
Cheese spaghetti bake, 1 (12 oz) 10
Cheesy spaghetti bake, 1 cup.....................8
Chicken a la king, 1 (11½ oz) 8
Chicken and broccoli pasta bake, 1
  (8 oz)...8
Chicken enchiladas, 1 (4¾ oz) 5
Chicken lasagna, 1 cup...............................7
Chicken Oriental, 1 5
Chicken pie, 1 (10 oz)...............................11
Chicken pie, 1 cup.....................................12
Chili with beans, 1 (8¾ oz).........................6
Creamed chicken, 1 (6½ oz).......................6
Creamed chipped beef, ½ cup....................4
Escalloped chicken and noodles, 1 cup 9
Escalloped chicken and noodles, 1
  (10 oz)...11
Fettucini alfredo, 1 (11½ oz) 12
Fettucini primavera, 1 (10 oz) 8
Five cheese lasagna, 1 (10¾ oz) 7
Grandma's chicken & vegetable rice
  bake, 1 cup 8
Homestyle baked chicken breast, 1............6
Homestyle beef pot roast and browned
  potatoes, 1...5
Homestyle beef stroganoff, 1 8
Homestyle breaded pork cutlet, 1
  (10 oz)...8
Homestyle chicken and dumplings, 1
  (10 oz)...6
Homestyle chicken breast in barbecue
  sauce, 1 (10 oz) 12
Homestyle chicken breast with
  mushroom gravy, 1 (10 oz) 8
Homestyle chicken fettucini, 1 (10½ oz) 8

Dinners, frozen
Stouffer's (con't)   POINTS

Homestyle chicken Parmigiana, 1
(12 oz) 10
Homestyle chunky beef and tomatoes,
1 (10 oz) 6
Homestyle fish fillet with macaroni and
cheese, 1 (9 oz) 10
Homestyle fried chicken breast, 1 8
Homestyle green pepper steak, 1
(10½ oz) 6
Homestyle meatloaf, 1 9
Homestyle roast turkey, 1 7
Homestyle salisbury steak, 1 8
Homestyle sliced beef brisket, 1 (10 oz) 8
Homestyle veal Parmigiana, 1 9
Lasagna bake, 1 (11½ oz) 10
Lasagna with meat sauce, 1 (10½ oz) 8
Lasagna with meat sauce, 1 cup 6
Lasagna with tomato sauce and
Italian sausage, 1 9
Macaroni and beef, 1 (11½ oz) 8
Macaroni and cheese, 1 cup 8
Macaroni and cheese with broccoli, 1
(10½ oz) 9
Meatloaf in gravy, 1 serving (5½ oz) 5
Noodles romanoff, 1 (12 oz) 11
Pasta shells and American cheese,
1 cup 6
Penne pasta & chicken bake, 1 (11½ oz) 7
Scalloped potatoes, ½ cup 3
Spaghetti with meat sauce, 1 (12 oz) 9
Spaghetti with meatballs in sauce, 1 8
Stuffed green peppers, 1 serving 4
Stuffed pepper, 1 (10 oz) 4
Swedish meatballs, 1 (11½ oz) 12
Tuna noodle casserole, 1 (10 oz) 9
Turkey pie, 1 (10 oz) 12
Turkey tetrazzini, 1 (10 oz) 9
Vegetable and chicken pasta bake, 1
(12 oz) 8
Vegetable lasagna, 1 (10½ oz) 9
Vegetable lasagna, 1 cup 7

POINTS

Stouffer's Hearty Portions
Beef pot roast, 1 (16 oz) 7
Chicken fettucini, 1 (16¾ oz) 14
Chicken pot pie, 1 serving (8 oz) 14
Country fried beef steak, 1 (16 oz) 12
Fried chicken breast, 1 11
Meatloaf with mashed potatoes, 1
(17 oz) 13
Pork and roasted potatoes, 1 10
Roast turkey breast, 1 (16 oz) 10
Salisbury steak with pasta shells, 1
(16 oz) 13
Veal Parmigiana, 1 (17½ oz) 11

Stouffer's Lean Cuisine
Cafe Classics
Baked chicken, 1 (8.63 oz) 5
Baked fish, 1 (9 oz) 6
Beef peppercorn, 1 (8¾ oz) 5
Beef portobello, 1 (9 oz) 5
Beef pot roast, 1 (9 oz) 4
Bow tie pasta & chicken, 1 (9½ oz) 4
Cheese lasagna with chicken scaloppini,
1 (10 oz) 5
Chicken & vegetables, 1 (10½ oz) 4
Chicken a l'orange, 1 (9 oz) 4
Chicken in peanut sauce, 1 (9 oz) 5
Chicken in wine sauce, 1 (8.1 oz) 4
Chicken medallions w/ creamy cheese
sauce, 1 (9.4 oz) 6
Chicken Mediterranean, 1 (10½ oz) 5
Chicken Parmesan, 1 (10.9 oz) 6
Chicken piccata, 1 (9 oz) 6
Chicken w/ basil cream sauce, 1 (8½ oz) 5
Country vegetables & beef, 1 (9 oz) 4
Fiesta chicken, 1 (9¼ oz) 5
Glazed chicken, 1 (8½ oz) 5
Glazed turkey tenderloins, 1 (9 oz) 5
Grilled chicken, 1 (9.4 oz) 5
Herb roasted chicken, 1 (8 oz) 3
Honey mustard chicken, 1 (8 oz) 5
Honey roasted chicken, 1 (8½ oz) 5
Honey roasted pork, 1 (9½ oz) 5

Meatloaf w/ whipped potatoes, 1
   (9.4 oz) **5**
Oriental beef, 1 (9¼ oz) **4**
Oven roasted beef, 1 (9¼ oz) **5**
Roasted turkey breast, 1 (9¾ oz) **5**
Salisbury steak, 1 (9½ oz) **5**
Shrimp and angel hair pasta, 1 (10 oz) **5**
Southern beef tips, 1 (8¾ oz) **5**

Stouffer's Lean Cuisine Everyday Favorites

Alfredo pasta primavera, 1 (10 oz) **6**
Angel hair pasta, 1 (10 oz) **4**
Cheese cannelloni, 1 (9.1 oz) **4**
Cheese lasagna casserole, 1 (10 oz) **5**
Cheese ravioli, 1 (8½ oz) **5**
Chicken chow mein, 1 (9 oz) **4**
Chicken enchilada suiza, 1 (9 oz) **5**
Chicken fettucini, 1 (9¼ oz) **5**
Chicken florentine, 1 (8 oz) **4**
Chicken lasagna, 1 (10 oz) **6**
Chicken pie, 1 (9½ oz) **6**
Classic cheese lasagna, 1 (11½ oz) **6**
Deluxe Cheddar potato, 1 (10.4 oz) **5**
Fettucini alfredo, 1 (9¼ oz) **6**
Fettucini primavera, 1 (10 oz) **5**
Homestyle turkey, 1 (9.4 oz) **5**
Hunan beef & broccoli, 1 (8½ oz) **5**
Lasagna w/ meat sauce, 1 (10½ oz) **6**
Macaroni & beef, 1 (10 oz) **5**
Macaroni & cheese, 1 (10 oz) **6**
Mandarin chicken, 1 (9 oz) **5**
Oriental style dumplings, 1 (9 oz) **6**
Penne pasta, 1 (10 oz) **5**
Roasted chicken, 1 (8.1 oz) **5**
Roasted potatoes with broccoli, 1
   (10¼ oz) **5**
Santa fe rice & beans, 1 (10.4 oz) **6**
Spaghetti w/ meat sauce, 1 (11½ oz) **5**
Spaghetti w/ meatballs, 1 (9½ oz) **5**
Stuffed cabbage, 1 (9½ oz) **4**
Swedish meatballs, 1 (9.1 oz) **6**
Teriyaki stir fry, 1 (10 oz) **5**
Three bean chili w/ rice, 1 (10 oz) **5**

Vegetable eggroll, 1 (9 oz) **6**
Vegetable lasagna, 1 (10½ oz) **5**

Stouffer's Lean Cuisine Family Style Favorites

Chicken lasagna, 1 ....**4**
Five cheese lasagna, 1 ....**4**

Stouffer's Lean Cuisine Hearty Portions

Cheese & spinach manicotti, 1 (15½ oz) **7**
Chicken & barbecue sauce, 1 (13.9 oz) **7**
Chicken fettucini w/ broccoli, 1
   (13.63 oz) **8**
Chicken florentine, 1 (13¼ oz) **7**
Glazed chicken, 1 (13 oz) **6**
Grilled chicken & penne pasta, 1 (14 oz) **7**
Homestyle beef stroganoff, 1 (14¼ oz) **7**
Jumbo rigatoni w/ meatballs, 1 (15.4 oz) **9**
Oriental glazed chicken, 1 (14 oz) **7**
Roasted chicken w/ mushrooms, 1
   (12½ oz) **6**
Roasted turkey breast, 1 (14 oz) **6**
Salisbury steak, 1 (15½ oz) **6**

Stouffer's Lean Cuisine Skillet Sensations

Beef teriyaki and rice, 1 serving (12 oz) **5**
Chicken alfredo (family size), 1 serving
   (12 oz) **6**
Chicken primavera, 1 serving (12 oz) **6**
Fiesta beef and rice, 1 serving (12 oz) **5**
Garlic chicken, 1 serving (12 oz) **6**
Herb chicken and roasted potatoes,
   serving (12 oz) **5**
Roasted turkey, 1 serving (12 oz) **4**
Savory beef and vegetables, 1 serving
   (12 oz) **6**
Three cheese chicken, 1 serving (12 oz) **8**

Stouffer's Skillet Sensations

Beef stroganoff, 1 serving (10 oz) **7**
Broccoli and beef, 1 serving (12½ oz) **6**
Cheddar beef, 1 serving (12½ oz) **14**
Chicken alfredo, 1 serving (12½ oz) **10**
Grilled chicken and vegetables,
   1 serving (12½ oz) **9**

D

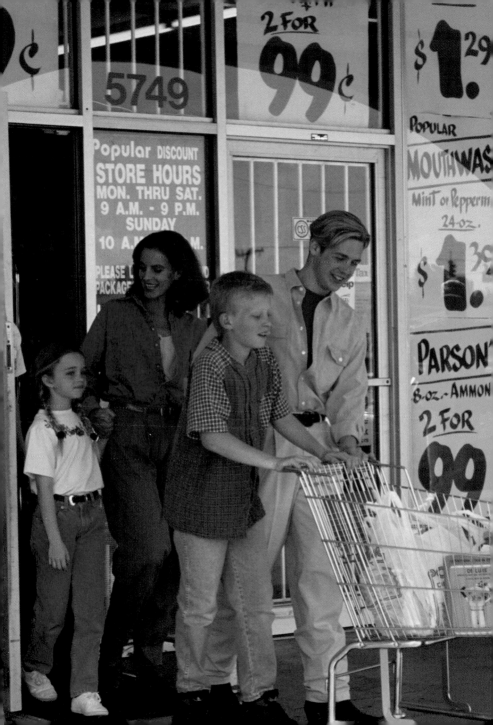

Dinners, frozen, Stouffer's Skillet Sensations (con't)

Homestyle beef, 1 serving (12½ oz)...........6
Homestyle chicken, 1 serving (12½ oz)......8
Savory chicken and rice, 1 serving
(10 oz)..6
Teriyaki chicken, 1 serving (12½ oz) 6

The Fillo Factory Spinach & cheese
fillo pie, ¼ pie (170 g)...........................7

Tyson
Beef fajita, 3½ fajitas (357 g) 12
Beef stir fry, 2¾ cups 8
Chicken broccoli and cheese, 1 piece
(168 g) 7
Chicken cordon bleu, 1 piece (168 g)........8
Chicken fajita, 3½ fajitas (374 g) 9
Chicken kiev, 1 piece (168 g) 11
Chicken stir fry, 2¾ cups 8
Chicken w/ wild rice and mushroom,
1 piece (168 g) 7

Weight Watchers **Smart Ones**

Weight Watchers Smart Ones
Angel hair pasta, 1 serving (283 g) 4
Broccoli & cheese baked potato,
1 serving (283 g) 5
Chicken enchiladas suiza, 1 serving
(255 g) 6
Chicken mirabella, 1 serving (260 g) 3
Chicken Oriental, 1 serving (255 g) 4
Creamy rigatoni with broccoli,
1 serving (255 g) 4
Fettucini alfredo, 1 serving (262 g)............5
Fiesta chicken, 1 serving (241 g) 4
Grilled salisbury steak & gravy,
1 serving (269 g) 6
Honey-dijon chicken, 1 serving (241 g) 4
Lasagna alfredo, 1 serving (255 g) 6
Lasagna bolognese, 1 serving (255 g)........4
Lasagna florentine, 1 serving (297 g) 6
Lemon herb chicken piccata, 1 serving
(255 g) 4
Macaroni & cheese, 1 serving (283 g)........4

Penne pasta, 1 serving (283 g)..................6
Radiatore Romano, 1 serving (294 g) 5
Ravioli florentine, 1 serving (241 g)...........4
Roast turkey medallions, 1 serving
(255 g) 4
Santa fe style & beans, 1 serving
(283 g) 6
Shrimp marinara, 1 serving (255 g) 3
Spaghetti bolognese, 1 serving (326 g)......5
Spaghetti marinara, 1 serving (255 g) 5
Spicy penne Mediterranean, 1 serving
(289 g) 5
Spicy szechuan style vegetables,
1 serving (255 g) 4
Swedish meatballs, 1 serving (258 g) 6
Three cheese macaroni, 1 serving
(255 g) 6
Three cheese ziti marinara, 1 serving
(255 g) 6
Traditional lasagna with meat sauce,
1 serving (297 g) 6
Tuna noodle gratin, 1 serving (269 g) 6

**Weight Watchers Smart Ones
Main Street Bistro**
Basil chicken, 1 serving (269 g)..................6
Chicken carbonara, 1 serving (269 g) 6
Chicken fettucini, 1 serving (283 g) 6
Fajita chicken supreme, 1 serving
(262 g) 6
Fillet of beef, 1 serving (269 g) 4
Fire-grilled chicken & vegetables,
1 serving (283 g) 6
Golden baked garlic chicken, 1 serving
(283 g) 6
Oven-roasted chicken, 1 serving (255 g) 6
Oven-roasted chicken primavera,
1 serving (283 g) 6
Penne pollo, 1 serving (283 g) 6
Pepper steak, 1 serving (283 g)................4
Roasted chicken with sour cream,
1 serving (269 g) 3
Slow-roasted turkey breast, 1 serving
(283 g) 5
Stuffed turkey breast, 1 serving (283 g) 5

D

D

Weight Watchers Smart Ones
Main Street Bistro Bowls
Bean & beef salsa verde bowl,
1 serving (311 g) 6
Beef & vegetable rice bowl, 1 serving
(311 g) 5
Chicken & vegetables Caribbean,
1 serving (311 g) 4
Gnocchi with grilled chicken, 1 serving
(311 g) 5
Pasta fagioli, 1 serving (311 g)..................5
Southwestern style chicken bowl,
1 serving (311 g) 4
Yukon gold potato & corn chowder,
1 serving (311 g) 5

Dinners, refrigerated
Foster Farms Fresh & Easy
Chicken & homestyle gravy, 1¼ cups.........9
Chicken alfredo, 1¼ cups..........................8
Chicken cacciatore, 1¼ cups 7
Teriyaki chicken, 1¼ cups 6
White wine & herb chicken, 1¼ cups.........8

Dinners, shelf
Chi-Chi's Dinner Kits
Burrito, 2 shells & seasoning (90 g)...........6
Fajita, 2 shells & seasoning (117 g)...........6
Soft taco, 2 shells & seasoning (16 g)........6
White, 2 shells & seasoning (62 g) 4
Yellow, 2 shells & seasoning (62 g) 4

Dinty Moore American Classics
Beef ravioli, 1 bowl (283 g) 6
Chicken & noodles, 1 bowl (283 g).............6
Chicken w/ potatoes, 1 bowl (283 g) 5
Lasagna, 1 bowl (283 g)...........................8
Pot roast, 1 bowl (283 g)..........................4
Roast beef w/ potatoes, 1 bowl (283 g) 5
Salisbury steak, 1 bowl (283 g) 6
Spaghetti w/ meatballs, 1 bowl (283 g) 6
Turkey & dressing, 1 bowl (283 g) 6
Turkey w/ potatoes, 1 bowl (284 g) 5

Dinty Moore Microwave Cups
Chicken & dumplings, 1 cup (213 g)........4

Hormel Microcup Meals
Chili mac, 1 cup 4
Lasagna, 1 cup 4
Macaroni and cheese, 1 cup 6
Noodles & chicken, 1 cup 5
Ravioli/tomato sauce, 1 cup.......................5
Scalloped potatoes flavored with ham,
1 cup 6
Spaghetti w/ meat sauce, 1 cup 5

Kid's Kitchen
Beans & wieners, 1 cup 6
Beefy macaroni, 1 cup...............................4
Cheezy mac & beef, 1 cup 6
Macaroni & cheese, 1 cup 6
Mini beef ravioli, 1 cup 5
Noodle rings & chicken, 1 cup 3
Pizza wedges 3 cheese, 1 cup 6
Pizza wedges cheese burger, 1 cup 5
Pizza wedges pepperoni, 1 cup 5
Spaghetti & meatballs, 1 cup 5
Spaghetti rings & franks, 1 cup 5
Spaghetti rings & meatballs, 1 cup............5

Dips
Breakstone
Bacon & onion, 2 Tbsp 2
Chesapeake clam, 2 Tbsp 1
French onion, 2 Tbsp 1
Toasted onion, 2 Tbsp 1

Breakstone Free
Creamy salsa, 2 Tbsp.................................0
French onion, 2 Tbsp 1
Ranch, 2 Tbsp 1

Chi-Chi's
Fiesta bean dip, 2 Tbsp 1
Fiesta cheese dip, 2 Tbsp 1

Frito-Lay
French onion, 2 Tbsp 2
Fritos bean dip, 2 Tbsp 1
Fritos hot bean dip, 2 Tbsp........................1
Jalapeño & Cheddar cheese, 2 Tbsp...........1
Mild Cheddar cheese, 2 Tbsp 2

Smart Ones is going to bowl you over.

Main Street Bistro Bowl Selections

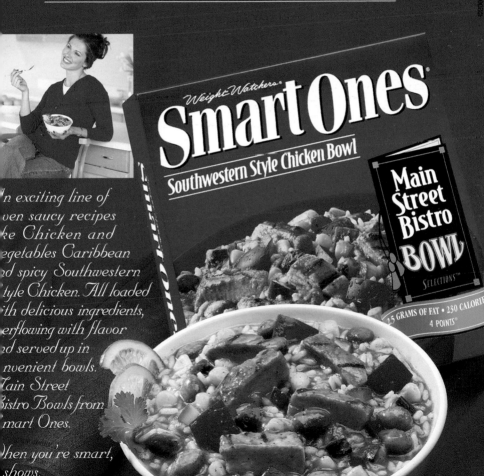

Weight Watchers® SmartOnes®
Southwestern Style Chicken Bowl

Main Street Bistro BOWL SELECTIONS™
2.5 GRAMS OF FAT • 230 CALORIES 4 POINTS®

An exciting line of even saucy recipes like Chicken and Vegetables Caribbean and spicy Southwestern style Chicken. All loaded with delicious ingredients, overflowing with flavor and served up in convenient bowls. Main Street Bistro Bowls from Smart Ones.

When you're smart, it shows.

Dips (con't)   POINTS

Fritos
Chili, 170.1 g...4
Chili cheese, 34 g...................................1
Sloppy Joe, 170.1 g................................4

Guiltless Gourmet
Mild black bean dip, 2 Tbsp.....................0
Spicy black bean dip, 2 Tbsp....................0

Hidden Valley Ranch
Fiesta, prepared, 2 Tbsp..........................2
French onion, prepared, 2 Tbsp 2
Garden vegetable, prepared, 2 Tbsp 2
Original, prepared, 2 Tbsp........................2
Reduced calorie original, prepared,
   2 Tbsp...2

Knudsen Free
Creamy salsa, 2 Tbsp...............................0
French onion, 2 Tbsp 1
Ranch, 2 Tbsp 1

Kraft
Avocado, 2 Tbsp 2
Bacon & horseradish, 2 Tbsp....................2
French onion, 2 Tbsp 2
Green onion, 2 Tbsp 2
Jalapeño, 2 Tbsp 2
Ranch, 2 Tbsp 2

Kraft Cheez Whiz
Medium cheese & salsa dip, 2 Tbsp...........3
Mild cheese & salsa dip, 2 Tbsp 3

Kraft Free
French onion, 2 Tbsp 1
Ranch, 2 Tbsp 1
Salsa, 2 Tbsp 0

Kraft Premium
Bacon & horseradish, 2 Tbsp....................2
Bacon & onion, 2 Tbsp 2
Clam, 2 Tbsp 1
French onion, 2 Tbsp 1
Ranch, 2 Tbsp 1

Naturally Fresh
Bleu cheese dip, 2 Tbsp 5
Chocolate peanut butter dip, 1 oz 2
Country garden dip, 2 Tbsp......................4
Dill dip, 2 Tbsp..4

POINTS

Fat-free bacon, tomato and chive dip,
   2 Tbsp...1
Fat-free caramel dip, 1 oz 2
Fat-free chocolate dip, 1 oz......................1
French onion dip, 2 Tbsp...........................3
Ranch dip, 2 Tbsp 3
Tropical fruit dip, 2 Tbsp 2

Old El Paso
Black bean, 2 Tbsp...................................0
Cheese 'n salsa, low fat, medium,
   2 Tbsp...1
Cheese 'n salsa, medium, 2 Tbsp..............1
Cheese 'n salsa, mild, 2 Tbsp 1
Chunky salsa, medium, 2 Tbsp 0
Chunky salsa, mild, 2 Tbsp.......................0
Jalapeño, 2 Tbsp 0

Taco Bell Home Originals Fat free
   black bean dip, 2 Tbsp 0

Tostitos
Low fat salsa con queso, 70 g...................1
Restaurant style salsa, 62 g......................0
Roasted garlic salsa, 68 g.........................0
Salsa con queso, 68 g 2
Salsa mild, medium or hot, 66 g 0

Doughnuts
Lance
Chocolate glazed donuts, 1 package
   (113 g)...11
Crunch gem donuts, 6 (71 g) 6
Sugar gem donuts, 6 (71 g) 7
Sugar glaze donuts, 1 package (106 g)....10

Dressings, salad
Best Foods
Caesar dressing (oil and vinegar), 2 Tbsp 3
Caesar dressing, fat free, 2 Tbsp...............1
Chardonny vinaigrette dressing, 2 Tbsp 1
Chunky blue cheese dressing, 2 Tbsp.........4
Cream ranch dressing, fat free, 2 Tbsp.......1
Creamy Caesar dressing, 2 Tbsp...............5
Creamy French dressing, 2 Tbsp 5
Creamy Italian dressing, 2 Tbsp 4
Creamy ranch dressing, 2 Tbsp..................4

Creamy thousand island dressing,
2 Tbsp..4

French style dressing, fat free, 2 Tbsp 1

Garlic ranch dressing, 2 Tbsp 4

Honey dijon dressing, fat free, 2 Tbsp........1

Italian dressing, 2 Tbsp...............................3

Italian dressing, fat free, 2 Tbsp 0

Italian herb ranch dressing, 2 Tbsp............4

Orange vinaigrette, 2 Tbsp.........................2

Raspberry vinaigrette dressing, fat free,
2 Tbsp..1

Roasted tomato and garlic balsamic
vinaigrette dressing, fat free, 2 Tbsp........0

Roasted tomato balsamic vinaigrette
dressing, 2 Tbsp.....................................3

Spring onion ranch dressing, 2 Tbsp 4

Best Foods Citrus Splash Dressing

Orange Oriental, 2 Tbsp 2

Ruby red ginger, 2 Tbsp 2

Tangerine balsamic, 2 Tbsp.......................2

Tangy tangerine, 2 Tbsp.............................2

Good Seasons

Cheese garlic, prepared as directed,
2 Tbsp..4

Fat free honey French, prepared as
directed, 2 Tbsp 0

Fat free honey mustard, prepared as
directed, 2 Tbsp 0

Fat free Italian, prepared as directed,
2 Tbsp..0

Fat free zesty herb, prepared as
directed, 2 Tbsp 0

Garlic and herbs, prepared as directed,
2 Tbsp..4

Gourmet Caesar, prepared as directed,
2 Tbsp..4

Gourmet Parmesan Italian, prepared as
directed, 2 Tbsp 4

Honey French, prepared as directed,
2 Tbsp..4

Honey mustard, prepared as directed,
2 Tbsp..4

Italian, prepared as directed, 2 Tbsp..........4

Mexican spice, 2 Tbsp 4

Mild Italian, prepared as directed,
2 Tbsp..4

Oriental sesame, prepared as directed,
2 Tbsp..4

Reduced calorie Italian, prepared as
directed, 2 Tbsp 1

Reduced calorie zesty Italian, prepared
as directed, 2 Tbsp.................................1

Roasted garlic, prepared as directed,
2 Tbsp..4

Zesty Italian, prepared as directed,
2 Tbsp..4

Hain Pure Foods

1000 island, 2 Tbsp 3

Creamy Italian, 2 Tbsp...............................5

Dijon creamy vinaigrette, 2 Tbsp 4

Poppyseed rancher's, 2 Tbsp 4

Harry & David

Italian dressing, 2 Tbsp...............................0

Pesto dried tomato dressing, 2 Tbsp...........0

Raspberry balsamic dressing, 2 Tbsp 0

Hellmann's

Caesar dressing (oil and vinegar), 2 Tbsp 3

Caesar dressing, fat free, 2 Tbsp................1

Chardonnay vinaigrette dressing,
2 Tbsp..1

Chunky blue cheese dressing, 2 Tbsp.........4

Cream ranch dressing, fat free, 2 Tbsp.......1

Creamy Caesar dressing, 2 Tbsp.................5

Creamy French dressing, 2 Tbsp 5

Creamy Italian dressing, 2 Tbsp 4

Creamy ranch dressing, 2 Tbsp...................4

Creamy thousand island dressing,
2 Tbsp..4

French style dressing, fat free, 2 Tbsp 1

Garlic ranch dressing, 2 Tbsp 4

Honey dijon dressing, fat free, 2 Tbsp........1

Italian dressing, 2 Tbsp...............................3

Italian dressing, fat free, 2 Tbsp 0

Italian herb ranch dressing, 2 Tbsp............4

Orange vinaigrette, 2 Tbsp.........................2

Raspberry vinaigrette dressing, fat free,
2 Tbsp..1

D

Dressings, salad, Hellmann's (con't)

POINTS

Roasted tomato and garlic balsamic
vinaigrette dressing, fat free, 2 Tbsp........0
Roasted tomato balsamic vinaigrette
dressing, 2 Tbsp......................................3
Spring onion ranch dressing, 2 Tbsp 4

Hellmann's Citrus Splash Dressing
Orange Oriental, 2 Tbsp 2
Ruby red ginger, 2 Tbsp 2
Tangerine balsamic, 2 Tbsp.......................2
Tangy tangerine, 2 Tbsp............................2

Hidden Valley Ranch
Bacon, prepared, 2 Tbsp 3
Blue cheese, prepared, 2 Tbsp...................3
Coleslaw, 2 Tbsp 1
Creamy Parmesan, fat-free, 2 Tbsp 1
French, 2 Tbsp 1
Honey dijon, 2 Tbsp 1
Honey dijon, prepared, 2 Tbsp...................3
Original, 2 Tbsp 1
Original buttermilk, prepared, 2 Tbsp 3
Original lowfat, prepared, 2 Tbsp 1
Original milk, prepared, 2 Tbsp 3
Original, reduced calorie, prepared,
2 Tbsp..2
Ranch Italian, prepared, 2 Tbsp.................4
Reduced calorie original ranch, 2 Tbsp 2
Reduced calorie ranch Italian, 2 Tbsp 1
Thousand island, 2 Tbsp 1

Hidden Valley Ranch, fat free
Blue cheese, 2 Tbsp..................................0
Honey dijon, 2 Tbsp 1
Italian Parmesan, 2 Tbsp...........................0

Kraft
Bacon & tomato, 2 Tbsp 4
Buttermilk ranch, 2 Tbsp...........................4
Caesar Italian, 2 Tbsp...............................3
Caesar ranch, 2 Tbsp................................3
Catalina, 2 Tbsp.......................................3
Catalina with honey, 2 Tbsp......................4
Classic Caesar, 2 Tbsp 3
Coleslaw, 2 Tbsp 4
Creamy French, 2 Tbsp 4
Creamy garlic, 2 Tbsp...............................3

POINTS

Creamy Italian, 2 Tbsp..............................3
Cucumber ranch, 2 Tbsp 4
Fat free mayonnaise dressing, 1 Tbsp 0
Garlic ranch, 2 Tbsp 5
Honey dijon, 2 Tbsp 3
House Italian with olive oil blend, 2 Tbsp ...3
Peppercorn ranch, 2 Tbsp 5
Presto Italian, 2 Tbsp................................3
Ranch, 2 Tbsp..5
Roka brand blue cheese, 2 Tbsp 4
Russian, 2 Tbsp..3
Sour cream & onion ranch, 2 Tbsp.............5
Thousand island, 2 Tbsp 3
Thousand island with bacon, 2 Tbsp..........4
Tomato & herb Italian, 2 Tbsp 3
Zesty Italian, 2 Tbsp 3

Kraft ⅓ Less Fat
Catalina, 2 Tbsp.......................................2
Cucumber ranch, 2 Tbsp 2
Italian, 2 Tbsp..2
Ranch, 2 Tbsp..3
Thousand island, 2 Tbsp 2

Kraft Free
Blue cheese flavored, 2 Tbsp.....................1
Caesar Italian, 2 Tbsp...............................1
Catalina, 2 Tbsp.......................................1
Classic Caesar, 2 Tbsp 1
Creamy Italian, 2 Tbsp..............................1
French style, 2 Tbsp..................................1
Garlic ranch, 2 Tbsp 1
Honey dijon, 2 Tbsp 1
Italian, 2 Tbsp..0
Peppercorn ranch, 2 Tbsp 1
Ranch, 2 Tbsp..1
Red wine vinegar, 2 Tbsp..........................0
Sour cream & onion ranch, 2 Tbsp.............1
Thousand island, 2 Tbsp 1

Kraft Miracle Whip
Light dressing, 1 Tbsp 1
Salad dressing, 1 Tbsp..............................2

Kraft Miracle Whip Free Nonfat
dressing, 1 Tbsp......................................0

Naturally Fresh

Bacon honey mustard dressing, 2 Tbsp......1
Bleu cheese dressing, 2 Tbsp 5
Caesar dressing, 2 Tbsp...........................4
Classic Caesar dressing, 2 Tbsp 5
Creamy cilantro dressing, 2 Tbsp...............4
Creamy Italian dressing, 2 Tbsp 5
Creamy Oriental dressing, 2 Tbsp 4
Fat-free balsamic vinaigrette dressing,
   2 Tbsp..0
Fat-free bleu cheese dressing, 2 Tbsp 1
Fat-free honey French dressing, 2 Tbsp 1
Fat-free honey mustard dressing, 2 Tbsp....1
Fat-free Italian dressing, 2 Tbsp 0
Fat-free lemon vinaigrette dressing,
   2 Tbsp..1
Fat-free ranch dressing, 2 Tbsp 0
Fat-free raspberry vinaigrette dressing,
   2 Tbsp..1
Fat-free thousand island dressing,
   2 Tbsp..0
Fat-free tomato basil vinaigrette, 2 Tbsp....0
Grilled Caesar dressing, 2 Tbsp 4
Honey French dressing, 2 Tbsp 3
Honey mustard dressing, 2 Tbsp.................4
Italian herb vinaigrette dressing, 2 Tbsp 3
Lite bleu cheese dressing, 2 Tbsp 3
Lite honey mustard dressing, 2 Tbsp..........2
Lite peppercorn ranch dressing, 2 Tbsp......2
Lite ranch dressing (no msg), 2 Tbsp 2
Lite ranch dressing (with msg), 2 Tbsp.......2
Olive oil & vinegar dressing, 2 Tbsp...........3
Pesto ranch dressing, 2 Tbsp.....................2
Poppy seed dressing, 2 Tbsp 4
Roasted garlic bleu cheese dressing,
   2 Tbsp..5
Slaw dressing, 2 Tbsp................................3
Thousand island dressing, 2 Tbsp 3
Wine & cheese dressing, 2 Tbsp 4

Newman's Own

Balsamic vinaigrette, 2 Tbsp 3
Caesar dressing, 2 Tbsp.............................4
Family recipe Italian dressing, 2 Tbsp 3

Light Italian dressing, 2 Tbsp 1
Olive oil & vinegar dressing, 2 Tbsp...........4
Parisienne dijon lime, 2 Tbsp.....................3
Ranch dressing, 2 Tbsp..............................4

San-J

Tamari mustard, 2 Tbsp 1
Tamari peanut, 2 Tbsp...............................1
Tamari sesame, 2 Tbsp 1
Tamari vinaigrette, 2 Tbsp..........................1

Seven Seas

2-cheese Italian, 2 Tbsp.............................2
Chunky blue cheese, 2 Tbsp.......................4
Classic Caesar, 2 Tbsp 3
Creamy Italian, 2 Tbsp...............................3
Green goddess, 2 Tbsp 4
Herb vinaigrette, 2 Tbsp 4
Herbs & spices, 2 Tbsp...............................3
Honey mustard, 2 Tbsp...............................3
Ranch, 2 Tbsp..5
Red wine vinegar & oil, 2 Tbsp 3
Viva Italian, 2 Tbsp 3
Viva Russian, 2 Tbsp..................................4

Seven Seas ⅓ Less Fat

Creamy Italian, 2 Tbsp...............................2
Italian with olive oil oil blend, 2 Tbsp 1
Ranch, 2 Tbsp..3
Red wine vinegar & oil, 2 Tbsp 1
Viva Italian, 2 Tbsp 1

Seven Seas Free

Creamy Italian, 2 Tbsp...............................1
Ranch, 2 Tbsp..1
Raspberry vinaigrette, 2 Tbsp.....................1
Red wine vinegar, 2 Tbsp...........................0
Viva Italian, 2 Tbsp ....:.0

Weight Watchers

Caesar salad dressing, 1 serving (21 g)......0
Caesar salad dressing, 1 serving (30 g)......0
Creamy Italian salad dressing,
   1 serving (30 g) 1
French style salad dressing, 1 serving
   (30 g) 1
Honey dijon salad dressing, 1 serving
   (30 g) 1

143

Dressings, salad
Weight Watchers (con't) — POINTS

Italian salad dressing, 1 serving (30 g) 0
Ranch salad dressing, 1 serving (30 g) 1
Ranch salad dressing, 1 serving (21 g) 1

Wish-Bone

Balsamic vinaigrette, 2 Tbsp 2
Berry vinaigrette, 2 Tbsp...........................1
Chunky blue cheese, 2 Tbsp.....................4
Classic Caesar, 2 Tbsp 3
Classic house Italian, 2 Tbsp 4
Creamy Caesar, 2 Tbsp 5
Creamy Italian, 2 Tbsp..............................3
Deluxe French, 2 Tbsp 3
Italian, 2 Tbsp..2
Olive oil vinaigrette, 2 Tbsp 2
Oriental, 2 Tbsp 2
Parmesan & onion, 2 Tbsp 3
Ranch, 2 Tbsp 5
Red wine vinaigrette, 2 Tbsp.....................2
Roasted garlic vinaigrette, 2 Tbsp.............2
Robusto Italian, 2 Tbsp..............................2
Russian, 2 Tbsp..3
Sun-dried tomato vinaigrette, 2 Tbsp.........1
Sweet 'n spicy French, 2 Tbsp....................4
Thousand island, 2 Tbsp 4
White wine vinaigrette, 2 Tbsp...................2

Wish-Bone Fat Free

Chunky blue cheese, 2 Tbsp......................1
Classic Caesar, 2 Tbsp 1
Creamy Italian, 2 Tbsp..............................1
Creamy roasted garlic, 2 Tbsp 1
Deluxe French, 2 Tbsp 0
Honey dijon, 2 Tbsp 1
Italian, 2 Tbsp..0
Parmesan & onion, 2 Tbsp 1
Ranch, 2 Tbsp 1
Red wine vinaigrette, 2 Tbsp.....................1
Sweet 'n spicy French, 2 Tbsp....................1
Thousand island, 2 Tbsp 1

Wish-Bone Lite

Chunky blue cheese, 2 Tbsp......................2
Italian, 2 Tbsp..1
Ranch, 2 Tbsp 3

POINTS

Eclair

Weight Watchers

SmartOnes®

Weight Watchers Smart Ones

Chocolate eclair, 1 serving (59 g) 3

Egg rolls
Chun King

Chicken mini egg rolls, 6 (2.9 oz) 5
Chicken restaurant style egg rolls, 1
(3 oz)..4
Pork & shrimp mini egg rolls, 6 (2.9 oz).....5
Shrimp mini egg rolls, 6 (2.9 oz) 4
Shrimp restaurant style egg rolls, 1
(3 oz)..4

LaChoy

Chicken mini egg rolls, 6 (2.9 oz) 5
Chicken restaurant style egg rolls, 1
(3 oz)..5
Pork & shrimp bite size egg rolls, 12
(3 oz)..5
Pork & shrimp mini egg rolls, 6 (2.9 oz).....5
Pork restaurant style egg rolls, 1 (3 oz)......5
Shrimp mini egg rolls, 6 (2.9 oz) 4
Shrimp restaurant style egg rolls, 1
(3 oz)..4
Sweet & sour chicken restaurant style
egg rolls, 1 (3 oz)...................................5
Vegetable with lobster mini egg rolls,
6 (2.9 oz) 4

Egg substitutes

Beatrice Foods Egg beaters, ¼ cup 1
Morningstar Farms
Better'n eggs, frozen, ¼ cup 0
Scramblers, frozen, ¼ cup.........................1
Second Nature Pasteurized fat free
egg product, ¼ cup................................1

E

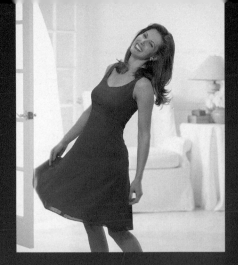

When you're smart, it shows.

Sinfully decadent chocolate eclairs from Smart Ones. So satisfying, you don't have to give up anything to feel this good. Smart Ones. When you're smart, it shows.

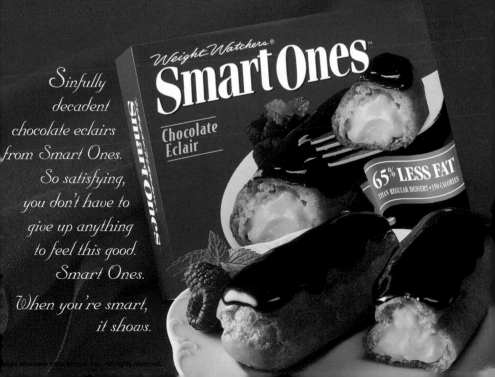

Weight Watchers®
SmartOnes™

Chocolate Eclair

65% LESS FAT
THAN REGULAR DESSERT • 150 CALORIES

Enchiladas
Patio Family Pack
Beef enchilads, 2 enchiladas (5.7 oz).........4
Cheese enchiladas, 2 enchiladas (5.7 oz)....4

Enchilada sauce
Chi-Chi's Enchilada sauce, ¼ cup.............1
Old El Paso
Enchilada sauce, hot, ¼ cup 0
Enchilada sauce, medium, ¼ cup...............0
Enchilada sauce, mild, ¼ cup 0
Green chilli enchilada sauce, ¼ cup...........1

Energy bars
Gatorade
Chocolate, 1 (65 g) 5
Mixed berry, 1 (65 g)..................................5
Orange, 1 (65 g) 5
Peanut butter, 1 (65 g) 5
PowerBar
Essentials energy bar, 1 (53 g) 3
Harvest energy bar, 1 (65 g) 4
Performance energy bar, 1 (65 g) 4
Protein plus protein bar, 1 (78 g)...............6

English muffins
Cobblestone Mill
Cinnamon raisin, 1 muffin (57 g) 2
Honey wheat, 1 muffin (57 g) 2
Original, 1 muffin (57 g)............................2

Falafel
Golden Grain Near East Falafel,
¼ cup 1

Figs
Tropical Nut & Fruit
Adriatic figs, ¼ cup 1
Black mission fig, ¼ cup.............................1
Calimyrna figs, ¼ cup................................1
Turkish figs, 2 pieces 2

Filberts
Tropical Nut & Fruit
Blanched filberts, 1 oz...............................5
Natural filberts, 1 oz 5

Fillo products
The Fillo Factory
Fillo dough, 3 sheets (57 g) 3
Fillo dough made with organic spelt
flour, 3 sheets (57 g) 3
Fillo hors d'oeuvre, portabello
mushroom & onion, 4 pieces (93 g) 4
Fillo hors d'oeuvre, potato & herb,
4 pieces (93 g) 5
Fillo hors d'oeuvre, spinach & cheese,
4 pieces (99 g) 4
Fillo hors d'oeuvre, spinach & tofu,
4 pieces (99 g) 4
Fillo hors d'oeuvre, vegetable medley,
4 pieces (93 g) 4
Fillo hors d'oeuvre, wild mushroom
& onion, 4 pieces (93 g) 4
Whole wheat fillo dough, 3 sheets
(57 g) 3

Fish
Fishery Products Healthy Bake
Bake 'r broil breaded fish fillets,
1 serving (112 g) 2
Schwan's
Alaskan BBQ salmon fillets, 1 fillet
with sauce (140 g)..................................3
Alaskan cod fillets, 4 oz.............................2
Alaskan ocean perch fillets, 4 oz 2
Alaskan salmon fillets (fillet only), 4 oz 2
Battercrisp cod, 1 piece (56 g) 3
Blue hake loins, 4 oz 1
Brd. blue hake portions, 1 piece (85 g) 4
Catfish fingers, 4 pieces raw (112 g) 4
Haddock squares, 1 piece (112 g) 4
Haddock sticks, 3 (84 g) 3

Flax seeds
Tropical Nut & Fruit Whole flax
seeds, 2 tsp...2

Flour
All Trump Flour, ¼ cup 1
Betty Crocker
All purpose, ¼ cup 2
Better for bread wheat blend, ¼ cup.........2

F

Organic – all purpose, ¼ cup 2
Self rising, ¼ cup 2
Unbleached, ¼ cup 2
Betty Crocker Softasilk Velvet cake
  flour, ¼ cup 2
La Piña Flour, ¼ cup 2
Martha White
All purpose bleached, ¼ cup.....................2
Self rising bleached, ¼ cup 2
Omega All purpose bleached, ¼ cup 2
Pillsbury
All purpose bleached, ¼ cup.....................2
All purpose unbleached, ¼ cup 2
Bread, ¼ cup 2
Medium rye, ¼ cup 2
Rye-wheat bohemian style, ¼ cup..............2
Self rising bleached, ¼ cup 2
Self rising unbleached, ¼ cup 2
Shake & blend, ¼ cup 2
Whole wheat, ¼ cup 2
Red Band
All purpose, ¼ cup 2
Better for bread, ¼ cup 2
Bread flour, ¼ cup 2
Self-rising, ¼ cup 2
Robin Hood
All purpose, ¼ cup 2
Self-rising, ¼ cup 2
Unbleached, ¼ cup 2
Whole wheat, ¼ cup 1
Wondra Flour, ¼ cup 2

Frankfurters
Boar's Head
Beef frankfurters – skinless, 1 (45 g) 3
Cocktail beef frankfurters, 5 (55 g)............5
Lite beef frankfurters, 1 (45 g) 2
Natural casing beef frankfurter giants,
  1 (57 g) 4
Natural casing pork & beef frankfurters,
  1 (57 g) 4
Pork & beef frankfurter, 1 (57 g) 4
Pork & beef frankfurter giants – natural
  casing, 1 (57 g) 4

Butterball Bunsize franks, 1 frank
  (57 g) 3
Healthy Choice
Low fat (bunsize) franks, 1 frank (50 g) 2
Low fat franks, 1 frank (40 g) 1
Low fat franks, 1 frank (50 g) 2
Healthy Choice Savory Selections
Low fat beef franks, 1 frank (50 g)..........2
Hebrew National
97% fat free beef franks, 1 (49 g) 1
Beef franks, 1 (49 g) 4
Dinner beef franks, 1 (113 g) 10
Reduced fat beef franks, 1 (48 g) 3
Louis Rich
Bun-length franks, made with turkey
  and chicken, 1 (57 g) 3
Cheese franks, made with turkey and
  chicken, 1 (45 g) 2
Franks, made with turkey and chicken,
  1 (43 g) 2
Franks, made with turkey and chicken,
  1 (45 g) 2
Oscar Mayer
Cheese hot dogs, made with pork,
  turkey & beef, 1 (45 g) 4
Franks, beef, 1 (45 g)................................4
Franks, beef jumbo, 1 (57 g) 5
Franks, beef, bun-length, 1 (57 g)..............5
Franks, beef, light, 1 (57 g) 3
Wieners, bun-length, made with pork
  & turkey, 1 (57 g)..................................5
Wieners, jumbo, made with pork &
  turkey, 1 (57 g) 5
Wieners, light, made with pork, turkey
  & beef, 1 (57 g) 3
Wieners, little, made with pork & turkey,
  6 (57 g) 5
Wieners, made with pork & turkey, 1
  (45 g) 4
Oscar Mayer Big & Juicy
Deli style beef franks, 1 (76 g) 6
Hot 'n spicy wieners, 1 (76 g)....................6
Original beef franks, 1 (76 g) 7

F

Frankfurters, Oscar Mayer
Big & Juicy (con't)   POINTS
Original wieners, 1 (76 g) 7
Quarter pound beef franks, 1 (114 g) 10
Smokie links wieners, 1 (76 g) 6

Oscar Mayer Free
Beef franks, 1 (50 g) 1
Hot dogs, 1 (50 g)....................................1

French fries
Ore-Ida
Fast food fries, 35 pieces (84 g) 3
Golden crinkles, 13 pieces (84 g) 2
Golden fries, 13 pieces (84 g) 2
Golden twirls, 17 pieces (84 g) 3
Shoestrings, 40 pieces (84 g) 3
Steak fries, 7 pieces (84 g)........................2

Schwan's Oven ready french fries, 3 oz 3

Frosting
Betty Crocker
Coconut pecan, mix, 3 Tbsp 3
Coconut pecan, prepared, 2 Tbsp 4
Fluffy white, mix, 3 Tbsp...........................2

Betty Crocker Whipped Deluxe
Chocolate, 2 Tbsp 2
Cream cheese, 2 Tbsp...............................2
Fluffy white, 2 Tbsp..................................2
Lemon, 2 Tbsp 2
Milk chocolate, 2 Thsp..............................2
Strawberry, 2 Tbsp 2
Vanilla, 2 Tbsp...2

Pillsbury Creamy Supreme
Banana creme, 2 Tbsp 4
Chocolate, 2 Tbsp 3
Chocolate fudge, 2 Tbsp 3
Chocolate mocha, 2 Tbsp 3
Coconut pecan, 2 Tbsp 4
Cookies & creme, 2 Tbsp 4
Cream cheese, 2 Tbsp...............................4
French vanilla, 2 Tbsp 4
Funfetti Easter, 2 Tbsp 4
Funfetti Halloween, 2 Tbsp 4
Funfetti holiday, 2 Tbsp 4
Funfetti pink vanilla, 2 Tbsp......................4
Funfetti valentines, 2 Tbsp 4
Funfetti vanilla, 2 Tbsp 4

POINTS

Hot fudge, 2 Tbsp 3
Lemon creme, 2 Tbsp 4
Milk chocolate, 2 Tbsp...............................3
Strawberry creme, 2 Tbsp 4
Vanilla, 2 Tbsp...4

Rich & Creamy
Butter cream, 2 Tbsp 3
Cherry, 2 Tbsp..3
Chocolate, 2 Tbsp 3
Chocolate w/ stars, 2 Tbsp 3
Coconut pecan, 2 Tbsp 3
Cream cheese, 2 Tbsp...............................3
Dark chocolate, 2 Tbsp 3
French vanilla, 2 Tbsp 3
Lemon, 2 Tbsp 3
Milk chocolate, 2 Tbsp...............................3
Milk chocolate w/ Reese's toppers,
  2 Tbsp...3
Rainbow chip, 2 Tbsp 3
Sour cream chocolate, 2 Tbsp 3
Sour cream white, 2 Tbsp 3
Strawberry cream cheese, 2 Tbsp 3
Vanilla, 2 Tbsp...3
Vanilla w/ stars, 2 Tbsp............................3
Vanilla with Hershey's toppers, 2 Tbsp.......3
White chocolate, 2 Tbsp 3

Sweet 'N Low
Chocolate frosting mix, 2 Tbsp 2
White frosting mix, 2 Tbsp........................1

Sweet Rewards
Chocolate, 2 Tbsp 3
Milk chocolate, 2 Tbsp...............................3
Vanilla, 2 Tbsp 3

Fruit & nut mix
EXPRESSnacks
Athlete's mix, ¼ cup 3
California mix, ¼ cup 2
Raisin nut mix, ¼ cup 3
Raisins & cashews, ¼ cup..........................2
Tropical snack, ¼ cup................................3

Tropical Nut & Fruit
Bazaar mix, ⅓ cup 2
Berry good, 1 oz 3

Berry natural, 30 g 3
Berry nutty, 1 oz 3
California ambrosia, ¼ cup.......................2
California mix, 1 oz...................................3
Diet delight, ¼ cup 3
Hawaiian mix, 1 oz 2
Hi-energy mix, 1 oz..................................2
Nutty tyme, 1 oz 4
Sienna cream crunch, 30 g 3
Sunburst, 1 oz 4
Sundance mix, 30 g 4
Tahitian gold, ¼ cup 3
Trail mix, 1 oz..3
Tropical's treasure, 1 oz...........................2

Fruit butters
Harry & David
Apple butter, 1 Tbsp................................1
Apricot butter, 1 Tbsp.............................1
Cherry butter, 1 Tbsp..............................1
Peach butter, 1 Tbsp...............................1
Pumpkin butter, 1 Tbsp...........................1

Smucker's
Cider apple butter, 1 Tbsp.......................1
Peach butter, 1 Tbsp...............................1
Spiced apple butter, 1 Tbsp.....................1

Fruit drinks
Capri Sun
Fruit punch, 1 (200 ml)............................2
Grape, 1 (200 ml) 2
Maui punch, 1 (200 ml)............................2
Mountain cooler, 1 (200 ml) 2
Orange, 1 (200 ml)...................................2
Pacific cooler, 1 (200 ml) 2
Red berry, 1 (200 ml) 2
Safari punch, 1 (200 ml)...........................2
Strawberry cooler, 1 (200 ml)...................2
Strawberry-kiwi, 1 (200 ml) 2
Surfer cooler, 1 (200 ml) 2
Wild cherry, 1 (200 ml) 2

Fruitopia
Berry lemonade, 8 fl oz 2
Fruit integration, 8 fl oz...........................2

Kiwiberry ruckus, 8 fl oz 2
Peachberry quencher, 8 fl oz 2
Strawberry passion awareness, 8 fl oz 2
The grape beyond, 8 fl oz 2
Tremendously tangerine, 8 fl oz 2
Tropical temptation, 8 fl oz.......................2

Koala
Black cherry, 1 bottle (11 fl oz) 3
Cranberry raspberry, 1 bottle (11 fl oz) 2
Grapefruit kiwi lime, 1 can (12 fl oz) 3
Orange mango, 1 can (12 fl oz) 2
Orange mango, 1 bottle (11 fl oz) 2
Orange passion fruit, 8 fl oz 2
Raspberry guava, 1 bottle (11 fl oz) 2
Raspberry guava, 1 can (12 fl oz)..............3
Strawberry kiwi peach, 8 fl oz...................2

Minute Maid
Concord punch, 8 fl oz 2
Cranberry apple raspberry blend, 8 fl oz 2
Fruit punch, 8 fl oz...................................2

Minute Maid Premium
Berry punch with vitamin c and
   calcium added, 1 drink box (200 ml) 2
Berry punch with vitamin c and
   calcium added, 8 fl oz 2
Citrus punch with vitamin c and
   calcium added, 8 fl oz 2
Fruit punch with vitamin c and
   calcium added, 1 drink box (200 ml) 2
Fruit punch with vitamin c and calcium
   added, 8 fl oz 2
Grape juice cocktail with vitamin c and
   calcium added, 8 fl oz...........................2
Grape punch with vitamin c and
   calcium added, 8 fl oz 2
Tropical punch with vitamin c and
   calcium added, 1 drink box (200 ml) 2
Tropical punch with vitamin c and
   calcium added, 8 fl oz 2

F

Ocean Spray Light
Cranberry juice cocktail, 8 fl oz 1
CranGrape, 8 fl oz....................................1
CranRaspberry, 8 fl oz 1

Schwan's Frozen Concentrates
Cranberry juice cocktail, prepared,
    1 cup 3
Lemonade, prepared, 1 cup 3
Orange juice with calcium, prepared,
    1 cup 2
Orange juice, prepared, 1 cup 2
Wild berry blend, prepared, 1 cup 2

Schwan's Non-Frozen Concentrates
Apple cherry berry, prepared, 1cup 2
Apple cranberry, prepared, 1 cup...............2
Apple, prepared, 1 cup 2
Black raspberry, prepared, 1 cup 2
Blue raspberry, prepared, 1 cup.................2
Fruit punch, prepared, 1 cup 2
Guava mango, prepared, 1 cup 2
Kiwi strawberry, prepared, 1 cup...............2
Orange strawberry banana, prepared,
    1 cup 2
Pineapple orange, prepared, 1 cup 2

Snapple
Attitude – persimmon, 1 serving
    (8 fl oz)..2
Bali blast, 1 can (11½ fl oz) 3
Bali blast, 1 serving (8 fl oz) 2
Black & blue berry, 1 WhipperSnapple
    (10 fl oz)..3
Cranberry grapefruit, 1 plastic container
    (8 fl oz)..2
Cranberry raspberry, 1 serving (8 fl oz) 2
Cranberry raspberry, 1 can (11½ fl oz) 3
Diet cranberry raspberry, 1 serving
    (8 fl oz)..0

Diet kiwi strawberry, 1 serving (8 fl oz) 0
Diet orange carrot, 1 serving (8 fl oz) 0
Diet ruby red, 1 serving (8 fl oz)................0
Diet white grape, 1 serving (8 fl oz) 0
Earth – grape cranberry, 1 serving
    (8 fl oz)..3
Fire – dragonfruit, 1 serving (8 fl oz) 2
Fruit punch, 1 serving (8 fl oz) 2
Fruit punch, 1 can (11½ fl oz) 3
Grapeade, 1 serving (8 fl oz)......................2
Grapeade, 1 can (11½ fl oz) 3
Gravity – carrot infusion, 1 serving
    (8 fl oz)..2
Island punch, 1 plastic container
    (8 fl oz)..2
Kiwi strawberry, 1 serving (8 fl oz) 2
Kiwi strawberry, 1 can (11½ fl oz) 3
Mango madness, 1 can (11½ fl oz) 3
Mango madness, 1 serving (8 fl oz)...........2
Meteor – tangelo, 1 serving (8 fl oz) 2
Orange dream, 1 WhipperSnapple
    (10 fl oz)..3
Orange tropic, 1 serving (8 fl oz)...............2
Orangeade, 1 serving (8 fl oz)....................2
Peach mango, 1 WhipperSnapple
    (10 fl oz)..3
Pineapple orange, 1 WhipperSnapple
    (10 fl oz)..3
Power berry, 1 WhipperSnapple
    (10 fl oz)..3
Power citrus, 1 WhipperSnapple
    (10 fl oz)..3
Rain – agave cactus, 1 serving (8 fl oz) 2
Raspberry peach, 1 serving (8 fl oz)...........2
Raspberry peach, 1 can (11½ fl oz) 3
Sky– passionfruit, 1 serving (8 fl oz)..........2
Strawberry banana, 1 WhipperSnapple
    (10 fl oz)..3
Summer peach, 1 (8 fl oz)..........................2
Sun – starfruit orange, 1 serving
    (8 fl oz)..2
Wild cherry, 1 WhipperSnapple (10 fl oz) 3

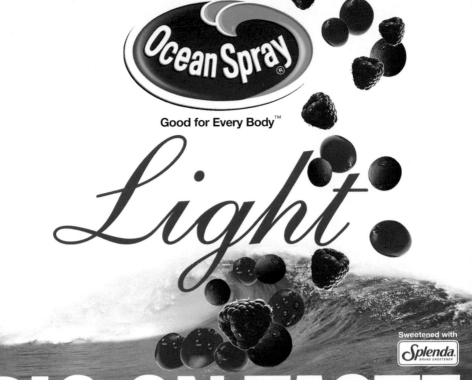

Ocean Spray®

Good for Every Body™

Light

Sweetened with **Splenda®** BRAND SWEETENER

BIG ON TASTE

SMALL ON CALORIES (2/3 FEWER)

Ocean Spray LIGHT has all the unique taste and goodness of
Ocean Spray cranberries, but with 2/3 fewer calories, and
only 10 grams of carbohydrates and sugar per 8 oz. serving. All that, plus
LIGHT cranberry juice cocktail helps you maintain your urinary tract health.

ONLY ONE DELICIOUS POINT®

Cranberry Juice
Cocktail

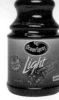
Cran•Grape®
Grape Cranberry
Juice Drink

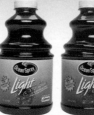
Cran•Raspberry®
Cranberry Raspberry
Juice Drink

For more information
on Ocean Spray® Juices
and Juice Drinks
visit us at

www.oceanspray.com

or call toll-free
1-800-662-3263
Mon-Fri, 9AM-4PM EST.

©2000 Ocean Spray Cranberries, Inc.

Fruit drinks (con't)   **POINTS**

Twister

Grape berry, 8 fl oz 3
Orange cranberry, 8 fl oz ....•........3
Orange, strawberry, banana, 8 fl oz...........3

V8 Splash

Apple medley, 1 cup 2
Berry blend, 1 cup 2
Citrus blend, 1 cup 2
Diet berry blend, 1 cup 0
Diet strawberry kiwi, 1 cup 0
Diet tropical blend, 1 cup.........................0
Fruit medley, 1 cup 2
Grape blend, 1 cup.................................2
Island blend, 1 cup 2
Kiwi melon, 1 cup 2
Strawberry banana, 1 cup 2
Strawberry kiwi, 1 cup............................2
Tropical blend, 1 cup 2

Fruit juices, combined

Dole

Orange peach mango, 8 fl oz....................2
Orange, strawberry, banana, 8 fl oz...........2
Pine-orange banana, 8 fl oz......................2
Pine-orange strawberry, 8 fl oz 3

Minute Maid Premium

Cherry with vitamin c and calcium
  added, 1 drink box (200 ml) 2
Grape with vitamin c and calcium
  added, 1 drink box (200 ml) 2
Orange passionfruit guava with calcium
  added, 8 fl oz 3
Orange tangerine with calcium added,
  8 fl oz..2
Ruby red grapefruit blend with calcium
  added, 8 fl oz 2

Snapple

Snapple farms cranberry apple, 1
  (12 fl oz)..4
Vitamin supreme, 1 (12 fl oz)....................3

Tropicana Pure Tropics

Orange kiwi passion, 8 fl oz 2
Orange peach mango, 8 fl oz....................2

POINTS

Orange pineapple, 8 fl oz 2
Orange, strawberry, banana, 8 fl oz...........2

Tropicana Season's Best

Cranberry medley, 8 fl oz.........................2
Fruit medley, 8 fl oz................................3
Orange pineapple, 8 fl oz 2
Strawberry orange, 8 fl oz 3

Fruit salad

Dole Tropical fruit salad in light syrup,
  canned, ½ cup.......................................1

Fruit snacks

Betty Crocker

Bugs Bunny, 1 pouch (25 g).....................2
Hawaiian punch, 1 pouch (25 g) 2
Lucky Charms, 1 pouch (25 g)...................2
Mini handouts, Scooby Doo, 2 pouches
  (23 g) 2
Pokemon, 1 pouch (25 g).........................2
Scooby Doo, 1 pouch (25 g).....................2
Shark bites, 1 pouch (25 g).......................2
Trix, 1 pouch (25 g).................................2
XL pouch, Bugs Bunny, 10 pieces (30 g).....2
XL pouch, Scooby Doo, 10 pieces (30 g) 2
Farley's Strawberry, 1 pouch (26 g) 2

Fruit by the Foot

Berry tie dye, 1 roll (21 g)........................2
Cherry, 1 roll (21 g).................................2
Color by the foot, 1 roll (21 g) 2
Endless party, 1 roll (21 g) 2
Flavor wave, 1 roll (21 g)..........................2
Pokemon, 1 roll (21 g).............................2
Strawberry, 1 roll (21 g)...........................2
Watermelon, 1 roll (21 g) 2

Fruit Gushers

Fruitomic punch, 1 pouch (25 g) 2
Sour berry blast, 1 pouch (25 g)................2
Strawberry splash, 1 pouch (25 g).............2
Tropical punch, 1 pouch (25 g)..................2
Watermelon blast, 1 pouch (25 g) 2
Wild cherry, 1 pouch (25 g)......................2

Fruit Roll-Ups

Cherry, 1 (14 g)......................................1
Crazy colors, 1 (14 g) 1

Double fruity, 1 (14 g) 1
Fun 'n games, 1 (14 g) 1
Galaxy blast, 1 (14 g)...............................1
Hot colors, 1 (14 g) 1
Mini handouts, strawberry, 2 (21 g)...........2
Peel 'n build, 1 (14 g) 1
Strawberry, 1 (14 g) 1
Stretchy faces, 1 (14 g).............................1
XL pouch – fun 'n games, 2 (34 g) 3
XL pouch – strawberry, 2 (34 g) 3
XL pouch peel 'n build, 2 (34 g) 3

Fruit String Thing
Bugs Bunny, 1 pouch (21 g).....................2
Scobby Doo!, 1 pouch (21 g) 2
Sneaky stripes, 1 pouch (21 g) 2
Strawberry split, 1 pouch (21 g) 2

Sunbelt Snacks & Cereals Fruit
jammers, 1 (28 g) 2

Fruit spreads
Brummel & Brown
Awesome apple & cinnamon, 1 Tbsp.........1
Blissfully blueberry, 1 Tbsp......................1
Simply strawberry, 1 Tbsp 1

Fruit, dried, mixed
Sunsweet
Orchard mix, ¼ cup 1
Tropical mix, ¼ cup.................................2

Tropical Nut & Fruit
Dale coconut roll, 1½ pieces (40 g) 2
Fruit medley, 40 g 2
Imperial mixed fruit, ¼ cup.......................1
Tropical medley, 40 g 2
Tropical mixed fruit, ¼ cup 2

Fruit, mixed
Del Monte
Chunky mixed fruits in heavy syrup,
½ cup..2
Fruit cocktail in heavy syrup, ½ cup..........2
Fruit naturals chunky mixed fruits in
fruit juice, ½ cup...................................1
Fruit naturals fruit cocktail in fruit
juices, ½ cup 1

Fruit naturals mixed fruit in fruit juices,
1 serving (4-oz cup) 1
Lie chunky mixed fruits in extra light
syrup, ½ cup...1
Lite fruit cocktail in extra light syrup,
½ cup 1
Tropical fruit salad in light syrup w/
passion fruit juice, ½ cup 1
Tropical fruit salad in pineapple &
passion fruit juices, ½ cup 1
Very cherry mixed fruit, 1 serving
(124 g) 2

Del Monte Fruit Cups
Fruit naturals mixed fruit in fruit juices,
4-oz cup 1
Lite mixed fruit in extra light syrup,
4-oz cup 1
Mixed fruit in heavy syrup, 4-oz cup..........2

Del Monte Fruit Rageous Crazy
cherry mixed fruit in cherry-flavored
light syrup, 4-oz cup 2

Del Monte Fruit To-Go
Banana berry peaches in natural
flavored light syrup, 4-oz cup 1
Fruity combo – mixed fruit in light
syrup, 4-oz cup......................................1
Wild berry jumble – peaches & pears
in light syrup, 4-oz cup..........................2

Del Monte Orchard Select
California mixed fruit in light syrup,
½ cup 2

EXPRESSnacks
Ambrosia, ¼ cup 2
Fruit fantasy, ¼ cup.................................1

Schwan's
Mixed fruit, frozen, 1¼ cups 1
Triple berry blend, frozen, 1 cup 1
Tropical fruit blend, frozen, 1 cup 1

Traverse Bay Fruit Co.
Berry & cherry blend, ⅓ cup 3
Retail fruit medley, ⅓ cup.........................2

Garlic bread

Marie Callender's

Original garlic bread, 1 piece (12 oz).........4

Parmesan & Romano garlic bread,
  1 piece (12 oz) 4

Gelatin desserts

Jell-O

Apricot, prepared, ½ cup 2

Berry black, prepared, ½ cup 2

Berry blue, prepared, ½ cup 2

Black cherry, prepared, ½ cup 2

Cherry, prepared, ½ cup 2

Cranberry raspberry, prepared, ½ cup 2

Cranberry strawberry, ½ cup 2

Cranberry, prepared, ½ cup........................2

Grape, prepared, ½ cup 2

Jell-O 1-2-3 brand strawberry, prepared,
  ⅔ cup..3

Lemon, prepared, ½ cup 2

Lime, prepared, ½ cup................................2

Mango, prepared, ½ cup 2

Mixed fruit, prepared, ½ cup 2

Orange, prepared, ½ cup 2

Peach passion fruit, prepared, ½ cup 2

Peach, prepared, ½ cup 2

Pineapple, prepared, ½ cup 2

Raspberry, prepared, ½ cup 2

Sparkling white grape, prepared, ½ cup.....2

Strawberry banana, ½ cup..........................2

Strawberry kiwi, prepared, ½ cup...............2

Strawberry, prepared, ½ cup......................2

Sugar-free cherry, prepared, ½ cup 0

Sugar-free cranberry, prepared, ½ cup 0

Sugar-free lemon, prepared, ½ cup............0

Sugar-free lime, prepared, ½ cup...............0

Sugar-free mixed fruit, prepared, ½ cup.....0

Sugar-free orange, prepared, ½ cup...........0

Sugar-free raspberry, prepared, ½ cup 0

Sugar-free strawberry banana, prepared,
  ½ cup 0

Sugar-free strawberry kiwi, prepared,
  ½ cup 0

Sugar-free strawberry, prepared, ½ cup 0

Sugar-free watermelon, prepared,
  ½ cup 0

Watermelon, prepared, ½ cup 2

Wild strawberry, prepared, ½ cup..............2

Jell-O Gelatin Snacks

Berry black, 1 (99 g)..................................1

Berry blue, 1 (99 g) 1

Cherry, 1 (99 g)..1

Orange, 1 (99 g) 1

Orange-strawberry-banana, 1 (99 g) 1

Raspberry, 1 (99 g).....................................1

Rhymin' lymon, 1 (99 g) 1

Strawberry, 1 (99 g) 1

Tropical fruit punch, 1 (99 g)......................1

Wild watermelon, 1 (99 g)..........................1

JELL-O®

BRAND

Jell-O Sugar Free Low Calorie
Gelatin Snacks

Orange, 1 (92 g) 0

Raspberry, 1 (92 g).....................................0

Strawberry, 1 (92 g) 0

Strawberry-kiwi, 1 (92 g)...........................0

Tropical berry, 1 (92 g) 0

Kraft Handi-Snacks

Blue raspberry, 1 (99 g) 2

Cherry, 1 (99 g)..2

Orange, 1 (99 g) 2

Strawberry, 1 (99 g) 2

Payaso Gelatin dessert, ⅛ package
  (25 g) 2

Ginger

Tropical Nut & Fruit Ginger,
  Australian, 1 oz 2

G

Your taste buds won't know what's missing.

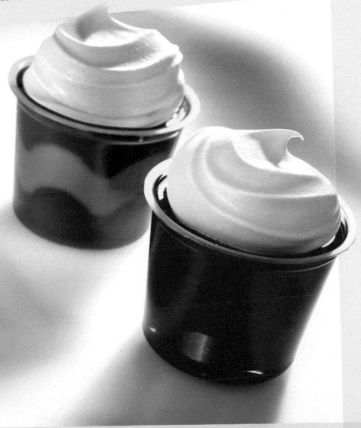

Fat Free Jell-O® meets Cool Whip® Free.™

Now, put them together for a snack so indulgent,
your taste buds won't know what's missing*

JELL-O Sugar Free Gelatin Snack: 0 **POINTS**, JELL-O Fat Free
Pudding Snack: 2 **POINTS**, COOL WHIP Free: 0 **POINTS**

*Pudding or Gelatin Snack with Topping is less than one gram of fat per serving.
© 2000 Kraft Foods, Inc.

Glazed fruit
Tropical Nut & Fruit
Diced orange peel glaze, 2 Tbsp................1
Glazed diced citron, 2 Tbsp......................1
Glazed green cherries, 1 piece (6 g)..........0
Glazed pineapple slice, ½ piece (28 g).......2
Glazed red cherries, 1 piece (5 g)..............0
Mello mix, 1 Tbsp 1

Granola bars
Health Valley Fat Free
Blueberry, 1 (42 g) 2
Chocolate chip, 1 (42 g) 2
Date almond, 1 (42 g) 2
Raisin, 1 (42 g) 2
Raspberry, 1 (42 g)...................................2
Strawberry, 1 (42 g) 2

Health Valley Moist & Chewy
Apple granola bar, 1 (29 g)........................2
Berry granola bar, 1 (29 g)........................2
Peanut granola bar, 1 (29 g) 2

Nature Valley
Cinnamon, 2 (42 g)...................................4
Oats 'n honey, 2 (42 g)..............................4
Peanut butter, 2 (42 g) 4

Quaker Oats
Chewy granola bar – chocolate chip,
  1 (28 g) 3
Chewy granola bar – low fat chocolate
  chunk, 1 (28 g)......................................2
Chewy granola bar – low fat cookies
  and cream, 1 (28 g) 2
Chewy granola bar – low fat oatmeal
  raisin, 1 (28 g)......................................2
Chewy granola bars – low fat s'mores,
  1 (28 g) 2
Granola dipps – chocolate chip, 1
  (35 g) 4
Low fat graham slam chocolate chip
  graham chewy granola bars, 1 (28 g)......2
Low fat graham slam cinnamon graham
  chewy granola bars, 1 (28 g) 2

Low fat graham slam honey graham
  chewy granola bars, 1 (28 g) 2
Low fat graham slam peanut butter
  graham chewy granola bars, 1 (28 g)......2
Reduced fat peanut butter chocolate
  chunk chewy granola bar, 1 (28 g)..........2

Sunbelt Snacks & Cereals
Chocolate chip chewy granola bars,
  1 (35 g) 3
Golden almond chewy granola bars,
  1 (28 g) 3
Oats & honey chewy granola bars,
  1 (28 g) 3

Grape juice
Tropicana Season's Best Grape
  juice, 1 can (11½ fl oz)...........................5

Grapefruit
Chiquita Grapefruit, ½ medium (154 g)....0
Dole Grapefruit, ½.....................................0

Grapefruit juice
Florida's Natural Ruby red grapefruit
  juice, 8 oz 2
Minute Maid Pink grapefruit blend,
  8 fl oz..2

Minute Maid Premium
Grapefruit juice with calcium added,
  8 fl oz..2

Tropicana Pure Premium
Golden grapefruit, 8 fl oz 2
Ruby red grapefruit, 1 carton (6 fl oz)........1
Ruby red grapefruit, 1 bottle (13 fl oz) 3
Ruby red grapefruit – Grovestand,
  8 fl oz..2
Ruby red grapefruit – original, 8 fl oz........2

Tropicana Season's Best
Grapefruit juice, 8 fl oz.............................2
Grapefruit juice, 10 fl oz...........................2
Grapefuit juice, 1 bottle (7 oz) 2

Grapes
Chiquita Grapes, 1½ cups 2
Dole Grapes, 1½ cups 1

G

Gravy

Dawn Fresh Brown gravy, ¼ cup 0

Durkee
  Mushroom in brown gravy mix, 2 tsp........0
  Onion in brown gravy mix, 2 tsp................0

French's
  Country gravy mix, 1⅓ tsp.....................1
  Country gravy, prepared, ¼ cup 1
  Sausage flavored country gravy mix,
    1⅓ Tbsp...1
  Sausage flavored country gravy,
    prepared, ¼ cup 1

Hain Pure Foods
  Brown gravy mix, 2 tsp 0
  Vegetarian chicken flavored gravy mix,
    2 tsp...1

Heinz
  Fat free beef gravy, ¼ cup 0
  Fat free chicken gravy, ¼ cup...................0
  Fat free turkey gravy, ¼ cup....................0

Heinz Homestyle
  Bistro style au jus, ¼ cup........................0
  Classic chicken gravy, ¼ cup 1
  Country sausage, ¼ cup 1
  Mushroom gravy, ¼ cup 1
  Onion gravy, ¼ cup 1
  Pork gravy, ¼ cup 1
  Roasted turkey gravy, ¼ cup 1
  Savory beef gravy, ¼ cup...........................1
  Zesty beef with roasted garlic, ¼ cup 1
  Zesty chicken with roasted garlic, ¼ cup 1

Lawry's Brown gravy mix, 2 tsp..............0

Pillsbury
  Brown, mix, 2 tsp....................................0
  Chicken style, mix, 2 tsp 0
  Homestyle, mix, 2 tsp 0

Tony Chachere's
  Brown gravy mix, 1½ tsp..........................0
  White gravy mix, 2 tsp 0

Gum, chewing

Icebreakers
  Cool mint, 1 (3 g) 0
  Hot cinnamon, 1 (3 g) 0
  Wintergreen, 1 (3 g)..................................0

Lance Double bubble, 1 piece (7 g)...........1

Life Savers
  Bubble yum, 1 piece (8 g).........................1
  Care free, 1 stick (2.5 g) 0

Wrigley's
  Big Red, 1 stick (3 g).................................0
  Doublemint, 1 stick (3 g)...........................0
  Juicy fruit, 1 stick (3 g)...............................0
  Spearmint, 1 stick (3 g)...............................0
  Winterfresh, 1 stick (3 g).............................0

Wrigley's Eclipse
  Spearmint, 2 pieces (3 g)............................0
  Winterfresh, 2 pieces (3 g)...........................0

Wrigley's Extra Sugarfree Gum
  Bubble gum, 1 stick (2.7 g)..........................0
  Cinnamon, 1 stick (2.7 g) 0
  Peppermint, 1 stick (2.7 g)...........................0
  Spearmint, 1 stick (2.7 g).............................0
  Winterfresh, 1 stick (2.7 g)...........................0

Wrigley's Freedent
  Peppermint, 1 stick (3 g) 0
  Spearmint, 1 stick (3 g) 0
  Winterfresh, 1 stick (3 g) 0

H

Ham

Boar's Head
  42% lower sodium ham, 2 oz 1
  Baby maple glazed ham honey coat
    ham, 3 oz...2
  Black forest brand smoked ham, 2 oz........1
  Boneless prosciutto, 1 oz...........................1
  Branded deluxe ham, 2 oz 1
  Cappy brand ham – natural casing, 2 oz 1
  Fiber cappy brand ham, 2 oz.....................1
  Gourmet pepper ham, 2 oz.......................1
  Honey coat, 2 oz.......................................1
  Maple glazed honey coat ham, 2 oz..........1
  Pepper brand ham, 2 oz 2
  Pesto Parmesan oven roasted ham, 2 oz....2
  Piccolo prosciutto boneless, 1 oz...............1
  Ready to eat ham, water added, 3 oz........2
  Rosemary & sundried tomato ham, 2 oz 2

Ham, Boar's Head (con't)   *POINTS*

Seasoned fresh roasted ham, 2 oz.............2
Semi-boneless smoked ham, 3 oz..............3
Skinless/shankless prosciutto, 1 oz 1
Smoked gourmet ham, 2 oz......................1
Smoked Virginia ham, 2 oz 1
Spiced ham, 2 oz 3
Square cappy brand ham, 2 oz.................1
Square cappy brand ham – whole, 2 oz.....1
Tavern ham, 2 oz 1
Virginia brand ham, 2 oz 1
Virginia ready to eat ham, 3 oz.................2
Whole smoked pork shoulder butt
    roast, 3 oz.......................................4

Farmland

97% fat free canned ham, 3 oz.................3
Canned ham patty, 2 oz 4
Cubed ham, 3 oz 3
Ham steak, 2.28 oz 1
Hickory smoked ham, 3 oz.......................6
Hickory smoked spiral sliced ham, 3 oz......4
Honey cured spiral sliced ham, 3 oz 4
Lean pit ham, 3 oz 3
Lower sodium ham, 2 oz 1
Maple river extra lean ham, 3 oz 5
Maple river lean ham, 3 oz......................3
Old fashioned pit ham, 3 oz.....................3
Skinless shankless ham, 3 oz...................3
Special select ham, 2 oz 1
Special select honey ham, 2 oz 0
Hormel Chunk ham, 2 oz.........................2

Louis Rich

Ham baked cooked, water added,
    1 slice (94 g) 2
Turkey ham, 15% water added, 2 oz
    (56 g) 2

Oscar Mayer

Ham slice, dinner, water added, 3 oz 2
Ham steaks, dinner, water added, 1
    (57 g) 1

Oscar Mayer Sweet Morsel

Smoked boneless pork shoulder butt,
    3 oz..5

Perdue

Honey smoked turkey ham, 2 oz 2
Tavern ham, 2 oz 1
Schwan's Ham, 2 oz 1

Hamburger bun

Nature's Own 100% whole grain
    wheat buns, 1 bun (53 g) 2
Wonder White hamburger buns, 1
    (43 g) 2
Wonder Light White hamburger
    buns, 1 (41 g).....................................1

Hash
Hormel

50% less fat corned beef hash, 1 cup........6
Corned beef hash, 1 cup...........................9
Roast beef hash, 1 cup.............................9
Sausage hash, 1 cup 10

Herring
Lascco

Premium roll mop herring, 2 oz.................2
Premium snack bit herring fillet, 2 oz 2
Premium sour cream herring fillet, 2 oz 3
Premium spiced cut herring, 2 oz 3
Premium wine snack herring fillet, 2 oz 2

Nathan's

Herring in cream sauce, ¼ cup 3
Herring in wine sauce, ¼ cup...................2
Herring tasti tidbits, ¼ cup 2
Lunch herring, ¼ cup 3
Old fashioned herring, ¼ cup...................3

Rite

Chopped herring salad, 2 Tbsp.................2
Creamy cajun herring, ¼ cup 3
Creamy dill herring, ¼ cup.......................3
Herring in cream, ¼ cup 3
Herring in mustard sauce, ¼ cup..............3
Herring in wine, ¼ cup 2

Hoisin sauce

House of Tsang Hoisin sauce, 1 tsp 0

Hominy

Faraon White hominy, ½ cup 1

Honey bun
Lance, Honey bun, 1 (85 g).......................7

Honeydew melon
Chiquita Honeydew melon, ¹⁄₁₀ medium
(134 g) 1
Dole Honeydew melon, ¹⁄₁₀ 1

Horseradish
Boar's Head
Horseradish and beets grated in
vinegar, 1 tsp 0
Horseradish grated in vinegar, 1 tsp 0
Pub style horseradish sauce –
squeezable, 1 tsp...................................0
Kraft
Cream style horseradish, 1 tsp 0
Horseradish sauce, 1 tsp............................1
Prepared horseradish, 1 tsp 0
Naturally Fresh Dijon horseradish
sauce, 2 Tbsp..3

Hot dogs (see Frankfurters)

Hot dog buns
Wonder White hot dog buns, 1 2
Wonder Light White hot dog buns,
1 (41 g) 1

Hot dog chili sauce
Austex
Hot dog chili sauce, 1 Tbsp 0
Hot dog chili sauce with onions, 1 Tbsp.....0
Castleberry's Hot dog chili sauce,
1 Tbsp..0

Hot sauce
Trappey's
Bull Louisiana hot sauce, 1 tsp..................0
Chef magic jalapeno sauces, 1 tsp 0
Indi-pep West Indian style hot sauce,
1 tsp...0
Mexi-pep hot sauce, 1 tsp 0
Red devil cayenne pepper sauce, 1 tsp 0
Red devil cayenne pepper sauce,
buffalo-style, 1 tsp.................................0

Hummus
Tribe of Two Sheiks
Bagel, 1 oz 1
Calamata olive, 1 oz 1
Classic, 1 oz 1
Cracked chili pepper, 1 oz.........................1
Dill, 1 oz 1
Forty spices, 1 oz 1
French onion, 1 oz 1
Garden vegetable, 1 oz 1
Jalapeno, 1 oz 1
Lemon, 1 oz 1
Roasted eggplant (baba), 1 oz 1
Roasted garlic, 1 oz 1
Roasted red pepper, 1 oz 1
Scallion, 1 oz...1
Sundried tomato & basil, 1 oz...................1

Hush puppies
Martha White Hushpuppy mix,
prepared, 1 serving (¹⁄₆ package)............7

Ice cream
Ben & Jerry's
Blondies are a swirls best friend,
low fat, ½ cup.......................................4
Bovinity divinity, ½ cup 7
Cherry garcia, ½ cup 7
Chocolate chip cookie dough, ½ cup 7
Chocolate fudge brownie, ½ cup...............6
Chubby hubby, ½ cup...............................9
Chunky monkey, ½ cup 7
Coconut cream pie, low fat, ½ cup 3
Coffee Heath bar crunch, ½ cup................8
Dilbert's world totally nuts, ½ cup.............8
Mint chocolate cookie, ½ cup 7
Mocha latte, low fat, ½ cup 3
New York super fudge chunk, ½ cup 7
Nutty waffle cone, ½ cup 8
Orange and cream, ½ cup 6
Peanut butter cup, ½ cup 9
Phish food, ½ cup 7

Ice Cream, Ben & Jerry's (con't)   POINTS

Pistachio pistachio, ½ cup 6
S'mores, low fat, ½ cup 4
Southern pecan pie, ½ cup 7
Triple caramel chunk, ½ cup 7
Vanilla caramel fudge, ½ cup....................7
Vanilla Heath bar crunch, ½ cup 8
Wavy gravy, ½ cup....................................8
World's best vanilla, ½ cup 6

Ben & Jerry's 2-Twisted Ice Cream

Entangled mints, ½ cup.............................7
Everything but the..., ½ cup 8
From Russia with buzz, ½ cup...................7
Half baked, ½ cup.....................................7
Jerry's jubilee, ½ cup 6
Monkey wrench, ½ cup 8
Pulp addiction, ½ cup 6
Urban jumble, ½ cup.................................8

Ben & Jerry's Special Batch Coffee
hazelnut swirl, ½ cup...............................7

Blue Bell

Banana fudge pie, ½ cup...........................4
Banana nut, ½ cup 4
Banana pudding, ½ cup 5
Banana split, ½ cup 4
Banana split light, ½ cup...........................2
Black walnut, ½ cup 4
Buttered pecan, ½ cup 5
Buttered pecan light, ½ cup......................3
Caramel sundae crunch, ½ cup 5
Cherry vanilla, ½ cup 4
Chocolate almond marshmallow, ½ cup 5
Chocolate cake, ½ cup 5
Chocolate chip, ½ cup 4
Chocolate chip cookie dough, ½ cup 5
Chocolate cream pie, ½ cup......................4
Chocolate pecan cheesecake, ½ cup..........5
Chocolate sundae, ½ cup 4
Coffee, ½ cup 4
Cookies & homemade vanilla, ½ cup..........4
Cookies n cream, ½ cup 4
Cookies n cream light, ½ cup....................3
Double dutch chocolate light, ½ cup 3
Dutch chocolate, ½ cup 4

POINTS

Fudge brownie nut, ½ cup.........................4
Fudge divinity, ½ cup 5
Homemade vanilla light, ½ cup.................3
Lemon, ½ cup...4
Milk chocolate, ½ cup 4
Mint chocolate chip, ½ cup.......................4
Natural vanilla bean, ½ cup.......................5
Neopolitan, ½ cup 4
No sugar fat free vanilla bean, ½ cup........2
No sugar lowfat cookies 'n cream, ½ cup ...2
No sugar lowfat country vanilla, ½ cup 2
No sugar lowfat rocky road, ½ cup.............2
Peaches & homemade vanilla, ½ cup 4
Peaches & homemade vanilla light,
  ½ cup 3
Pecan pralines 'n cream, ½ cup.................5
Peppermint, ½ cup 4
Pineapple & homemade vanilla, ½ cup......4
Pistachio almond, ½ cup 4
Rocky road, ½ cup 4
Rocky road light, ½ cup.............................2
Strawberries & homemade vanilla,
  ½ cup 4
Strawberries & homemade vanilla
  light, ½ cup 3
Strawberry, ½ cup 4
Strawberry cheesecake, ½ cup 4
Vanilla, ½ cup 4
White chocolate almond, ½ cup..................5

Breyers

Butter almond, ½ cup 4
Butter pecan, ½ cup..................................5
Caramel praline crunch, ½ cup..................4
Chocolate, ½ cup 4
Chocolate chip, ½ cup 4
Chocolate chip cookie dough, ½ cup 4
Chocolate rainbow, ½ cup 3
Coffee, ½ cup 4
Cookies in cream, ½ cup 4
Dulce de leche, ½ cup 4
French vanilla, ½ cup 4
Fruit rainbow, ½ cup 3

Mint chocolate chip, ½ cup......................4

Natural cherry vanilla, ½ cup 4

Natural peach, ½ cup 3

Natural strawberry, ½ cup 3

Natural vanilla, ½ cup 4

Natural vanilla & chocolate, ½ cup............4

Natural vanilla & orange sherbet, ½ cup 3

Rocky road, ½ cup 4

Vanilla fudge twirl, ½ cup 4

Vanilla, chocolate, strawberry, ½ cup........4

Viennetta, triple chocolate, 1 slice
(68 g) 5

Viennetta, vanilla, 1 piece (74 g)...............6

Viennetta, vanilla, 1 slice (68 g) 5

Breyers All Natural Calcium Rich

Natural vanilla, ½ cup...............................3

Breyers All Natural Light

French chocolate, ½ cup 3

French vanilla, ½ cup 3

Mint chocolate chip, ½ cup......................3

Natural vanilla, ½ cup 3

Pralines & caramel with pecans &
almonds, ½ cup 3

Rocky road, ½ cup 3

Strawberry, ½ cup 3

Vanilla, chocolate, strawberry, ½ cup........3

Breyers Fat Free Vanilla, ½ cup.............2

Breyers Homemade

Butter pecan, ½ cup.................................4

Double chocolate fudge, ½ cup.................4

Fudge brownie, ½ cup..............................4

Neapolitan, ½ cup 4

Vanilla, ½ cup 4

Breyers Ice Cream Parlor

Apple pie with cinnamon, ½ cup...............4

Banana split, ½ cup 4

Black forest, ½ cup 4

Candy bar sundae, ½ cup 4

Chocolate ice cream with Hershey's
chocolate almond bar pieces, ½ cup 4

Coffee & cream, ½ cup.............................4

Double chocolate malt, ½ cup 4

English toffee, ½ cup 4

Ice cream sandwich, ½ cup......................4

Marble mint chip, ½ cup 4

Mississippi mud, ½ cup 4

Peanut butter ice cream with Reese's
peanut butter cup pieces, ½ cup 4

Raspberry cobbler, ½ cup.........................4

Strawberry shortcake, ½ cup.....................4

Vanilla ice cream with Chips Ahoy,
½ cup 4

Vanilla ice cream with Oreo cookie
pieces, ½ cup 4

Breyers Light Vanilla, ½ cup 3

Breyers No Sugar Added

Vanilla, ½ cup 2

Vanilla Fudge Twirl, ½ cup.......................2

Vanilla, chocolate, strawberry, ½ cup.........2

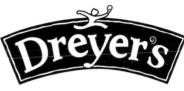

Dreyer's

Almond praline, ½ cup 4

Black cherry vanilla, ½ cup 4

Butter pecan, ½ cup.................................4

Chocolate, ½ cup.....................................4

Chocolate chips!, ½ cup...........................4

Coffee, ½ cup 3

Cookie dough, ½ cup 4

Cookies 'n cream, ½ cup 4

Double fudge brownie, ½ cup...................4

Dulce de leche, ½ cup 4

French vanilla, ½ cup 4

Ice cream sandwich, ½ cup......................4

Mint chocolate chips!, ½ cup....................4

Mocha almond fudge, ½ cup 4

Neapolitan, ½ cup 3

Real strawberry, ½ cup.............................3

Rocky road, ½ cup 4

Toasted almond, ½ cup 4

Triple chocolate thunder, ½ cup 4

Ice Cream, Dreyer's (con't)   POINTS

Vanilla, ½ cup 4
Vanilla bean, ½ cup 3

Dreyer's Fat Free

Caramel praline crunch, ½ cup.................2
Chocolate fudge, ½ cup...........................2
Chocolate peanut butter, ½ cup 2
Cookie chunk, ½ cup................................2
Raspberry marble chunk, ½ cup 2
Vanilla, ½ cup 2

Dreyer's Fat Free, No Sugar Added

Blueberry cobbler, ½ cup 2
Chocolate fudge, ½ cup...........................2
Raspberry vanilla swirl, ½ cup 2
Vanilla, ½ cup 2
Vanilla chocolate swirl, ½ cup.................2
Vanilla 'n caramel, ½ cup 2

Dreyer's Light

Butter pecan light ice cream, ½ cup 3
Chocolate fudge mousse light
  ice cream, ½ cup 2
Chocolate raspberry escape, ½ cup 3
Coffee mousse crunch light ice cream,
  ½ cup 3
Cookie dough light ice cream, ½ cup 3
Cookies 'n cream light ice cream, ½ cup....3
Crazy for caramel light ice cream,
  ½ cup 3
Espresso fudge chip light ice cream,
  ½ cup 3
French silk light ice cream, ½ cup 3
Mint chocolate chips! light ice cream,
  ½ cup 3
Peanut butter cups! light ice cream,
  ½ cup 3
Rocky road light ice cream, ½ cup.............3
S'mores n' more, ½ cup............................3
Vanilla light ice cream, ½ cup 2

Dreyer's No Sugar Added

All About PB, ½ cup 3
Butter pecan, ½ cup.................................3
Chips n' swirls, ½ cup 2
Double fudge brownie, ½ cup 2

POINTS

Strawberry, ½ cup.....................................2
Triple chocolate, ½ cup.............................2
Vanilla, ½ cup 2

Edy's

Almond praline, ½ cup 4
Black cherry vanilla, ½ cup 4
Butter pecan, ½ cup..................................4
Chocolate, ½ cup 4
Chocolate chips!, ½ cup 4
Coffee, ½ cup 3
Cookie dough, ½ cup 4
Cookies 'n cream, ½ cup 4
Double fudge brownie, ½ cup 4
Dulce de leche, ½ cup 4
French vanilla, ½ cup 4
Ice cream sandwich, ½ cup.......................4
Mint chocolate chips!, ½ cup 4
Mocha almond fudge, ½ cup 4
Neapolitan, ½ cup 3
Real strawberry, ½ cup..............................3
Rocky road, ½ cup 4
Toasted almond, ½ cup 4
Triple chocolate thunder, ½ cup 4
Vanilla, ½ cup 4
Vanilla bean, ½ cup 3

Edy's Fat Free

Caramel praline crunch, ½ cup..................2
Chocolate fudge, ½ cup.............................2
Chocolate peanut butter, ½ cup 2
Cookie chunk, ½ cup.................................2
Raspberry marble chunk, ½ cup 2
Vanilla, ½ cup 2

Edy's Fat Free, No Sugar Added

Blueberry cobbler, ½ cup 2
Chocolate fudge, ½ cup.............................2
Raspberry vanilla swirl, ½ cup 2

Vanilla, ½ cup 2
Vanilla chocolate swirl, ½ cup...................2
Vanilla 'n caramel, ½ cup 2

Edy's Light
Butter pecan light ice cream, ½ cup 3
Chocolate fudge mouse light ice cream,
  ½ cup 2
Chocolate raspberry escape, ½ cup 3
Coffee mousse crunch light ice cream,
  ½ cup 3
Cookie dough light ice cream, ½ cup 3
Cookies 'n cream light ice cream,
  ½ cup 3
Crazy for caramel light ice cream,
  ½ cup 3
Espresso fudge chip light ice cream,
  ½ cup 3
French silk light ice cream, ½ cup 3
Mint chocolate chips! light ice cream,
  ½ cup 3
Peanut butter cups! light ice cream,
  ½ cup 3
Rocky road light ice cream, ½ cup.............3
S'mores n' more, ½ cup..............................3
Vanilla light ice cream, ½ cup 2

Edy's No Sugar Added
All About PB, ½ cup 3
Butter pecan, ½ cup...................................3
Chips n' swirls, ½ cup 2
Double fudge brownie, ½ cup 2
Strawberry, ½ cup......................................2
Triple chocolate, ½ cup..............................2
Vanilla, ½ cup 2

Eskimo Pie
Reduced fat butter pecan ice cream
  sweetened with aspartame, ½ cup..........3
Reduced fat chocolate marshmallow
  ice cream sweetened with aspartame,
  ½ cup 3
Reduced fat fudge ripple ice cream
  sweetened with aspartame, ½ cup..........3
Reduced fat neapolitan, ½ cup 3

Reduced fat vanilla ice cream
  sweetened with aspartame, ½ cup..........3

Haagen-Dazs
Butter pecan, ½ cup...................................8
Cherry vanilla, ½ cup 6
Chocolate, ½ cup 7
Chocolate chocolate chip, ½ cup...............7
Chocolate chocolate fudge, ½ cup.............7
Chocolate, low fat, ½ cup..........................4
Coffee, ½ cup 7
Coffee fudge, low fat, ½ cup.....................4
Coffee mocha chip, ½ cup 7
Cookie dough chip, ½ cup 8
Cookies & cream, ½ cup............................7
Creme caramel pecan, ½ cup 8
Dulce de leche caramel, ½ cup 7
Macademia brittle, ½ cup 8
Mango, ½ cup 6
Mint chip, ½ cup..8
Pineapple coconut, ½ cup..........................6
Pistachio, ½ cup 7
Rum raisin, ½ cup 7
Strawberry, ½ cup 6
Strawberry, low fat, ½ cup 3
Vanilla, ½ cup 7
Vanilla chocolate chip, ½ cup 8
Vanilla fudge, ½ cup 7
Vanilla swiss almond, ½ cup......................8
Vanilla, low fat, ½ cup 4

Healthy Choice
Butter pecan crunch, ½ cup 2
Cappuccino chocolate chunk, ½ cup..........2
Cappuccino mocha crunch, ½ cup 2
Cherry chocolate chunk, 1 cup 2
Chocolate chocolate chunk, ½ cup 2
Coconut cream pie, ½ cup 2
Cookie crème de mint, ½ cup 3
Cookies 'n cream, ½ cup 2
Fudge brownie, ½ cup...............................2
Mint chocolate chip, ½ cup.......................2
Old fashioned blueberry hill, ½ cup 2
Old fashioned butterscotch blondie,
  ½ cup 3
Old fashioned cherry vanilla, ½ cup...........2

Old fashioned strawberry, ½ cup 2
Peanut butter cup, ½ cup 2
Praline & caramel, ½ cup 3
Praline caramel cluster, ½ cup..................3
Rocky road, ½ cup 3
Turtle fudge cake, ½ cup 2
Vanilla, ½ cup 2
Vanilla bean, ½ cup 2
Wild raspberry truffle, ½ cup 2

Schwan's

Blackjack cherry, ½ cup 4
Butter pecan, ½ cup.................................4
Cherry nut, ½ cup 3
Cherry vanilla, ½ cup 3
Chip and mint, ½ cup...............................4
Chocolate, ½ cup 3
Chocolate almond, ½ cup.........................3
Chocolate chip, ½ cup..............................4
Chocolate chip cookie dough, ½ cup.........4
Chocolate double fudge brownie, ½ cup 4
Chocolate fudge ripple, ½ cup 3
Chocolate malt twist, ½ cup 4
Chocolate marshmallow ripple, ½ cup 3
Cookies & cream, ½ cup...........................4
Dark sweet cherry, ½ cup 3
Maple nut, ½ cup 4
Peaches & cream, ½ cup 3
Pecan caramel quake, ½ cup.....................4
Pecan praline sundae, ½ cup 4
Rainbow sherbet, ½ cup...........................2
Raspberry rumble, ½ cup 4
Rocky road, ½ cup 4
Summer's dream, ½ cup 3
Vanilla, ½ cup 3
Vanilla ice cream cups, 1 (54 g) 3

Schwan's Lowfat Ice Cream

Butter crunch, ½ cup................................2
Praline almondine sundae, ½ cup..............3
Lowfat Ice Cream, Vanilla, ½ cup 2

Weight Watchers Smart Ones

Chocolate chip cookie dough,
1 serving (75 g) 4

         POINTS

Ice cream novelties

Ben & Jerry's

Berry wild whirl, 1 serving........................7
Cherry garcia yogurt pop, 1 serving...........6
Cookie dough pop, 1 serving 10
Passionfruit smooch, 1 serving.................8
Phish stick, 1 serving...............................7
S'mores pop, 1 serving 8
Totally nuts pop, 1 serving......................10
Vanilla heath bar crunch pop, 1 serving.....8
Vanilla pop, 1 serving..............................8

Dreyer's

Creamy banana whole fruit bar,
chocolate dipped, 1 5
Creamy strawberry whole fruit bar,
chocolate dipped, 1 4
Lemonade whole fruit bar, 1 2
Lime whole fruit bar, 1 2
Peach whole fruit bar, 1............................2
Strawberry whole fruit bar, 1 2
Tangerine whole fruit bar, 1 2
Wild berry whole fruit bar, 1 2

Edy's

Creamy banana whole fruit bar,
chocolate dipped, 1 5
Creamy strawberry whole fruit bar,
chocolate dipped, 1 4
Lemonade whole fruit bar, 1 2
Lime whole fruit bar, 1 2
Peach whole fruit bar, 1............................2
Strawberry, 1 2
Tangerine whole fruit bar, 1 2
Wild berry whole fruit bar, 1 2

Eskimo Pie

Fudge bars, 1 (55 g)................................1
Reduced fat vanilla ice cream bars
dipped in a dark chocolate flavored
coating, 1 (49 g)...................................3
Reduced fat vanilla ice cream bars
dipped in a milk chocolate flavored
coating with crisped rice, 1 (47 g)..........3

Reduced fat vanilla ice cream with
   cookie wafers, 1 (65 g).............................3
Vanilla ice cream cones topped with
   reduced fat milk chocolate flavored
   coating and peanuts, 1 (74 g).................5

Good Humor
Popsicle, 1 (57 g) 1
Strawberry shortcake, 1 (59 g) 4
Sugar free popsicle, 1 (55 g) 0

Haagen-Dazs
Chocolate & almonds, multi-pack,
   1 (87 g) 8
Chocolate & almonds, single pack,
   1 (106 g)..9
Chocolate & dark chocolate, multi-pack,
   1 (83 g) 7
Chocolate & dark chocolate, single
   pack, 1 (102 g) 9
Chocolate peanut butter swirl,
   multi-pack, 1 (82 g) 8
Chocolate sorbet, 1 (76 g) 1
Coffee & almond crunch, multi-pack,
   1 (87 g) 8
Coffee & almond crunch, single pack,
   1 (106 g)..10
Cookies & cream crunch, multi-pack,
   1 (88 g) 8
Cookies & cream crunch, single pack,
   1 (104 g)..10
Dulce de leche caramel, multi-pack,
   1 (86 g) 8
Dulce de leche caramel, single pack,
   1 (105 g)..9
Orange sorbet & vanilla ice cream,
   1 (71 g) 3
Raspberry sorbet & vanilla yogurt,
   1 (71 g) 2
Strawberry sorbet & vanilla ice cream,
   1 (71 g) 3
Tropical coconut, single pack, 1 (100 g).....9
Vanilla & almonds, multi-pack, 1 (87 g).....8
Vanilla & almonds, single pack, 1
   (206 g) 10

Vanilla & dark chocolate, multi-pack,
   1 (83 g) 7
Vanilla & dark chocolate, single pack,
   1 (102 g)..9
Vanilla & milk chocolate, multi-pack,
   1 (82 g) 7
Vanilla & milk chocolate, single pack,
   1 (100 g)..9

Klondike
Krispy krunch, 1 (96 g) 8
Original, 1 (93 g) 7
Reduced fat, no sugar added, 1 (78 g).......4

Nabisco SnackWell's, Ice cream
sandwiches, 1 (44 g) 2

Schwan's
Acapulco pops, 1 (55 g)............................1
Assorted twin pops, 1 (92 g).....................1
Banana pops, 1 (53 g) 1
Bomb pop, jr., 1 (52 g) 1
Caramel apple treats, 1 (57 g) 2
Chocolate malt push-ems, 1 (55 g)...........2
Chocolate sundae cups, 1 (55 g) 3
Fudge stick, 1 (79 g) 2
Ice cream sandwiches, 1 (63 g) 4
Lemon freeze cup, ½ cup..........................3
Orange sherbet push-ems, 1 (64 g) 2
Rainbow stick, 1 (62 g) 2
Rasp./orange Healthy Creations creme
   bars, 1 (64 g)..1
Root beer float bars, 1 (64 g)....................2
Schwan's pops, 1 (52 g) 0
Strawberry fruit bars, 1 (52 g)...................1
Strawberry sundae cups, 1 (55 g) 3
Trim Creations choc. fudge stick,
   1 (53 g) 1

Weight Watchers Smart Ones
Chocolate mousse, 1 serving (41 g)...........1
Chocolate treat, 1 serving (87 g)...............2
English toffee crunch, 1 serving (40 g).......3
Orange vanilla treat, 1 serving (41 g) 1
Vanilla sandwich, 1 serving (65 g).............3

Ice pops

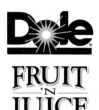

Dole
Fruit dips, banana fruit bar, 1 (2.7 fl oz) 4
Fruit dips, strawberry fruit bar, 1
  (2.7 fl oz) 4
Fruit'n juice, lemonade, 1 bar, 1 (77 g) 1
Fruit'n juice, raspberry, 1 bar, 1 (76 g) 1
Fruit'n juice, strawberry, 1 bar, 1 (76 g) 1
Fruit juice, variety pack, grape, 1 bar
  (1¾ fl oz) 1
Fruit juice, variety pack, raspberry, 1 bar
  (1¾ fl oz) 1
Fruit juice, variety pack, strawberry, 1 bar
  (1¾ fl oz) 1
Fruit juice, no sugar added, variety pack,
  grape, 1 bar (1¾ fl oz) 1
Fruit juice, no sugar added, variety pack,
  raspberry, 1 bar (1¾ fl oz) 1
Fruit juice, no sugar added, variety pack,
  strawberry, 1 bar (1¾ fl oz) 1
Minute Maid Fruit juice bar variety
  pack (cherry, grape, orange) with
  vitamin c added, 1 (66 ml) 1

Mr. Freeze
Assorted flavors, 2 (85 ml) 1
Tropical flavors, 2 (85 ml) 1

Italian ice
Luigi's
Real Italian ice variety pack (lemon/
  strawberry), 6 fl oz 2
Real Italian ice, cherry, 6 fl oz 2
Real Italian ice, lemon, 6 fl oz 2
Mama Tish's Fruttuoso Sorbetto
Premium Italian ices, cherry, 4 fl oz 2
Premium Italian ices, lemon, 4 fl oz 2

Jams
E.D.Smith
Apricot jam, 1 Tbsp 1
Black currant jam, 1 Tbsp 1
Blueberry jam, 1 Tbsp 1
Midnight raspberry jam, 1 Tbsp 1
Passionate fruits jam, 1 Tbsp 1
Peach jam, 1 Tbsp 1
Raspberry jam, 1 Tbsp 1
Seedless raspberry jam, 1 Tbsp 1
Strawberry jam, 1 Tbsp 1
Three fruit jam, 1 Tbsp 1
Smucker's
Blackberry, 1 Tbsp 1
Blackberry (seedless), 1 Tbsp 1
Black raspberry (seedless), 1 Tbsp 1
Boysenberry (seedless), 1 Tbsp 1
Grape, 1 Tbsp 1
Red plum, 1 Tbsp 1
Red raspberry (seedless), 1 Tbsp 1
Strawberry, 1 Tbsp 1
Strawberry (seedless), 1 Tbsp 1

Jelly
E.D.Smith
Apple jelly, 1 Tbsp 1
Mint jelly, 1 Tbsp 1
Red currant jelly, 1 Tbsp 1
Harry & David Pepper jelly, 1 Tbsp 1
Smucker's
Apple, 1 Tbsp 1
Blackberry, 1 Tbsp 1
Black raspberry, 1 Tbsp 1
Cherry, 1 Tbsp 1
Cinnamon apple, 1 Tbsp 1
Currant, 1 Tbsp 1
Elderberry, 1 Tbsp 1
Grape, 1 Tbsp 1
Guava, 1 Tbsp 1
Mint apple, 1 Tbsp 1
Mixed fruit, 1 Tbsp 1
Plum, 1 Tbsp 1
Quince, 1 Tbsp 1
Red raspberry, 1 Tbsp 1
Strawberry, 1 Tbsp 1

J

Ketchup
Del Monte, Ketchup, 1 Tbsp 0
Heinz
  Hot ketchup made with tabasco, 1 Tbsp 0
  Light harvest ketchup, 1 Tbsp....................0
  Tomato ketchup, 1 packet (7 g) 0
  Tomato ketchup, 1 Tbsp............................0
  Tomato ketchup, no salt added, 1 Tbsp......0

Kiwi
Dole Kiwi, 2 1

Knockwurst
Boar's Head Beef knockwurst,
    1 (113 g)..8
Hebrew National Beef knockwurst,
    1 (85 g) 7

Lemon
Dole Lemon, 1 0

Lemon juice
Minute Maid Premium Pure lemon
    juice, frozen from concentrate, 1 fl oz......0

Lemonade
Minute Maid Premium
  Country style lemonade, 8 fl oz..................2
  Lemonade, 8 fl oz 2
  Lemonade iced tea, 8 fl oz.........................2
  Pink lemonade, 8 fl oz...............................2
  Raspberry lemonade, 8 fl oz 2
  Soft frozen lemonade, 1 tube (118 ml) 2
  Tropical lemonade, 8 fl oz..........................2
Newman's Own
  Lemonade (carton), 8 fl oz.........................2
  Lemonade (glass), 1 bottle (295 ml) 3
Snapple
  Diet pink lemonade, 1 serving (8 fl oz) 0
  Lemonade, 1 serving (8 fl oz)....................2
  Pink lemonade, 1 can (11½ fl oz) 3
  Pink lemonade, 1 serving (8 fl oz) 2
  Raspberry lemonade, 1 plastic container
    (8 fl oz)..2
  Sun lemonade, 1 plastic container
    (8 fl oz)..2

Lentils
Faraon Lentils, uncooked, ¼ cup 2

Lettuce
Dole
  Chopped romaine, 3 oz 0
  Classic & romaine blend, 3 oz...................0
  Iceberg lettuce, 3 oz.................................0

Limeade
Minute Maid Premium Limeade,
    8 fl oz..2

Liver
Tyson Chicken livers, 4 oz 3

Liverwurst
Boar's Head
  Lite braunschweiger liverwurst, 2 oz 3
  Liverwurst pâté, 2 oz................................4
  Smoked liverwurst, 2 oz 5
  Strassburger liverwurst, 2 oz.....................5

Luncheon meat
Boar's Head
  Baby black forest brand ham, 3 oz 2
  Baby maple glazed honey coat sweet
    slice ham, 3 oz 2
  Baby sweet slice boneless smoked
    ham, 3 oz..2
  Black forest brand smoked ham, 3 oz........2
  Dutch brand loaf, 2 oz...............................4
  Fully cooked beef tongue, 3 oz..................7
  Junior beef salami, 2 oz.............................3
  Maple glazed honey coat sweet slice
    ham, 3 oz..2
  Natural casing head cheese, 2 oz 2
  Olive loaf, 2 oz 4
  Pickle & pepper loaf, 2 oz.........................4
  Sweet slice boneless smoked ham with
    natural juices, 3 oz................................2
  Tongue & bloodwurst, 2 oz.......................5
  USDA choice corned beef brisket –
    uncooked, 2.4 oz 5
Butterball
  Deli thin sliced smoked turkey breast,
    6 slices (54 g)..1

L

POINTS

Honey roasted & smoked turkey breast,
  6 slices (54 g)..1
Oven roasted chicken breast, 6 slices
  (54 g) 1
Oven roasted turkey breast, 6 slices
  (54 g) 1
Smoked chicken breast, 6 slices (54 g).......1

Butterball Turkey Variety Pack

Bologna, 3 slices (64 g) 4
Cooked turkey salami, 3 slices (64 g).........3
Smoked white turkey, 3 slices (64 g)..........3
Turkey ham, 3 slices (64 g) 3

Carl Buddig

Beef, 1 package 3
Chicken, 1 package 3
Corned beef, 1 package.............................2
Ham with natural juices, 1 package...........3
Honey ham with natural juices,
  1 package 3
Honey turkey, 1 package 3
Oven roasted turkey, 1 package 3
Pastrami, 1 package..................................2
Turkey breast with white meat,
  1 package 3
Turkey ham, 1 package..............................3

Carl Buddig Lean Slices

Brown sugar ham, 1 package (71 g)..........2
Honey roasted turkey breast, 1 package
  (71 g) 1
Honey smoked chicken breast,
  1 package (71 g) 1
Oven roasted honey ham, 1 package
  (71 g) 2
Oven roasted turkey breast, 1 package,
  (71 g) 1
Roasted chicken breast, 1 package
  (71 g) 1
Smoked ham, 1 package (71 g)..................2
Smoked turkey breast, 1 package
  (71 g) 1

Farmland

98% fat free turkey breast variety pack,
  1½ oz 1

Deli style cooked ham & water product,
  1 oz...1
Deli style cooked roast beef, 1 oz..............1
Deli style smoked turkey breast, 1 slice
  (28 g) 1
Smoked turkey breast, 2 oz.......................1
Turkey and ham variety pack, 2 oz 1

Healthy Choice Deli Traditions

Cooked ham, 6 slices (54 g).....................1
Cooked ham, oven roasted turkey
  breast, 6 slices (54 g).............................1
Cooked ham, oven roasted turkey
  breast, 6 slices (54 g).............................1
Oven roasted turkey breast, 6 slices
  (54 g) 1
Smoked ham, 6 slices (54 g) 1

Healthy Choice Sandwich Singles

Honey ham, 1 package..............................1
Honey maple ham, 1 package....................2
Honey roasted & smoked turkey breast,
  1 package 2
Oven roasted turkey breast, 1 package......2
Roast beef, 1 package 1
Smoked turkey breast, 1 package..............2

Healthy Choice Savory Selections

Honey ham, 6 slices (54 g) 1
Honey ham, honey roasted & smoked
  turkey breast, 6 slices (54 g)....................1
Honey maple ham, 6 slices (54 g) 1
Honey mustard ham, 6 slices (54 g) 1
Honey roasted & smoked chicken
  breast, 6 slices (54 g).............................2
Honey roasted & smoked turkey breast,
  6 slices (54 g)..1
Mesquite flavored smoked turkey
  breast, 6 slices (54 g).............................1
Pastrami, 6 slices (54 g) 2

Louis Rich

Chicken breast & white chicken,
  oven roasted, 1 slice (28 g) 1
Chicken breast, oven roasted deluxe,
  1 slice (28 g) 1
Chicken, white, oven roasted, 1 slice
  (35 g) 1

L

Ham, honey & water product, 40% added ingredients, 2 slices (47 g)............1

Ham, smoked & water product, 40% added ingredients, 2 slices (49 g)............1

Turkey breast & white turkey, hickory smoked, 1 slice (28 g) 1

Turkey breast & white turkey, oven roasted, 1 slice (28 g) 1

Turkey breast, hickory smoked, 1 slice (28 g) 1

Turkey breast, oven roasted, 1 slice (28 g) 1

Turkey breast, oven roasted, deli-thin, 4 slices (52 g)..............................1

Turkey ham, 15% water added, 1 slice (28 g) 1

Turkey ham, chopped, 15% water added, 1 slice (28 g) 1

Turkey ham, honey cured, 15% water added, 1 slice (28 g) 1

Turkey ham, honey cured, 15% water added, 1 slice (28 g) 1

Turkey pastrami, 1 slice (28 g) 1

Turkey salami cooked, 1 slice (28 g) 1

Turkey salami cotto, 1 slice (28 g) 1

Turkey, white, smoked, 1 slice (28 g)..........1

Oscar Mayer

Braunschweiger, liver sausage, 1 slice (28 g) 3

Braunschweiger, liver sausage, 2 oz 5

Canadian-style bacon, made from pork sirloin tips, 2 slices (46 g) 1

Ham and cheese loaf, 1 slice (28 g)...........2

Ham chopped, water added, 1 slice (28 g) 1

Ham, baked cooked, water added, 3 slices (63 g)..............................2

Ham, boiled, water added, 3 slices (63 g) 1

Ham, honey, water added, 3 slices (63 g) 2

Ham, lower sodium, water added, 3 slices (63 g)..............................2

Ham, smoked cooked, water added, 3 slices (63 g)..............................1

Head cheese, 1 slice (28 g) 1

Liver cheese, pork fat wrapped, 1 slice (38 g).................................3

Luncheon loaf, spiced, 1 slice (28 g) 2

New England brand sausage, 2 slices (46 g) 1

Old fashioned loaf, 1 slice (28 g)...............2

Olive loaf, made with chicken, pork and turkey, 1 slice (28 g) 2

Pickle and pimiento loaf, made with chicken, pork and turkey, 1 slice (28 g)....2

Turkey, white, oven-roasted, 1 slice (28 g) 1

Turkey, white, smoked, 1 slice (28 g)..........1

Oscar Mayer Free

Chicken breast, oven roasted, 4 slices (52 g) 1

Ham, baked cooked & water product, 3 slices (47 g) 1

Ham, honey & water product, 3 slices (47 g) 1

Ham, smoked & water product, 3 slices (47 g) 1

Turkey breast, oven roasted, 4 slices (52 g) 1

Turkey breast, smoked, 4 slices (52 g)........1

Spam

Less salt luncheon meat, 2 oz 5

Lite luncheon meat, 2 oz 3

Regular luncheon meat, 2 oz 5

Smoked Spam, 2 oz.................................5

Underwood Deviled ham spread, ¼ cup 4

Luncheon meat lunches
Oscar Mayer Lunchables

Bologna/American, no drink, 1 (128 g) 12

Bologna/American/cookies (4.15 oz), no drink, 1 (118 g)...............................12

Bologna/Wild cherry, with drink, 1 (318 g) 13

Chicken/turkey, 1 (145 g) 10

L

Luncheon meat lunches, Oscar Mayer Lunchables (con't)

Extra cheesy pizza, no drink, 1 (128 g) 7
Extra cheesy/fruit punch, with drink, 1 (347 g)..10
Ham/Cheddar, no drink, 1 (128 g) 9
Ham/Cheddar/cookies (4½ oz), no drink, 1 (129 g) 10
Ham/fruit punch (96g & 200ml), with drink, 1 (306 g) 7
Ham/fruit punch, with drink, 1 (318 g) 10
Ham/surfer cooler juice drink (164 g & 200 ml), 1 (374 g) 9
Ham/swiss, no drink, 1 (128 g)..................8
Ham/swiss, reduced fat, no drink, 1 (120 g) 6
Pepperoni pizza, no drink, 1 (128 g) 7
Pepperoni/orange, with drink, 1 (347 g) 10
Turkey Cheddar, reduced fat, no drink, 1 (120 g)..6
Turkey/American/cookies (4.2 oz), no drink, 1 (119 g) 9
Turkey/Cheddar, no drink, 1 (128 g)..........8
Turkey/ham, 1 (145 g) 9
Turkey/Pacific cooler juice drink, 1 (318 g) 10
Turkey/Pacific cooler juice drink (147 g & 200 ml), 1 (359 g)..................8
Turkey/surfer cooler juice drink, 1 (318 g) 10

Luncheon meat, lean
Louis Rich Carving Board

Chicken breast classic baked, 2 slices (45 g) 1
Chicken breast grilled, 2 slices (945 g).......1
Ham baked cooked, water added, 2 slices (45 g)......................................1
Ham honey glazed water added, thin carved, 6 slices (60 g)......................2
Ham honey glazed, water added, traditional carved, 2 slices (45 g) 1
Ham smoked cooked, water added, 2 slices (45 g)....................................1
Turkey breast hickory smoked, 2 slices (45 g) 1

Turkey breast oven roasted, thin carved, 6 slices (60 g) 1
Turkey breast oven roasted, traditional carved, 2 slices (45 g) 1
Turkey breast rotisserie flavor, 2 slices (45 g) 1

Louis Rich Deli-Thin

Chicken breast, oven roasted, 4 slices (52 g) 1
Turkey breast & white turkey, hickory smoked, 4 slices (52 g)..........................1
Turkey breast & white turkey, oven roasted, 4 slices (52 g) 1

Macadamia nuts
Planters Mauna Loa Macadamia nuts, 3 Tbsp..4
Tropical Nut & Fruit Macadamia nuts, 1 oz..5

Macaroni and cheese
Kraft

All shapes, prepared, 1 cup.....................10
Original, light, prepared, 1 cup.................6
Original, prepared, 1 cup 10

Kraft Deluxe

Four cheese blend, prepared, 1 cup 7
Light deluxe macaroni & cheese dinner, prepared, 1 cup 6
Original, prepared, 1 cup 7

Kraft Premium

Cheesy alfredo, prepared, 1 cup 9
Mild white Cheddar, prepared, 1 cup.......10
Thick 'n creamy, prepared, 1 cup 10
Three cheese, prepared, 1 cup...................9

Kraft Velveeta

Bacon, prepared, 1 cup 8
Original, prepared, 1 cup 8
Salsa, prepared, 1 cup 8

Mandarin oranges
Del Monte Mandarin oranges in light syrup, ½ cup..2

Del Monte Fruit Cups Mandarin oranges in light syrup, 4-oz cup (113 g) ..1
Dole Mandarian oranges in light syrup, canned, ½ cup 1

Mangos
Dole Mango, ½ cup 1
Tropical Nut & Fruit Mango slices, 3 slices (44 g)..3

Manicotti
Rosetto Cheese manicotti, 2 pieces (145 g) 6

Margarine
Brummel & Brown
Spread soft, 1 Tbsp 1
Spread, stick, 1 Tbsp 3
Hain Pure Foods
Safflower oil margarine, 1 Tbsp.................3
Soft safflower oil margarine, 1 Tbsp 3
I Can't Believe It's Not Butter
Easy squeeze, 1 Tbsp..............................2
Fat Free, 1 Tbsp.....................................0
Light, soft, 1 Tbsp 1
Light, stick, 1 Tbsp 2
Soft, 1 Tbsp 3
Stick, 1 Tbsp 3
Unsalted, stick, 1 Tbsp............................3
Imperial
⅓ less fat, 1 Tbsp...................................2
Light, 1 Tbsp...2
Soft, 1 Tbsp 2
Stick, 1 Tbsp 3
Mrs. Filbert's
Soft, 1 Tbsp 2
Stick golden quarters, 1 Tbsp 2
Promise
Buttery light, soft, 1 Tbsp 1
Buttery light, stick, 1 Tbsp 2
Reduced calorie spread, 1 Tbsp.................2
Soft, 1 Tbsp 2
Stick, 1 Tbsp 3
Ultra, 1 Tbsp..1

Ultra fat free soft, 1 Tbsp...........................0
Ultra fat free squeeze, 1 Tbsp 0
Ultra fat free stick, 1 Tbsp 0
Shedd's
Spread, stick, 1 Tbsp 2
Spread, whipped, 1 Tbsp 1
Shedd's Country Crock
Churn style, 1 Tbsp..................................2
Churn style, soft, 1 Tbsp 2
Cinnamon spread, 1 Tbsp 2
Easy squeeze, 1 Tbsp...............................2
Honey spread, 1 Tbsp 2
Light, 1 Tbsp..1
Natual canola oil blend, 1 Tbsp..................2
Soft, 1 Tbsp 2
Spreadable sticks, 1 Tbsp..........................2
Shedd's Willow Run Stick, 1 Tbsp 3
Take Control Soft, 1 Tbsp 2

Marinades
A1
Steak marinade – classic steakhouse, 1 Tbsp...0
Steak marinade – hickory, 1 Tbsp 0
Steak marinade – Italian herb, 1 Tbsp 0
Durkee Grill Creations
Asian marinade, 1 tsp 0
Smokey chipotle marinade, 1 tsp...............0
Tomato garlic pesto marinade, 1 tsp..........0
House of Tsang Mandarin marinade, 1 Tbsp...1
Lawry's
Herb & garlic marinade with lemon juice, 1 Tbsp 0
Lemon pepper marinade with lemon juice, 1 Tbsp 0
Mesquite marinade with lime juice, 1 Tbsp...0
Teriyaki marinade with pineapple juice, 1 Tbsp 1

Marmalade
Smucker's Sweet orange, 1 Tbsp 1

M

Marshmallows
Jet-Puffed
Marshmallows, mini, ½ cup 2
Marshmallows, regular, 4 pieces (28 g)......2

Mayonnaise

Best Foods®

Best Foods
Light mayonnaise, 1 Tbsp 1
Mayonnaise dressing low fat, 1 Tbsp.........1
Real mayonnaise, 1 Tbsp 3
Hain Pure Foods
Canola mayonnaise, 1 Tbsp 3
Eggless mayonnaise dressing, 1 Tbsp 3
Lite safflower mayonnaise, 1 Tbsp.............1
Safflower mayonnaise, 1 Tbsp...................3

HELLMANN'S®

Hellmann's
Light mayonnaise, 1 Tbsp 1
Mayonnaise dressing low fat, 1 Tbsp.........1
Real mayonnaise, 1 Tbsp 3
Kraft
Light mayonnaise, 1 Tbsp 1
Real mayonnaise, 1 Tbsp 3

Meal replacement drinks
Balanced
Chocolate, 1 can (325 ml)........................4
Strawberry, 1 can (325 ml) 4
Vanilla, 1 can (325 ml) 4
Kids Balanced
Choco-chocolate, 1 drink box (236 ml) 3
Very vanilla, 1 drink box (236 ml) 3

Milk
Alba Nonfat dry milk, prepared, 8 fl oz......2
Foremost
Lowfat milk, 1%, 1 cup 2

Reduced fat milk, 2%, 1 cup.....................3
Vitamin D milk, 1 cup...............................4
Golden Guernsey
Lowfat milk, 1%, 1 cup 2
Reduced fat milk, 2%, 1 cup.....................3
Vitamin D milk, 1 cup...............................4
Morning Glory
Lowfat milk, 1%, 1 cup 2
Reduced fat milk, 2%, 1 cup.....................3
Vitamin D milk, 1 cup...............................4
Pet
Evaporated milk, regular, 2 Tbsp 1
Evaporated milk, skimmed, 2 Tbsp 0

Milk flavorings
Nesquik
Chocolate powder, 2 Tbsp........................2
No sugar added chocolate powder,
2 Tbsp...0
Strawberry powder, 2 Tbsp 2

Milk, flavored
Hershey's
Chocolate fat free milk ultra-pasteurized,
1 cup..3
Chocolate flavored drink, 1 drink box
(240 ml)..3
Chocolate milk, 1 cup 5
Chocolate reduced fat milk ultra-
pasteurized, 1 cup 4
Strawberry reduced fat milk ultra-
pasteurized, 1 cup 4
Nesquik
Banana reduced fat, 1 cup........................4
Chocolate, 1 cup......................................5
Fat free chocolate, 1 cup 3
Strawberry, 1 cup.....................................5

Mixers
Campbell's Bloody Mary mix, 1 serving
(349 g) 1
Del Monte
Snap-E-Tom tomato and chile cocktail,
10 fl oz...2
Snap-E-Tom tomato and chile cocktail,
6 fl oz...1

M

Naturally Fresh
Classic bloody mary mixer, 6 fl oz 0
Classic grenadine mixer, 1 fl oz 2
Classic margarita mixer, 4 fl oz 2
Classic pina colada mixer, 4 fl oz 5
Classic strawberry daiq. mixer, 4 fl oz 5
Classic whiskey sour, 4 fl oz 1

Molasses
Brer Rabbit
Molasses – blackstrap, 1 Tbsp 1
Molasses, full flavored, 1 Tbsp 1
Molasses, mild flavored, 1 Tbsp 1

Mousse
Sans Sucre Sugar Free
Cheesecake mousse mix, ½ cup 2
Chocolate cheesecake mousse mix,
  ½ cup 2
Chocolate mousse mix, ½ cup 1
French vanilla mousse mix, ½ cup 2
Key lime pie & mousse mix, ½ cup 2
Lemon mousse mix, ½ cup 2
Mocha cappuccino mousse mix, ½ cup......1
Strawberry mousse mix, ½ cup 2
Weight Watchers Smart Ones
Chocolate mousse, 1 serving (77 g).........4

Mozzarella, breaded, frozen
Giorgio Italian breaded mozzarella
sticks, 2 (37 g).......................................3

Muffins
Betty Crocker
Apple cinnamon mix (pouch),
  prepared, 1 3
Apple streusel mix (box), no-cholesterol/
  low fat recipe, prepared, 1.....................4
Apple streusel mix (box), prepared, 1 5
Banana nut mix (box), 1 4
Banana nut mix (box), no-cholesterol/
  low fat recipe, prepared, 1.....................3
Banana nut mix (pouch), 1 4
Blueberry mix (pouch), prepared, 1 4
Chocolate chip mix (pouch), prepared, 1 4
Corn muffin mix (pouch), prepared, 1 4

Cranberry orange mix (box), no-
  cholesterol/low fat recipe, prepared, 1.....3
Cranberry orange mix (box), prepared, 1 3
Double chocolate mix (box), 1 5
Double chocolate mix (box), no-
  cholesterol recipe, prepared, 1 4
Lemon poppyseed mix (box), no-
  cholesterol/low fat recipe, prepared, 1.....3
Lemon poppyseed mix (box), prepared,
  1 4
Lemon poppyseed mix (pouch),
  prepared, 1 4
Twice the blueberry mix (box), no-
  cholesterol/low fat recipe, prepared, 1.....3
Twice the blueberry mix (box), prepared,
  1 3
Wild blueberry mix (box), no-cholesterol/
  low fat recipe, prepared, 1.....................3
Wild blueberry mix (box), prepared, 1........4
Gladiola Corn muffin mix, prepared,
1 (⅕ recipe) 4
Hostess
Banana walnut mini muffins, 3 (34 g)........4
Blueberry mini muffins, 3 (34 g) 4
Chocolate chip mini muffins, 3 (34 g) 4
Kellogg's
Toaster muffin, cinnamon, 1 piece
  (46 g) 3
Toaster muffin, strawberry, 1 piece
  (46 g) 3
Kellogg's Eggo Toaster muffins,
blueberry, 1 piece (45 g).........................3
Martha White
Apple cinnamon, prepared, 1 (⅕ recipe) 3
Banana nut, prepared, 1 (⅕ recipe) 4
Blackberry, prepared, 1 (⅕ recipe) 4
Blueberry, prepared, 1 (⅕ recipe) 4
Chocolate chip, prepared, 1 (⅕ recipe) 4
Cinnamon, prepared, 1 (⅕ recipe) 4
Double blueberry, prepared, 1 (⅐ recipe)....3
Honey bran, prepared, 1 (⅙ recipe) 3
Lemon poppyseed, prepared, 1
  (⅙ recipe) 3

M

Low fat apple cinnamon, prepared, 1 (⅕ recipe) 3

Low fat blueberry, prepared, 1 (⅕ recipe) 3

Low fat strawberry, prepared, 1 (⅕ recipe) 3

Strawberry, prepared, 1 (⅕ recipe) 4

Wildberry, prepared, 1 (⅕ recipe) 4

Yellow corn, prepared, 1 (⅕ recipe) 4

Otis Spunkmeyer

Almond poppy seed, ½ muffin (2 oz).........5

Apple cinnamon, ½ muffin (2 oz)...............5

Apple cinnamon, 1 muffin (2¼ oz) 6

Apple cinnamon, low fat, ½ muffin (2 oz)...6

Apple cinnamon, low-fat, 1 muffin (2¼ oz)...4

Banana mini muffins, 3 muffins (1½ oz)...4

Banana nut, ½ muffin (2 oz)......................6

Banana nut, 1 muffin (2¼ oz) 7

Banana nut, low fat, ½ muffin (2 oz).........4

Banana nut, low-fat, 1 muffin (2¼ oz).......4

Blueberry mini muffins, 3 muffins (1½ oz)...4

Cheese streusel, ½ muffin (2 oz) 5

Chocolate chip, ½ muffin (2 oz) 6

Chocolate chocolate chip, 1 muffin (2¼ oz)...6

Chocolate chocolate chip, ½ muffin (2 oz)...6

Chocolate chocolate chip mini muffins, 3 muffins, 1½ oz.....................................4

Chocolate chocolate chip, low-fat, ½ muffin, 2¼ oz 4

Chocolate chocolate chip, low-fat, 1 serving (2 oz) 4

Cinnamon spice ½ muffin (2 oz) 5

Corn, ½ muffin (2 oz)................................6

Harvest bran, 1 muffin (2¼ oz) 5

Harvest bran, ½ muffin (2 oz) 4

Lemon, ½ muffin (2 oz) 5

Orange, ½ muffin (2 oz) 6

Pineapple, ½ muffin (2 oz).........................5

Wild blueberry, 1 muffin (2¼ oz) 5

Wild blueberry, ½ muffin (2 oz).................5

Wild blueberry, low-fat, 1 muffin, 2¼ oz 4

Wild blueberry, low-fat, ½ muffin (2 oz) 4

Pillsbury

Apple cinnamon mix, baked, 1 (⅙ recipe) 4

Banana nut mix, baked, 1 (⅙ recipe) 4

Blueberry mix, baked, 1 (⅙ recipe) 4

Chocolate chip mix, baked, 1 (⅙ recipe) 4

Cinnamon, 1 (⅙ recipe) 4

Strawberry mix, baked, 1 (⅙ recipe) 4

Wildberry mix, baked, 1 (⅙ recipe)............4

Sara Lee

Blueberry muffins, 1 5

Corn muffins, 1 6

Sweet Rewards

Apple cinnamon, fat free recipe, prepared, 1 2

Apple cinnamon, prepared, 1 3

Wild blueberry, fat free recipe, prepared, 1 2

Wild blueberry, prepared, 1 3

Weight Watchers Smart Ones

Banana muffins, 1 serving (71 g) 3

Blueberry muffins, 1 serving (71 g)............3

Mushrooms

B in B

Pieces & stems, canned, 1 can (120 g).......0

Sliced with garlic, canned, 1 can (120 g) 1

Sliced, canned, 1 can (120 g) 0

Whole, canned, 1 can (120 g) 0

Brandywine

Mushrooms, canned, ½ cup 0

Mushrooms, no salt, canned, ½ cup 0

Giorgio

Chunky portabella mushrooms, canned, ½ cup...0

Homestyle breaded mushrooms, frozen, 3 oz...2

Italian breaded mushrooms, frozen, 3 oz...2

M

Marinated portabella caps, frozen,
1 cap (113 g) 1
Mushrooms, canned, ½ cup (130 g) 0
Mushrooms, frozen, ¾ cup (85 g) 0
Mushrooms, no salt, canned, ½ cup
(130 g) 0

Green Giant
Pieces & stems, canned, ½ cup (120 g)......0
Sliced mushrooms, canned, ½ cup
(120 g) 0
Whole mushrooms, canned, ½ cup
(120 g) 0

PA Dutchman
Chunky portabella mushrooms,
canned, ½ cup (130 g) 0
Mushrooms, canned, ½ cup (130 g) 0
Mushrooms, no salt, canned, ½ cup
(130 g) 0

Mustard
Best Foods Honey mustard dressing,
1 tsp...0

Boar's Head
Decatessen style mustard, 1 tsp 0
Honey mustard, 1 tsp 0
Squeezable delicatessen style mustard,
1 tsp...0

Grey Poupon
Classic deli mustard, 1 tsp 0
Country dijon mustard, 1 tsp 0
Dijon mustard, 1 tsp 0
Honey mustard, 1 tsp 0
Spicy brown mustard, 1 tsp 0

Harry & David
Champagne/honey mustard, 1 tsp..............0
Honey dill mustard, 1 tsp 0
Hot & sweet orange mustard, 1 tsp...........0

Heinz
Dijon mustard, 1 packet (12 g)..................0
Honey mustard, 1 packet (12 g) 0
Mild mustard, 1 Tbsp 0
Spicy brown mustard, 1 tsp 0

Hellmann's Honey mustard dressing,
1 tsp...0

Kraft
Horseradish mustard, 1 tsp 0
Prepared mustard, 1 tsp 0

N

Nachos
Totino's
Beef & cheese, 6 (87 g) 5
Grande, 6 (87 g) 5
Nacho cheese, 6 (87 g)............................5
Taco, 6 (87 g) 5

Nectars
Libby's
Apple, 1 can (11½ fl oz) 4
Apricot, 1 can (5½ fl oz)...........................2
Apricot, 1 can (11½ fl oz) 4
Banana, 1 can (11½ fl oz) 4
Guava, 1 can (11½ fl oz) 4
Mango, 1 can (11½ fl oz) 4
Papaya, 1 can (11½ fl oz) 4
Peach, 1 can (5½ fl oz) 2
Peach, 1 can (11½ fl oz) 4
Pear, 1 can (5½ fl oz) 2
Pear, 1 can (11½ fl oz) 4
Strawberry banana, 1 can (11½ fl oz)........4
Strawberry kiwi, 1 can (11½ fl oz).............4

Nectarines
Dole Nectarine, 1 1
Tropical Nut & Fruit Nectarines,
¼ cup 1

Noodle mixes, flavored
Kraft Noodle Classics
Cheddar cheese, prepared, 1 cup 9
Savory chicken, prepared, 1 cup 7
Lipton Noodles & Sauce
Alfredo broccoli, prepared, ⅔ cup 5
Alfredo, prepared, ⅔ cup.........................5
Beef flavor, prepared, ⅔ cup....................4
Butter & herb, prepared, ⅔ cup 5
Butter, prepared, ⅔ cup...........................5
Chicken broccoli, prepared, ⅔ cup 5
Chicken flavor, prepared, ⅔ cup...............5

Noodle mixes, flavored
Lipton Noodles & Sauce
(con't)   **POINTS**

Creamy chicken, prepared, ⅔ cup 5
Parmesan, prepared, ⅔ cup 5
Sour cream & chive, prepared, ⅔ cup........5
Stroganoff, prepared, ⅔ cup 4

Nuts, mixed
EXPRESSnacks Mixed nuts, salted,
  1 package (1¾ oz) 8
Planters
Deluxe mixed nuts, 1 oz 4
Dry roasted mixed nuts, 1 oz 4
Honey roasted mixed nuts (oil roasted),
  1 oz...4
Lightly salted mixed nuts, 1 oz..................4
Select mix cashews with almonds and
  macadamias, 1 oz..................................4
Select mix cashews with almonds and
  pecans, 1 oz 4
Sweet roasts cinnamon, almonds,
  peanuts & pecans, 1 oz 4
Sweet roasts honey, peanuts &
  cashews, 1 oz (28 g) 4
Sweet roasts honey, peanuts &
  cashews, 1 package (42 g) 6
Sweet roasts honey, peanuts &
  cashews, 1 package (57 g) 8
Sweet roasts vanilla, almonds, cashews
  & peanuts, 1 oz 4
Unsalted mixed nuts, 1 oz (28 g)...............4
Tropical Nut & Fruit
Imperial mixed nuts, 1 oz 5
Mixed nuts and peanuts, 1 oz...................5
Select mixed nuts, 30 g 5
Sundae nut topping, 15 g........................2

Oils
Faraon Olive oil, 1 Tbsp..........................3
Hain Pure Foods
Almond oil, 1 Tbsp...................................4
Canola oil, 1 Tbsp 4
Extra virgin olive oil, 1 Tbsp.....................4
Garlic flavored oil, 1 Tbsp........................4

Light in taste olive oil, 1 Tbsp...................4
Peanut oil, 1 Tbsp 4
Safflower oil, 1 Tbsp 4
Sesame oil, 1 Tbsp 4
Sunflower oil, 1 Tbsp 4
Walnut oil, 1 Tbsp....................................4
House of Tsang
Hot chili sesame oil, 1 tsp 1
Mongolian fire oil, 1 tsp...........................1
Pure sesame oil, 1 tsp 1
Singapore curry oil, 1 tsp.........................1
Wok oil, 1 Tbsp..4
Mazola
Corn oil, 1 Tbsp 4
Right blend canola and corn oil, 1 Tbsp....4
Naturally Fresh
Olive oil, 2 Tbsp 8
Salad oil, 2 Tbsp 8
Progresso
Extra mild olive oil, 1 Tbsp 4
Extra virgin olive oil, 2 Tbsp.....................4
Olive oil (Riviera blend), 1 Tbsp 4

Okra
Trappey's Cocktail okra, hot, 30 g 0

Olives
Faraon
Olives stuffed pim, 5 (15 g) 1
Spanish olives, 7 (15 g) 1

Onions
Boar's Head Sweet Vidalia onions in
  sauce, 1 Tbsp 0
Dole Vidalia onion, ½ cup 0
Green Giant Whole onions, canned,
  ½ cup..0

Onion rings
Ore-Ida
Gourmet onion rings, 4 pieces (86 g) 5
Onion ringers, 6 pieces (90 g) 5

Orange
Dole Orange, 1 0

O

Orange juice

Florida's Natural Orange juice, 8 oz......2

Minute Maid

Orange blend, 8 fl oz 2

Orange juice, 8 fl oz................................2

Orange juice with calcium, 8 fl oz 2

Minute Maid Premium

Country style orange juice, 8 fl oz 2

Home squeezed style orange juice,
8 fl oz..2

Home squeezed style orange juice
with calcium added, 8 fl oz 2

Low acid orange juice, 8 fl oz 2

Orange juice with vitamin c and
calcium added, 1 drink box (200 ml) 2

Original orange juice, 8 fl oz...................2

Original orange juice with calcium
added, 8 fl oz 2

Pulp free orange juice, 8 fl oz 2

Payaso Orange juice, 1 bottle (8.45 oz) ...3

Snapple Snapple Farms orange grove,
12 fl oz 3

Tropicana Original Orange juice,
1 carton (8 fl oz) 2

Tropicana Pure Premium

Grovestand, 1 carton (6 fl oz) 2

Grovestand, 1 carton (8 fl oz) 2

Grovestand, 1 carton (10 fl oz) 3

Homestyle, 1 carton (6 fl oz)...................2

Homestyle, 1 carton (8 fl oz)...................2

Homestyle, 1 carton (10 fl oz).................3

Original, 1 carton (6 fl oz) 2

Original, 1 carton (10 fl oz) 3

Original, 1 bottle (13 fl oz) 4

Tropicana Season's Best

Orange juice, 1 bottle (7 fl oz) 2

Orange juice, 8 fl oz................................2

Orange juice, 10 fl oz 3

Orange juice, 1 can (11.5 fl oz) 3

Pancakes

Betty Crocker

Complete buttermilk mix (box),
prepared, 3 4

Complete buttermilk mix (pouch),
prepared, 3 4

Complete original mix (box),
prepared, 3 4

Original mix (pouch), prepared, 3.............5

Bisquick Shake 'N Pour

Blueberry, 3 4

Buttermilk, 3 4

Original, 3...5

Kellogg's Eggo Buttermilk, 3 (116 g) 6

Martha White

Flapstax pancake mix, ½ cup 5

Pancake & waffle mix, prepared,
1 serving...7

Pillsbury Hungry Jack

Blueberry, 3 (116 g) 5

Buttermilk, 3 (116 g)...............................6

Buttermilk complete mix, ⅓ cup 3

Buttermilk mini's, 11 (112 g) 6

Buttermilk, mix, ⅓ cup 3

Extra light & fluffy complete, mix,
⅓ cup 3

Extra light & fluffy, mix, ⅓ cup...............3

Original, 3 (116 g) 6

Original, mix, ⅓ cup...............................4

Schwan's Buttermilk pancakes, 3
(120 g) 8

Sweet 'N Low Pancake mix, 4 servings
(45 g) 3

Pancake and sausage

State Fair Original pancake'n
sausage, 1 (2½ oz) 6

Papaya

Dole Papaya, ½ cup 0

EXPRESSnacks Papaya chunks, dried,
¼ cup 3

Tropical Nut & Fruit Papaya chunks,
40 g 3

P

Pasta
Di Giorno
Angel's hair, 2 oz 3
Fettuccini, 2½ oz 4
Herb linguine, 2½ oz..............................4
Linguine, 2½ oz 4
Red bell pepper fettuccine, 2½ oz 4
Spinach fettuccine, 2½ oz........................4
Faraon
Pasta concha shells, uncooked, 1 cup 5
Pasta fideo cambry, uncooked, ½ cup 4
Harry & David
Fusilli, 2 oz...4
Spinach fettuccini, 2 oz 4
Tomato fettuccini, 2 oz.............................4
Tri-color shells, 2 oz 4
Mueller's
Angel hair, 2 oz 4
Bow ties, 2 oz...4
Dumplings, 2 oz..4
Elbows, 2 oz...4
Fettuccine, 2 oz 4
Fideos fidelini, 2 oz..................................4
Hearty egg noodles, extra wide, 2 oz........4
Jumbo shells, 2 oz 4
Lasagne, 2 oz 4
Linguine, 2 oz...4
Munchen egg noodles, 2 oz......................4
Old fashioned egg noodles, fine, 2 oz.......4
Old fashioned egg noodles, medium,
   2 oz...4
Old fashioned egg noodles, wide, 2 oz 4
Orzo pasta, 2 oz.......................................4
Pasta ruffle, 2 oz......................................4
Penne rigate, 2 oz....................................4
Ready cut, 2 oz...4
Ridged elbows, 2 oz..................................4
Ridged mostaccioli, 2 oz 4
Ridged ziti, 2 oz.......................................4
Rigatoni, 2 oz...4
Rotini, 2 oz 4
Ruffle trio, 2 oz...4
Salad macaroni, 2 oz 4

Sea shells, 2 oz..4
Small sea shells, 2 oz 4
Spaghetti, 2 oz...4
Thin spaghetti, 2 oz 4
Tri-color bow ties pasta, 2 oz...................4
Tri-color orzo pasta, 2 oz.........................4
Twist trio, 2 oz...4
Twists, 2 oz 4
Vermicelli, 2 oz..4
Yolk free noodle style pasta, wide, 2 oz....4
Yolk free noodle style pasta, medium,
   2 oz...4
Ziti, 2 oz 4
Mueller's Micro Quick
Elbows, 2 oz...4
Spaghetti, 2 oz...4
Twists, 2 oz 4
Ziti, 2 oz 4

Pasta mixes, flavored
Betty Crocker
Cheddar & broccoli rice mix, reduced-fat
   recipe, prepared, 1 cup..........................6
Chicken herb risotto mix, reduced-fat
   recipe, prepared, 1 cup..........................5
Creamy garlic & herb rotini mix,
   prepared, 1 cup 5
Creamy garllc & herb rotini mix,
   reduced-fat recipe, prepared, 1 cup........7
Creamy herb risotto mix, reduced-fat
   recipe, prepared, 1 cup..........................6
Creamy homestyle chicken pasta mix,
   low-fat recipe, prepared, 1 cup 4
Creamy homestyle chicken pasta mix,
   prepared, 1 cup 4
Garden vegetable pilaf mix, low-fat
   recipe, prepared, 1 cup..........................4
Garlic alfredo fettuccine mix, prepared,
   1 cup...8
Garlic alfredo fettuccine mix, reduced-
   fat recipe, prepared, 1 cup.....................6
Long grain & wild rice pilaf mix,
   reduced-fat recipe, prepared, 1 cup........4

P

Roasted chicken vegetable penne mix,
prepared, 1 cup 4

Roasted chicken vegetable penne mix,
reduced-fat recipe, prepared, 1 cup 4

Southwestern rice mix, reduced-fat
recipe, prepared, 1 cup 5

Three cheese gemelli mix, prepared,
1 cup 6

Three cheese gemelli mix, reduced-fat
recipe, prepared, 1 cup 6

Tomato Parmesan pasta mix, prepared,
1 cup 4

Tomato Parmesan pasta mix, reduced-
fat recipe, prepared, 1 cup 4

Kraft Spaghetti Classics

Mild Italian, prepared, 1 cup 4

Spaghetti with meat sauce, prepared,
1 cup 7

Tangy Italian, prepared, 1 cup 4

Zesty cheese, prepared, 1 cup 4

Lipton Pasta & Sauce

3 cheese rotini, prepared, ¾ cup 5

Bow tie chicken primavera, prepared,
¾ cup 4

Bow tie Italian cheese, prepared, ¾ cup ...5

Cheddar broccoli, prepared, ⅔ cup 5

Creamy garlic, prepared, ⅔ cup 6

Creamy mushroom, prepared, ¾ cup 5

Creamy tomato Parmesan, prepared,
¾ cup 5

Mild Cheddar cheese, prepared, ¾ cup 4

Roasted garlic & olive oil with tomatoes,
prepared, ¾ cup 4

Roasted garlic chicken flavor, prepared,
¾ cup 4

Zesty Cheddar, prepared, ¾ cup 5

Spice Islands Pasta Gourmet

Alfredo sauce, mix, 1⅓ Tbsp 1

Alfredo, prepared,1 cup 8

Garlic herb, dry mix, 2 tsp 0

Garlic herb, prepared, 1 cup 5

Pesto, dry mix, 2 tsp 0

Pesto, prepared, 1 cup 5

Zatarain's New Orleans Style Pasta Dinner Mixes

Black beans & bow ties, prepared, 1 cup ..2

Creole garlic, prepared, 1 cup 2

Gumbo, prepared, 1 cup 2

Jambalaya, prepared, 1 cup 2

Red beans & twists, prepared, 1 cup 2

The big cheesy, prepared, 1 cup 3

Pasta sauces

Amy's Organic

Family marinara pasta sauce, ½ cup 0

Garlic mushroom pasta sauce, ½ cup 2

Tomato basil pasta sauce, ½ cup 3

Classico

D'Abbruzzi (Italian sausage with
green peppers & onions), ½ cup 1

Di capri (sun dried tomatoes), ½ cup 2

Di firenze (spinach & cheese florentine),
½ cup 2

Di genoa (spicy tomato & pesto), ½ cup ...2

Di liguria (tomato alfredo), ¼ cup 1

Di napoli (tomato & basil), ½ cup 1

Di palermo (pecorino romano & herb),
½ cup 1

Di parma (tomato and four cheeses),
½ cup 2

Di roma arrabbiata (spicy red pepper),
½ cup 1

Di sicilia (mushroom & ripe olives),
½ cup 1

Di siena (fire roasted tomato and garlic),
½ cup 1

Di sorrento (roasted garlic), ½ cup 1

Di toscana (portobello mushroom),
½ cup 1

Del Monte

Four cheese, ½ cup 1

Tomato & basil, ½ cup 1

Traditional, ½ cup 1

With garlic and onion, ½ cup....................1

With green peppers and mushrooms,
½ cup 1

With meat, ½ cup 1

With mushrooms, ½ cup..........................1

P

Pasta sauces (con't)   *POINTS*

Del Monte Chunky
Garlic & herb, ½ cup 1
Italian herb, ½ cup..................................1
Basil pesto sauce, ¼ cup 9

Di Giorno
Marinara sauce, ½ cup.............................1
Plum tomato & mushroom sauce, ½ cup...1
Plum tomato cream sauce, ½ cup 4
Roasted red bell pepper cream sauce,
   ¼ cup..4

Five Brothers
Fresh tomato & basil, ½ cup 1
Grilled summer vegetable, ½ cup..............2
Imported Romano & garlic, ½ cup.............2
Marinara with burgundy wine, ½ cup.......1
Mushroom & garlic grill, ½ cup.................1
Oven roasted garlic & onion, ½ cup 1
Tomato alfredo, ¼ cup 1

Hain Pure Foods Spaghetti sauce
mix, 1 Tbsp 0

Newman's Own
Bombolina, ½ cup.....................................2
Marinara style ventian, ½ cup 1
Marinara style ventian with
   mushrooms, ½ cup 1
Roasted garlic & red and green
   peppers, ½ cup......................................1
Say cheese, ½ cup 1
Sockarooni, ½ cup 1
Spicy summer sauce – diavolo, ½ cup 1

Prego
Authentic Italian sausage, 1 serving
   (130 g) 2
Chicken parmesan pasta sauce, 1 serving
   (130 g) 2
Diced onion & garlic, 1 serving (125 g).....2
Flavored with meat, 1 serving (130 g)......3
Hamburger, 1 serving (125 g) 2
Italian sausage & garlic, 1 serving
   (125 g) 2
Made with mushrooms, 1 serving
   (125 g) 3
Marinara, 1 serving (125 g) 2

POINTS

Mushroom Parmesan, 1 serving (125 g) ...2
No salt added, 1 serving (125 g)..............2
Pepperoni, 1 serving (125 g)....................2
Roasted chicken pasta sauce, 1 serving,
   (130 g) 2
Roasted chicken with peppers & grilled
   onions, 1 serving (130 g).......................2
Roasted garlic & herb, 1 serving (125 g)...2
Roasted red pepper & garlic, 1 serving
   (125 g) 2
Three cheese pasta sauce, 1 serving
   (125 g) 1
Tomato & basil, 1 serving (125 g) 2
Tomato & basil & garlic, 1 serving
   (125 g) 2
Tomato Parmesan, 1 serving (125 g) 2
Traditional, 1 serving (125 g) 3

Prego Extra Chunky
Garden combination, 1 serving (130 g) 1
Garlic supreme, 1 serving (125 g) 2
Mushroom & diced tomatoes, 1 serving
   (125 g) 2
Mushroom & garlic, 1 serving (125 g) 2
Mushroom & green peppers, 1 serving
   (130 g) 2
Mushroom supreme, 1 serving (130 g) 2
Mushroom with extra spice, 1 serving
   (130 g) 2
Olive and garlic, 1 serving (125 g) 1
Roasted garlic Parmesan, 1 serving
   (130 g) 2
Tomato onion & garlic, 1 serving
   (125 g) 2
Tomato supreme, 1 serving (125 g) 2

Progresso Marinara (authentic), ½ cup...2

Ragu Chunky Gardenstyle
Garden combination, ½ cup 2
Mushroom & green pepper, ½ cup...........2
Mushroom & roasted garlic, ½ cup 2
Roasted red pepper & onion, ½ cup.........2
Super chunky mushroom, ½ cup 2
Super garlic, ½ cup 2
Super vegetable primavera, ½ cup 2

P

Tomato, basil & Italian cheese, ½ cup.......2
Tomato, garlic & onion, ½ cup 2
Tomato, spinach & cheese, ½ cup.............2

Ragu Light

Chunky mushroom & garlic, ½ cup 1
No sugar added tomato & basil, ½ cup 1
Roasted garlic primavera, ½ cup..............1
Tomato & basil, ½ cup 1

Ragu Old World Style

Flavored with meat, ½ cup......................1
Marinara, ½ cup 2
Mushroom, ½ cup....................................1
Traditional, ½ cup...................................1

Ragu Robusto

7-herb tomato, ½ cup 1
Chopped tomato, olive oil & garlic,
  ½ cup 2
Parmesan & Romano, ½ cup....................2
Red wine & herbs, ½ cup 1
Roasted garlic, ½ cup..............................2
Sautéed beef, onion & garlic, ½ cup.........2
Sautéed onion & garlic, ½ cup.................2
Sautéed onion & mushroom, ½ cup 2
Spicy red pepper, ½ cup 2
Sweet Italian sausage & cheese, ½ cup 2

Pastrami

Boar's Head

Cap off top round pastrami – USDA
  choice, 2 oz...2
Pastrami navel, 2 oz...............................5
Pastrami round, 2 oz...............................2
USDA choice pastrami brisket, 2 oz..........4
Louis Rich Turkey pastrami, 2 oz.............2
Perdue Pastrami, 1 serving (2 oz)............2

Peaches

Del Monte

Halves, lite peaches in extra light syrup
  (yellow cling), ½ cup..............................1
Halves, melba peaches in heavy syrup
  (yellow cling), ½ cup..............................2
Halves, peaches in heavy syrup (yellow
  cling), ½ cup 2

Halves, peaches in heavy syrup (yellow
  freestone), ½ cup 2
Sliced, fruit nat. peaches in pear &
  peach juices (yellow cling), ½ cup..........1
Sliced, lite peaches in extra light syrup
  (yellow freestone), ½ cup......................1
Sliced, peaches in heavy syrup (yellow
  cling), ½ cup 2
Sliced, peaches in heavy syrup (yellow
  freestone), ½ cup 2
Sliced, peaches in natural raspberry
  flavored light syrup (yellow cling),
  ½ cup 2
Sliced, spiced peaches in light syrup
  (yellow cling), ½ cup.............................2
Sweet cinnamon chunky-cut peaches
  in light syrup (yellow cling), ½ cup 1
Whole, spiced peaches in heavy syrup
  (yellow cling), ½ cup.............................2

Del Monte Fruit Cups

Diced peaches in heavy syrup, 4-oz cup....2
Fruit naturals diced peaches in pear
  and peach juices, 4-oz cup 1
Lite diced peaches in extra light syrup,
  4-oz cup 1

Del Monte Fruit Pleasures Raspberry
  flavored peaches in naturally-flavored
  light syrup, ½ cup.................................2

Del Monte Fruit Rageous

Peachy pie peaches in a naturally-
  flavored sauce, 4-oz cup 2
Wild raspberry flavored peaches in
  light syrup, 4-oz cup 2

Del Monte Fruit To-Go Peachy
  peaches in peach-flavored light syrup,
  4-oz cup 1

Del Monte Orchard Select Sliced,
  yellow cling peaches in light syrup,
  ½ cup 2
Dole Peach, 2 1
Tropical Nut & Fruit Dried peaches,
  ¼ cup 1

P

Peanut butter

Laura Scudder's Reduced fat peanut
butter, 2 Tbsp 5

Reese's Creamy peanut butter, 2 Tbsp 5

Skippy

Peanut butter spread reduced fat,
creamy, 2 Tbsp 4

Peanut butter spread reduced fat,
super chunk, 2 Tbsp......................4

Peanut butter, creamy, 2 Tbsp 5

Peanut butter, super chunk, 2 Tbsp...........5

Roasted honey nut peanut butter,
creamy, 2 Tbsp 5

Roasted honey nut peanut butter, super
chunk, 2 Tbsp 5

Smucker's Reduced fat natural peanut
butter, 2 Tbsp 5

Peanuts

Frito-Lay

Hot peanuts, 3 Tbsp 5

Salted peanuts, 3 Tbsp 5

Lance

BBQ peanuts, ¼ cup 4

Honey toasted peanuts, ¼ cup.................4

Long tube salted peanuts, ¼ cup 4

Roasted peanuts, ¾ cup......................4

Salted in shell roasted peanuts, ⅔ cup 4

Salted peanuts, 1 package (32 g)..............4

Salted peanuts, 1 package (28 g)..............4

Salted peanuts, 1 package (25 g)..............3

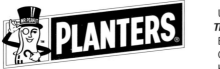

Planters

Cocktail peanuts, 1 oz......................4

Dry roasted peanuts, 1 bag (14 g)............2

Dry roasted peanuts, 1 package (28 g) 4

Dry roasted peanuts, 1 oz......................4

Dry roasted peanuts lightly salted,
1 package (7 g) 1

Dry roasted peanuts lightly salted,
1 package (49 g) 7

Dry roasted peanuts lightly salted, 1 oz....4

Dry roasted peanuts lightly salted,
1 package (14 g) 2

Dry roasted peanuts unsalted, 1 oz 4

Honey roasted peanuts (oil roasted),
1 oz......................4

Honey roasted peanuts (oil roasted),
1 package (28 g) 4

Honey roasted peanuts, dry roasted,
1 package (14 g) 2

Honey roasted peanuts, dry roasted,
1 oz......................4

Honey roasted peanuts, dry roasted,
1 package (28 g) 4

Honey roasted peanuts, dry roasted,
1 package (49 g) 6

Honey roasted peanuts, dry roasted,
1 package (57 g) 7

Lightly salted cocktail peanuts, 1 oz 4

Lightly salted cocktail peanuts,
1 package (57 g) 7

Lightly salted peanuts, 1 package
(49 g) 7

Salted peanuts, 1 oz 4

Salted peanuts, 1 package (28 g) 4

Salted peanuts, 1 package (49 g) 7

Salted peanuts, 1 package (57 g) 9

Sweet 'n crunchy peanuts, 1 oz...............3

Sweet 'n crunchy peanuts, 2 packages
(28 g) 3

Unsalted cocktail peanuts, 1 oz 4

Tropical Nut & Fruit

Blanched peanuts, 1 oz 3

Granulated peanuts, 1 oz 4

Honey roasted peanuts, ¼ cup.................4

In-shell peanuts, 1 oz......................4

In-shell peanuts, roasted, salted, 1 oz.......4

Peanut butter stock, 1 oz 4

Peanuts, sugar toasted, 1 oz...................4

Redskin peanuts, 1 oz 5

Redskin peanuts, raw, 1 oz 4

P

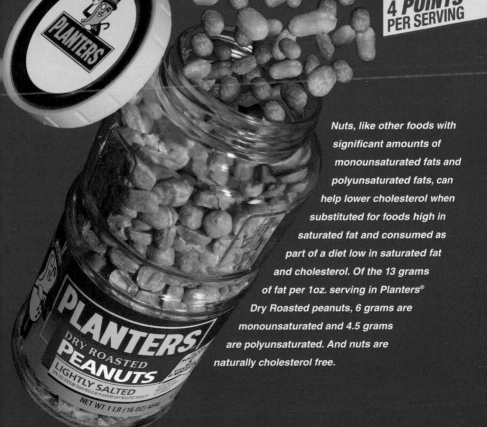

Did you know Nuts

Can help lower cholesterol?

4 POINTS® PER SERVING

PLANTERS

Nuts, like other foods with significant amounts of monounsaturated fats and polyunsaturated fats, can help lower cholesterol when substituted for foods high in saturated fat and consumed as part of a diet low in saturated fat and cholesterol. Of the 13 grams of fat per 1oz. serving in Planters® Dry Roasted peanuts, 6 grams are monounsaturated and 4.5 grams are polyunsaturated. And nuts are naturally cholesterol free.

PLANTERS
DRY ROASTED
PEANUTS
LIGHTLY SALTED
50% LESS SODIUM THAN REGULAR PLANTERS DRY ROASTED PEANUTS
NET WT 1 LB (16 OZ) 454g

Peanuts, Tropical Nut & Fruit (con't)

POINTS

Roasted peanuts, 1 oz.............................4
Spanish peanuts, 1 oz 5
Wow nuts (ale nuts), ¼ cup....................5
Weight Watchers Honey roasted
  peanuts, 1 serving (20 g)......................2

Pears
Del Monte
Cinnamon flavored pear halves in light
  syrup, ½ cup 1
Halves, fruit naturals pears in pear juice,
  ½ cup 1
Halves, lite pears in extra light syrup,
  ½ cup 1
Halves, pear in heavy syrup, ½ cup...........2
Natural ginger flavor pear halves, ½ cup ..2
Sliced, lite pears in extra light syrup,
  ½ cup 1

Del Monte Fruit Cups
Diced pears in heavy syrup, 4-oz cup........2
Lite diced pears in extra light syrup,
  4-oz cup 1

Del Monte Orchard Select Sliced,
  bartlett pears in light syrup, ½ cup 1
Dole Pear, 1...1

Tropical Nut & Fruit
Pears, ¼ cup...1
Pears, natural, ¼ cup 1

Peas
Del Monte
Peas, sweet, ½ cup 0
Peas, sweet, no salt added, ½ cup............0
Peas, sweet, very young small, ½ cup.......0

Faraon
Black eye peas, uncooked, ¼ cup 1
Split peas, uncooked, ¼ cup 2
Whole green peas, uncooked, ¼ cup 2

Green Giant
Blackeye peas, canned, ½ cup..................1
Sugar snap peas, frozen, ¾ cup 0
Sweet peas, 50% less sodium, canned,
  ½ cup 1
Sweet peas, canned, ½ cup 0
Sweet peas, frozen, ⅔ cup 1

POINTS

Green Giant Harvest Fresh
Sugar snap peas, frozen, ⅔ cup 0
Sweet peas & pearl onions, frozen,
  ½ cup 0

Hain Pure Foods
Chick peas, ½ cup...................................2
Sweet peas, ½ cup 1
Hanover Sweet peas, ⅔ cup 0

Hanover The Gold Line
Petite peas, ⅔ cup 1
Snow peas, 1 cup 0
Sugar snap peas, ¾ cup 0

Joan of Arc Blackeye peas, canned,
  ½ cup 1

LeSueur
Baby early peas, frozen, ¾ cup 1
Baby sweet peas, frozen, ⅔ cup 0
Baby sweet peas, frozen, ¾ cup 1
Early June peas, frozen, ⅔ cup.................0
Early peas, 50% less sodium, canned,
  ½ cup 0
Early peas, canned, ½ cup 1

LeSueur Harvest Fresh
Baby sweet peas, frozen, ⅔ cup 1
Early June peas, frozen, ⅔ cup.................1

Schwan's
Peas, ⅔ cup 1
Sugar snap peas, ⅔ cup 0

Pecans
Tropical Nut & Fruit
Pecan halves, 1 oz 5
Pecan pieces, 1 oz...................................5
Pecans, roasted & salted, 1 oz 6
Roasted pecans, 1 oz 6

Peppers
Chi-Chi's
Green chilies diced, 2 Tbsp 0
Green chilies whole, ¾ 0

Chiquita Bell pepper, 1 medium serving
  (148 g) 0

Faraon
Chile peppers, 2 Tbsp 0
Chili jalapenos, 3 pieces (30 g) 0

Hanover Diced green peppers, ¾ cup 0
Harry & David
  Fire roasted peppers, ½ (30 g) 0
  Mustard red pepper cilantro, 1 tsp 0
Old El Paso
  Green chillies, chopped (peeled),
    21 pieces (30 g) 0
  Green chillies, whole (peeled), 1 (35 g).....0
  Jalapeno slices (pickled), drained,
    21 (31 g) 0
  Jalapenos, whole (peeled), 3 (30 g) 0
  Jalapenos, whole (pickled), 2 (26 g) 0
Pancho Villa Diced green chillies,
    2 Tbsp 0
Progresso
  Peppers, cherry, sliced & so hot (drained),
    2 Tbsp 0
  Peppers, hot cherry (drained), 1 (28 g)......0
  Peppers, roasted (drained), 1 piece (28 g) ..0
  Peppers, sweet fried with onions
    (drained), 2 Tbsp 0
  Peppers, Tuscan (drained), 3 (28 g)...........0
Rosa D'oro Stuffed cherry peppers,
    2 oz..2
Trappey's
  Banana peppers – mild, 1 serving (28 g) ...0
  Cherry peppers, mild, 32 g.......................0
  Jalapeno peppers – sliced, 28 g 0
  Tabasco peppers in vinegar, 1 serving
    (28 g) 0
  Tempero peppers – golden green
    pepperoncini, 1 serving (28 g) 0
  Torrido peppers – Santa fe grande,
    1 serving (36 g) 0

Pepperoni
Boar's Head
  Natural casing pepperoni – single
    stick, 1 oz 4
  Pre-sliced pouch pepperoni, 16 slices
    (28 g) 4
  Sandwich style pepperoni, 1 oz................4
Hormel
  Chunk pepperoni, 1 oz 4

  Sliced pepperoni, 15 slices (28 g).............4
  Twin pepperoni, 1 oz................................4
Hormel Pillow Pack
  Pepperoni, 16 slices (28 g) 4
  Turkey pepperoni, 17 slices (30 g) 2
Oscar Mayer Pepperoni, 15 slices
    (30 g) 4

Persimmons
Dole Persimmons, 1 medium 1

Picante sauce
Chi-Chi's
  Picante hot, 2 Tbsp 0
  Picante medium, 2 Tbsp 0
  Picante mild, 2 Tbsp................................0
Old El Paso
  Thick 'n chunky picante, hot, 2 Tbsp 0
  Thick 'n chunky picante, medium, 2 Tbsp ..0
  Thick 'n chunky picante, mild, 2 Tbsp........0
Taco Bell Home Originals
  Picante sauce, medium, 2 Tbsp 0
  Picante sauce, mild, 2 Tbsp.....................0

Pickles
B&G
  Bread & butter chips, 1 oz......................1
  Crunchy kosher dills, 1 oz.......................0
  Deluxe kosher dill spears, 1 oz 0
  Dill gherkins, 1 oz 0
  Hamburger dill chips, 1 oz 0
  Kosher dill chips, 1 oz 0
  Kosher dill spears, 1 oz............................0
Claussen
  Chips, bread 'n butter, 4 slices (28 g)........0
  Halves, kosher dills, ½ (28 g) 0
  Hearty garlic deli style, 2 slices (34 g) 0
  Kosher dills, 2 (34 g) 0
  Mini dills, kosher, 1 (23 g) 0
  Sandwich slices, bread 'n butter, 2 slices
    (34 g) 1
  Spears, kosher dills, 1 (34 g) 0
  Super slices for burgers, 1 slice (24 g) 0
  Whole, half sours New York deli style,
    ½ (28 g) 0

P

Whole, hearty garlic deli style, ½
(28 g) 0
Whole, kosher dills, ½ (28 g)....................0

Del Monte
Dill hamburger chips, 5½ (28 g)...............0
Dill pickle halves, ¼ (28 g) 0
Dill whole pickles, 1½ (28 g) 0
Sweet gherkin pickles, 2 (28 g) 1
Sweet midgit pickles, 3 (28 g)..................1
Sweet pickle chips, 5 (28 g) 1
Sweet whole pickles (12 oz jar), 1
(28 g) 1
Sweet whole pickles (8 & 22 oz jar),
2 (28 g) 1
Tiny kosher dill pickles, 2½ (28 g) 0

Heinz
Bread & butter sandwich slices, 1 oz........1
Dill pickles, 1 oz 0
Genuine dill pickles, 1 oz.........................0
Hamburger dill chips, 1 oz.......................0
Kosher dill sandwich slices, 1 oz 0
Kosher dills, 1 oz 0
Old fashioned bread and butter pickles,
1 oz..0
Sweet gherkins, 1 oz...............................1
Sweet pickles, 1 oz 1

Pico de gallo
Chi-Chi's Pico de gallo, 2 Tbsp 0

Pies
Banquet
Banana cream pie, 1 serving (⅓ pie) 8
Chocolate cream pie, 1 serving (⅓ pie).....8
Coconut cream pie, 1 serving (⅓ pie) 8
Lemon cream pie, 1 serving (⅓ pie)..........8

Lance
Coconut pies, 1 (85 g)..............................8
Fried apple pies, 1 (85 g).........................8
Fried cherry pies, 1 (85 g) 8
Pecan pie, 1 (85 g)..................................8

Mrs. Smith's
Apple pie, 1 serving (⅛ pie) 8
Apple pie, reduced fat, 1 serving (⅙ pie)....4

Banana cream pie, 1 serving (¼ pie) 7
Blueberry pie, 1 serving (⅛ pie) 7
Boston cream pie, 1 serving (⅛ pie) 4
Cherry pie, 1 serving (⅛ pie)....................8
Chocolate cream pie, 1 serving (¼ pie).....8
Coconut cream pie, 1 serving (¼ pie) 7
Coconut custard pie, 1 serving (⅛ pie) 6
Dutch apple crumb pie, 1 serving (⅛ pie)..7
Hearty pumpkin pie, 1 serving (⅛ pie) 5
Key lime pie, 1 serving (⅑ pie) 10
Lemon cream pie, 1 serving (¼ pie)..........7
Lemon meringue pie, 1 serving (⅛ pie).....7
Mince pie, 1 serving (⅛ pie) 9
Peach pie, 1 serving (⅛ pie).....................7
Peanut butter cream pie, 1 serving
(¼ pie)...9
Pecan pie, ⅕ pie (136 g)........................12
Pecan pie, ⅛ pie (128 g)........................12
Pumpkin custard pie, 1 serving (⅛ pie).....5
Red raspberry pie, 1 serving (⅛ pie) 8
Sweet potato pie, 1 serving (⅛ pie)..........7

Mrs. Smith's Restaurant Classics
Cookies & cream pie, 1 serving (⅑ pie).....9
French silk chocolate pie, 1 serving
(⅑ pie)...14
Peanut butter silk pie, 1 serving (⅑ pie)...15

Mrs. Smith's Special Recipe
Deep dish apple pie, 1 serving (1/12 pie).....7
Deep dish cherry pie, 1 serving (1/12 pie)....8
Deep dish cherry-berry pie, 1 serving
(1/12 pie)...8
Deep dish peach pie, 1 serving (1/12 pie) 7
Homemade pumpkin pie, 1 serving
(1/10 pie)...6
Southern pecan pie, 1 serving (⅛ pie) 13

Pet-Ritz
Apple homestyle pie, 1 serving (⅙ pie)....8
Banana cream homestyle pie, 1 serving
(⅓ pie)..8
Cherry homestyle pie, 1 serving (⅙ pie)....7
Chocolate cream homestyle pie,
1 serving (⅓ pie) 8

P

Coconut cream homestyle pie, 1 serving
(⅓ pie)..8
Deep dish 9", frozen, ⅛ (21 g).................2
Dutch apple homestyle pie, 1 serving
(⅙ pie)..8
Extra large 9⅝", frozen, ⅛ (27 g) 3
Key lime cream homestyle pie, 1 serving
(⅓ pie)..8
Lemon cream homestyle pie, 1 serving
(⅓ pie)..8
Pumpkin homestyle pie, 1 serving (⅙ pie)..5
Regular 9", frozen, ⅛ (18 g) 2
Veg. deep dish, frozen, ⅛ (21 g) 2
Veg. regular 9", frozen, ⅛ (19 g) 2

Sara Lee
Blueberry pie, ⅛ pie 8
French silk cream pie, ⅕ pie 11
Lemon meringue cream pie, ⅙ pie 6
Peach pie, ⅛ pie 7
Raspberry pie, ⅛ pie 9
Tropical coconut cream pie, ⅕ pie 11

Sara Lee Oven Fresh
Apple pie, ⅛ pie 8
Cherry pie, ⅛ pie 7
Dutch apple pie, ⅛ pie 8

Sara Lee Signature Selections
Caramel applenut pie, ⅑ pie....................9
Cinnamon French apple pie, ⅒ pie 8
Fruits of the forest pie, ⅑ pie 8

Weight Watchers Smart Ones
Mississippi mud pie, 1 serving (69 g) 3

Pie crust
Betty Crocker
Pie crust mix (box), 1 serving
(⅛ of 9" crust) 3
Pizza crust mix (pouch), 1 serving
(¼ crust) 3

Keebler
Chocolate ready crust, ⅛ crust (21 g) 2
Graham cracker ready crust, ⅛ crust
(21 g) 2

Reduced fat ready pie crust, ⅛ crust
(21 g) 2
Shortbread ready crust, ⅛ crust (21 g)......3

Mrs. Smith's
9" pie crust, deep dish, 1 serving
(⅛ pie crust) 3
9" pie crust, regular, 1 serving
(⅛ pie crust) 3

Oronoque Orchards
6" pie crust, ready to bake, 1 serving
(¼ shell) 3
9" pie crust, deep dish, ready to bake,
1 serving (⅛ pie crust) 3
9" pie crust, regular, ready to bake,
1 serving (⅛ pie crust) 2

Pillsbury
All ready pie crust, refrigerated, ⅛ crust
(27 g) 3
Pie crust mix, 2 Tbsp 3

Pie fillings
Durkee
Lemon pie filling, 1 Tbsp 1
Lemon pie filling, prepared, ⅓ cup 2

E.D.Smith Light and Fruity
Apple pie filling, ⅓ cup 2
Blueberry pie filling, ⅓ cup 2
Cherry fruit filling, 90 ml 2
Cherry pie filling, ⅓ cup 2
Cherry/cranberry pie filling, ⅓ cup 3
Lemon pie filling, ⅓ cup 3
Mixed berry pie filling, ⅓ cup 3
Peach/passion fruit pie filling, ⅓ cup 2
Pumpkin pie filling, ⅓ cup 2
Raisin pie filling, ⅓ cup 2
Raspberry pie filling, ⅓ cup 2
Rhubarb/strawberry pie filling, ⅓ cup.......2
Strawberry pie filling, ⅓ cup....................2

Lucky Leaf
Apple pie filling, no sugar added,
⅓ cup 0
Cherry pie filling, no sugar added,
⅓ cup 1

P

Pierogies

Giorgio

Giorgio
Mini breaded potato & cheese, 2
(72 g) 4
Mini breaded potato & onion, 2
(72 g) 4
Potato & cheese, 3 (122 g) 3
Potato & cheese mini, 5 (132 g)...............4
Potato & mushroom, 5 (132 g) 4
Potato & onion, 3 (122 g).........................4
Potato & onion mini, 5 (132 g) 4
Potato, cheese & bacon, 5 (132 g)............5

Mrs. T's
Potato & Cheddar pierogies, 3 (120 g)......3
Potato & onion pierogies, 3 (120 g).........3

Schwan's Pierogies, 3 (120 g) 3

Pilaf
Golden Grain Near East
Barley pilaf mix, 2 oz 3
Lentil pilaf, 2 oz......................................3
Wheat pilaf mix, 2 oz..............................3

Pine nuts
Tropical Nut & Fruit Pine nuts
(pignolias), ¼ cup..................................4

Pineapples
Del Monte
Chunks, pineapple in heavy syrup,
½ cup 2
Chunks, pineapple in its own juice,
½ cup 1
Crushed pineapple in heavy syrup,
½ cup 2

Crushed pineapple in its own juice,
½ cup 1
Sliced, pineapple in heavy syrup,
2 slices (117 g)....................................2
Sliced, pineapple in its own juice,
2 slices (114 g)....................................1
Spears, pineapple in its own juice,
½ cup 1
Tidbits, pineapple in its own juice,
½ cup 1
Wedges, pineapple in its own juice,
½ cup 1

Del Monte Fruit Cups Pineapple
tidbits in pineapple juice, 4-oz cup.........1

Dole
Pineapple, 2 slices 1
Pineapple chunks in juice, ½ cup 1
Pineapple chunks in syrup, ½ cup 2
Pineapple crushed in juice, canned,
½ cup 1
Pineapple crushed in syrup, canned,
½ cup 2
Pineapple slices in juice, canned,
2 slices (114 g)....................................1
Pineapple slices in syrup, canned,
2 slices (117 g)....................................2
Pineapple tidbits in juice, canned,
½ cup 1
Pineapple tidbits in syrup, canned,
½ cup 2

EXPRESSnacks Pineapple snacks,
dried, 9 pieces (40 g) 2

Tropical Nut & Fruit
Natural pineapple, 2 pieces 2
Pineapple wedge, 10 pieces (40 g)...........2

Pineapple juice
Del Monte
Pineapple juice from concentrate, 6 fl oz ..2
Pineapple juice from concentrate, 8 fl oz ..3
Pineapple juice not from concentrate,
8 oz..2

Pistachios

EXPRESSnacks Pistachios natural,
salted, 1 package (1¾ oz)....................7

Lance
Pistachios, 1 package (43 g) 3
Pistachios, long tube, ¼ cup 2

Planters
Dry roasted pistachios (uncolored),
½ cup..4
Dry roasted pistachios (uncolored),
1 package (25 g) 3
Dry roasted pistachios (uncolored),
1 package (31 g) 5
Dry roasted pistachios (uncolored),
1 package (32 g) 5

Tropical Nut & Fruit
Natural pistachios, ¼ cup 4
Red pistachios, ¼ cup 4
Shelled pistachios, 1 oz 4
Shelled raw pistachios, 1 oz 4

Pizza

Amy's
Cheese pizza, 1 serving (4⅓ oz)...............7
Mushroom and olive pizza, 1 serving
(4⅓ oz)..5
Pesto pizza with tomato and broccoli,
1 serving (4½ oz) 7
Roasted vegetable pizza, 1 serving (4 oz)...5
Spinach pizza, 1 serving (4⅔ oz) 7
Veggie combo pizza, 1 serving (4½ oz).....5

Di Giorno Rising Crust
Chicken supreme, 8", ⅓ pizza (137 g) 6
Four cheese, 12", ⅛ pizza (139 g)............7
Four cheese, 8", ⅓ pizza (114 g)..............6
Italian sausage, 8", ⅓ pizza (124 g)........7
Pepperoni, 12", ⅛ pizza (148 g) 8
Pepperoni, 8", ⅓ pizza (120 g) 7
Spinach, 8", ⅓ pizza (123 g) 5
Supreme, 12", ⅛ pizza (165 g) 8
Supreme, 8", ⅓ pizza (135 g) 7
Three meat, 12", ⅛ pizza (154 g)..............8
Three meat, 8", ⅓ pizza (126 g) 7
Vegetable, 12", ⅛ pizza (159 g)...............6
Vegetable, 8", ⅓ pizza (130 g) 5

Healthy Choice Meals To Go
Cheese French bread pizza, 1 (6 oz) 6
Pepperoni French bread pizza, 1 (6 oz) 6
Sausage French bread pizza, 1 (6 oz) 6
Supreme French bread pizza, 1 (6.35 oz) ..6
Vegetable French bread pizza, 1 (6 oz) 5

Jacks Great Combinations
Double cheese, 9", ½ pizza (158 g)........10
Double cheese, 12", ¼ pizza (140 g) 9
Pepperoni, 12", ¼ pizza (149 g) 9
Pepperoni & mushroom, 12", ¼ pizza
(137 g) 8
Pepperoni & sausage, 9", ½ pizza
(146 g) 9
Sausage, 12", ¼ pizza (153 g) 9
Sausage & mushroom, 12", ¼ pizza
(140 g) 7
Sausage & pepperoni, 12", ¼ pizza
(137 g) 8
Supreme, 12", ¼ pizza (149 g) 8
Bacon cheeseburger, 12", ¼ pizza
(135 g)..8

Jacks Naturally Rising Pizza
Bacon cheeseburger, 12", ⅙ pizza
(143 g) 8
Canadian style bacon, 12", ⅙ pizza
(141 g) 6
Cheese, 9", ⅓ pizza (135 g)....................6
Cheese, 12", ⅙ pizza (129 g)...................6
Combination with sausage & pepperoni,
9", ¼ pizza (121 g) 7
Combination with sausage & pepperoni,
12", ⅙ pizza (148 g)..............................8
Pepperoni, 9", ⅓ pizza (147 g) 8
Pepperoni, 12", ⅙ pizza (141 g) 8
Pepperoni supreme, ⅙ pizza (146 g)........8
Sausage, 9", ⅓ pizza (154 g) 8
Sausage, 12", ⅙ pizza (146 g) 8
Spicy Italian sausage, ⅙ pizza (145 g) 7
The works, 9", ¼ pizza (128 g) 6
The works, 12", ⅙ pizza (151 g) 7

Jack's Original
Canadian style bacon, 12", ¼ pizza
(124 g) 6

P

Pizza, Jack's Original (con't)

POINTS

Cheese, 12", ⅓ pizza (142 g)....................8
Hamburger, 12", ¼ pizza (125 g) 7
Pepperoni, ¼ pizza (122 g) 7
Pepperoni, 9", ½ pizza (142 g) 9
Sausage, ¼ pizza (123 g) 7
Sausage, 9", ½ pizza (144 g) 8
Spicy Italian sausage, ¼ pizza (123 g) 6

Jack's Pizza Bursts
Combination sausage & pepperoni,
  6 pieces (85 g) 6
Pepperoni, 6 pieces (85 g) 6
Sausage, 6 pieces (85 g) 6
Supercheese, 6 pieces (85 g)....................6
Supreme, 6 pieces (85 g) 6

Jeno's Crisp 'N Tasty
Canadian style bacon, 1 serving (195 g) ..10
Cheese, 1 serving (95 g) 10
Combination, 1 serving (198 g)..............12
Hamburger, 1 serving (206 g) 11
Pepperoni, 1 serving (192 g)...................12
Sausage, 1 serving (198 g) 12
Supreme, 1 serving (204 g)......................12
Three meat, 1 serving (198 g) 12

Kid Cuisine Muchers
Backpacking pizza snacks, 6 pieces
  (2.7 g) 5
Fire chief cheese pizza, 1 (5.2 g) 7
Poolside pepperoni pizza, 1 (5.2 g) 8

Marie Callender's
Cheese French bread pizza, 1 (7.2 oz) 12
Pepperoni French bread pizza, 1 (7½ oz)..13
Supreme French bread pizza, 1 (7½ oz) ..11

Schwan's Self-Rising Pizza
Cheese, ⅕ pizza (152 g) 9
Pepperoni, ⅙ pizza (133 g) 8
Supreme, ⅙ pizza (145 g) 8

Schwan's Special Recipe Pizza
Four cheese, ⅓ pizza (140 g) 10
Pepperoni, ⅓ pizza (154 g) 11
Sausage, ¼ pizza (128 g) 9
Sausage & pepperoni, ¼ pizza (126 g) 9
Supreme, ¼ pizza (130 g) 9

POINTS

Stouffer's
Cheese, ½ (5.2 oz) 8
Deluxe, ½ (6.2 oz)....................................9
Extra cheese, ½ (5.9 oz) 9
Five cheese, ½ (5.1 oz) 9
Grilled vegetable, ½ (5.8 oz)....................7
Pepperoni, ½ (5.6 oz)...............................8
Pepperoni and mushroom, ½ (6.1 oz).....10
Sausage, ½ (6 oz) 9
Sausage and pepperoni, ½ (6.1 oz) 11
Three meat, ½ (6.1 oz) 10
White, ½ (5.1 oz) 10

Stouffer's Lean Cuisine
Cheese pizza, 1 (6 oz) 6
Deluxe pizza, 1 (6.1 oz)............................6
Pepperoni pizza, 1 (5¼ oz) 6
Sun dried tomatoes, 1 (6 oz)....................7

Tombstone Double Top
Pepperoni, ⅙ pizza (127 g) 8
Sausage, ⅙ pizza (132 g) 7
Sausage & pepperoni, ⅙ pizza (132 g) 8
Supreme, ⅙ pizza (133 g) 8
Two cheese, ⅙ pizza (149 g)....................9

Tombstone For One
½ less fat cheese pizza, 1(184 g) 7
½ less fat vegetable pizza, 1 (206 g) 7
Extra cheese, 1 (198 g)...........................12
Pepperoni, 1 (198 g) 13
Supreme, 1 (215 g) 13

Tombstone Light
Supreme pizza, ⅕ pizza (138 g) 6
Vegetable pizza, ⅕ pizza (131 g) 5

Tombstone Original
Canadian style bacon, 12", ¼ pizza
  (156 g) 8
Deluxe, 9", ⅓ pizza (125 g) 6
Deluxe, 12", ⅕ pizza (136 g) 7
Extra cheese, 9", ½ pizza (159 g)............8
Extra cheese, 12", ¼ pizza (145 g)..........8
Hamburger, ⅓ pizza, (113 g)....................6
Hamburger, ⅕ pizza (125 g) 7
Pepperoni, 9", ⅓ pizza (113 g) 7
Pepperoni, 12", ¼ pizza (152 g) 9

P

Pepperoni & sausage, 9", ⅓ pizza
(118 g) 7
Sausage, ⅕ pizza (125 g) 7
Sausage, 9", ⅓ pizza (114 g) 6
Sausage & mushroom, 12", ⅕ pizza
(131 g) 7
Sausage & pepperoni, 12", ⅕ pizza
(125 g) 7
Supreme, 9", ⅓ pizza (125 g) 7
Supreme, 12", ⅕ pizza (130 g) 7

Tombstone Oven Rising
Italian sausage, ⅙ pizza (144 g)..............7
Pepperoni, ⅙ pizza (141 g) 8
Supreme, ⅙ pizza (146 g) 7
Three cheese, ⅙ pizza (138 g)..................7
Three meat, ⅙ pizza (146 g) 8

Tombstone Thin Crust
Four meat combo, ¼ pizza (143 g) 9
Italian sausage, ¼ pizza (143 g)...............9
Pepperoni, ¼ pizza (138 q) 10
Supreme, ¼ pizza, (149 g) 9
Supreme taco, ¼ pizza (145 g)..................9
Three cheese, ¼ pizza (134 g)..................9

Totino's Family Size
Cheese, ⅓ pizza (160 g) 8
Combination, ¼ pizza (125 g)...................7
Pepperoni, ⅓ pizza (160 g) 10
Sausage, ¼ pizza (128 g) 7

Totino's Party Pizza
Bacon burger, ½ pizza (149 g) 9
Canadian style bacon, ½ pizza
(147 g) 7
Cheese, ½ pizza (139 g) 7
Combination, ½ pizza (152 g)...................9
Hamburger, ½ pizza (155 g) 9
Pepperoni, ½ pizza (145 g) 9
Sausage, ½ pizza (153 g) 9
Sausage & mushroom, ½ pizza
(153 g) 8
Sausage & sliced pepperoni, ½ pizza
(152 g) 9
Sliced pepperoni, ½ pizza (145 g) 9
Supreme, ½ pizza (155 g) 9

Three meat, ½ pizza (149 g) 8
Zesty Italiano, ½ pizza (152 g)................9

Totino's Pizza For One
Cheese, 1 pizza (104 g) 6
Combination, 1 pizza (119 g)...................8
Pepperoni, 1 pizza (113 g)........................7
Sausage, 1 pizza (116 g) 7
Supreme, 1 pizza (121 g) 7

Weight Watchers Smart Ones
Deluxe combo, 1 serving (186 g)..............8
Pepperoni pizza, 1 serving (157 g) 8

Pizza crust
Betty Crocker Italian herb pizza
crust mix (pouch), ¼ crust (46 g) 3
Martha White
Pizza crust mix, deep pan, prepared,
⅕ package 3
Pizza crust mix, prepared, ¼ package.......3
Pillsbury Pizza crust, ⅕ loaf (57 g)..........3

Pizza sauce
Contadina
Pizza sauce, ¼ cup...................................0
Pizza sauce, flavored with pepperoni,
¼ cup 1
Pizza sauce, four cheese, ¼ cup 1
Pizza squeeze, ¼ cup 0
Progresso Pizza, ¼ cup...........................0

Pizza snacks
Banquet
Cheese pizza snack, 6 pieces (3 oz)..........4
Pepperoni & sausage pizza snack,
6 pieces (3 oz).....................................5
Pepperoni pizza snack, 6 pieces (3 oz)......5
Totino's Pizza Rolls
Cheese, 6 rolls (85 g) 5
Combination, 6 rolls (85 g) 5
Pepperoni, 6 rolls (85 g) 6
Pepperoni supreme, 6 rolls (85 g)............5
Sausage, 6 rolls (85 g).............................5
Supreme, 6 rolls (85 g).............................5
Three meat, 6 rolls (85 g) 5

P

POINTS

Plums
Dole Plum, 2 1

Pomegranates
Dole Pomegranates, 1 medium 2

Popcorn
Act II
96% fat free, popped, 5 cups...................2
Butter, popped, 5 cups 4
Light natural, popped, 5 cups 2
Light butter, popped, 5 cups 2
Natural, popped, 5 cups 4
Bachman Lite popcorn, 5 cups 2
Boston's
Caramel popcorn, fat free, ⅔ cup.............2
White Cheddar, 2¾ cups 3
Chester's Popcorn
Butter – prepopped, 3 cups 4
Cheddar cheese – prepopped, 3 cups.......4
Microwave – butter, 5 cups 4
Cracker Jack
Fat free butter toffee popcorn, ¾ cup.......2
Fat free caramel popcorn, ¾ cup 2
Original popcorn, ½ cup...........................2

Jolly Time
American's best, microwave-popped,
  5 cups 1
Blast o butter light, microwave-popped,
  4 cups 2
Blast o butter, microwave-popped,
  3½ cups...3
Butter-licious light, microwave-popped,
  5 cups 2
Butter-licious, microwave-popped,
  4 cups 3
Cheddar cheese flavor, microwave-
  popped, 3 cups.....................................3

POINTS

Crispy 'n white light, microwave-popped,
  5 cups 2
Crispy 'n white, microwave-popped,
  4 cups 3
Healthy pop, microwave-popped, 5 cups....1
White & buttery butter flavor white,
  microwave-popped, 4 cups...................3
White pop corn, air popped, 5 cups..........1
Yellow pop corn, air popped, 5 cups.........1
Lance
Plain popcorn, 2 cups...............................1
Spicy cheese popcorn, 2 cups 4
White Cheddar cheese popcorn,
  1 package (⅝ oz) 2
White Cheddar cheese popcorn,
  1 package (⅞ oz) 4
White Cheddar cheese popcorn, 1 oz 4
White Cheddar cheese popcorn,
  1 package (1½ oz)..................................6
Newman's Own
Butter flavored microwave popcorn,
  3½ cups...4
Light butter flavored microwave
  popcorn, 3½ cups 2
Light natural microwave popcorn,
  3½ cups...2
Natural flavored microwave popcorn,
  3½ cups...4
Popcorn jar, unpopped, 3 Tbsp 2
Pop-Secret
94% fat free butter, popped, 6 cups 2
94% fat free natural, 6 cups....................2
Butter (snack size) (with Real Land O
  Lakes butter), popped, 1 cup 1
Butter (with Real Land O Lakes butter),
  popped, 1 cup 1
Butter, popped, 4 cups 3
Cheddar cheese, popped, 5 cups 3
Homestyle, popped, 1 cup 1
Jumbo pop butter, popped, 1 cup.............1
Jumbo pop movie theater butter,
  popped, 1 cup 1
Light butter (snack size), 1 cup 0

P

192

Light butter, popped, 6 cups 2
Light natural, popped, 6 cups 2
Movie theater butter, popped, 1 cup 1
Natural, popped, 4 cups 3

Smartfood
Reduced fat golden butter, 3⅓ cups 2
Reduced fat white Cheddar cheese,
　3 cups 3
White Cheddar cheese, 2 cups 4

Tropical Nut & Fruit
Black popcorn, 2 Tbsp 1
Golden caramel corn, 1 oz 3
Golden nut crunch, 1 oz 3
Poppin' nut crunch, 1 oz 3

Weight Watchers
Butter flavored, 1 serving (19 g) 1
Butter toffee popcorn, 1 serving (26 g) 2
Caramel popcorn, 1 serving (26 g) 2
White Cheddar cheese, 1 serving (19 g) ... 2

Popcorn cakes
Hain Pure Foods
Barbeque flavor, mini, 6 corn cakes
　(15 g) 1
Butter flavor, 1 corn cake (9 g) 1
Butter flavor, mini, 7 corn cakes
　(15 g) 1
Caramel flavor, 1 corn cake (13 g) 1
Caramel flavor, mini, 6 corn cakes
　(15 g) 1
Mild Cheddar flavor, mini, 6 corn cakes
　(15 g) 1
Plain, 1 corn cake (9 g) 1
Plain, mini, 8 corn cakes (15 g) 1
White Cheddar flavor, mini, 6 corn cakes
　(15 g) 1

Quaker Oats
Blueberry crunch corn cakes, 1 (13 g) 1
Butter flavor corn grain cakes, 1 (9 g) 1
Corn cakes – caramel apple, 3 (14 g) 1
Corn cakes – caramel chocolate chip,
　1 (15 g) 1
Corn cakes – caramel flavored, 1
　(13 g) 1

Mild white Cheddar corn grain cakes,
　1 (11 g) 1
Strawberry crunch corn cakes, 1 (13 g) 1

Pork
Farmland
Extra tender AHA certified boneless
　center cut pork loins, 4 oz 3
Extra tender AHA certified boneless
　pork tenderloin, 4 oz 3
Extra tender boneless chef's prime
　rib end roast, 4 oz 3
Extra tender boneless picnic roast, 4 oz.... 3
Extra tender boneless pork sirloin, 4 oz 3
Extra tender boneless ultra-supreme
　center cut pork loin, 4 oz 4
Extra tender boneless ultra-supreme
　pork spare ribs, 4 oz 8

Schwan's
Boneless pork filets, 1 (124 g) 3
Boneless pork loin chops, 1 (168 g) 6
Center cut pork loin chops, 1 (160 g) 6
Herb/garlic boneless pork roast, 4 oz 3

Pork skins
Baken-ets
BBQ, 9 pieces (14 g) 2
Hot n' spicy, 7 pieces (14 g) 2
Hot n' spicy cracklins, 8 pieces (14 g) 2
Regular, 9 pieces (14 g) 2
Regular cracklins, 8 pieces (14 g) 1

Lance
BBQ pork skins, 8 pieces (12 g) 2
BBQ pork skins, 19 pieces (28 g) 4
Plain pork skins, 9 pieces (12 g) 2
Plain pork skins, 22 pieces (28 g) 4

Pot pies
Amy's
Broccoli pot pie, 1 (7½ oz) 10
Country vegetable pie, 1 (7½ oz) 8
Mexican tamale pie, 1 (8 oz) 4
Shepherd's pie, 1 (8 oz) 3
Vegetable pot pie, 1 (7½ oz) 9
Vegetable pot pie – non-dairy, 1
　(7½ oz) 6

P

Pot Pies (con't) POINTS

Banquet
Beef, 1 (7 oz)..10
Cheesy potato & broccoli with ham,
   1 (7 oz)..10
Chicken, 1 (7 oz)....................................9
Chicken & broccoli, 1 (7 oz)....................8
Macaroni and cheese, 1 (6½ oz) 4
Turkey, 1 (7 oz) 8
Vegetable cheese, 1 (7 oz)......................8

Marie Callender's
Beef, 1 cup...13
Beef, 1 (9½ oz) 17
Chicken, 1 cup......................................15
Chicken, 1 (9½ oz) 17
Chicken & broccoli, 1 cup 16
Chicken & broccoli, 1 (9½ oz) 16
Chicken au gratin, 1 cup 14
Chicken au gratin, 1 (9½ oz)..................17
Turkey, 1 cup 15
Turkey, 1 (9½ oz) 17

Morton
Macaroni & cheese, 1 (6½ oz) 4
Vegetable pie with beef, 1 (7 oz) 8
Vegetable pie with chicken, 1 (7 oz).........8
Vegetable pie with turkey, 1 (7 oz)...........7

Potatoes
Boston Markets
Garlic dill new potatoes, 1 serving
   (127 g) 3
Mashed potatoes, 1 serving (140 g) 4

Budget Gourmet
Cheddared potatoes, 1 serving (155 g) 6
Cheddared potatoes & broccoli,
   1 serving (141 g) 3

Del Monte
Sliced, new potatoes, ⅔ cup....................1
Whole, new potatoes, 2 pieces
   (approx 2 medium w/ liquid) (158 g)......1

Marie Callender's Skillet Meals
Au gratin potatoes, ⅔ cup 4

Ore-Ida
Golden patties, 1 (63 g) 3
Potato wedges with skin, 8 pieces
   (84 g) 2

POINTS

Potatoes O'Brien, ¾ cup 1
Tater tots, 9 pieces (86 g) 4
Twice baked potatoes, butter, 1 piece
   (141 g) 3
Twice baked potatoes, Cheddar cheese,
   1 piece (141 g) 4
Twice baked potatoes, garlic Parmesan,
   1 piece (141 g) 4
Twice baked potatoes, sour cream
   & chives, 1 piece (141 g) 4
Whipped potatoes, bacon & cheese,
   1 tray (140 g).......................................4
Whipped potatoes, cheese, 1 tray
   (140 g) 4
Whipped potatoes, sour cream and
   chives, 1 tray (140 g) 4

Schwan's
Baked potato w/ broccoli & cheese, 1
   (284 g) 9
Baked potato w/ ham & cheese, 1
   (284 g) 10
Deluxe potato Cheddar, ½ cup 3
Mashed potato nuggets, 10 pieces
   (140 g) 2
Quick Taters, 13 pieces (85 g) 3
Seasoned potato curls, 3 oz (84 g) 4
Stuffed potatoes, 1 (142 g)......................4

Stouffer's
Potatoes au gratin, ½ cup 3
Scalloped potatoes, ½ cup......................4

Potato chips
Hain Pure Foods
Louisiana barbeque flavor baked
   crisps, 12 chips (1 oz) 2
Original flavor baked crisps,
   12 chips (1 oz) 2

Harry's
Baked potato crisps, 1 oz 2
Hampten recipe potato chips, 1 oz...........4
Hampten recipe potato chips, 1¼ oz 5

Lance
BBQ potato chips, 22 chips (28 g)............4
BBQ potato chips, 24 chips (28 g)............4
BBQ potato chips, 35 chips (43 g)............5

P

Plain potato chips, 20 chips (25 g) 3
Plain potato chips, 23 chips (28 g) 4
Plain potato chips, 24 chips (28 g) 4
Plain potato chips, 35 chips (43 g) 6
Ripple potato chips, 15 chips (28 g) 4
Ripple potato chips, 23 chips (43 g) 5
Salt & vinegar potato chips, 22 chips
 (28 g) 4
Salt & vinegar potato chips, 33 chips
 (43 g) 6
Sour cream & onion potato chips,
 22 chips (28 g) 4
Sour cream & onion potato chips,
 23 chips (28 g) 4
Sour cream & onion potato chips,
 33 chips (43 g) 6

Lays

Baked KC masterpiece B.B.Q.,
 11 chips (1 oz) 2
Baked original, 11 chips (1 oz) 2
Baked sour cream & onion, 12 chips
 (1 oz) 2
Classic, 20 chips (1 oz) 4
Cracker barrell cheese, 17 chips (1 oz) 9
Deli style original, 17 chips (1 oz) 4
Flamin' hot, 17 chips (1 oz) 4
KC masterpiece B.B.Q., 15 chips (1 oz) 4
Limon, 17 chips (1 oz) 4
Salt & vinegar, 17 chips (1 oz) 4
Sour cream & onion, 17 chips (1 oz).........4
Spicy B.B.Q., 17 chips (1 oz)....................4
Toasted onion & cheese, 17 chips (1 oz) ...4
Unsalted, 19 chips (1 oz) 4
Wavy original, 11 chips (1 oz)..................4

Lays Wow

Mesquite B.B.Q., 20 chips (1 oz)...............1
Original, 20 chips (1 oz) 1
Sour cream & chive, 19 chips (1 oz) 1

Miss Vickie's

Country BBQ, 14 chips (1 oz) 3
Jalapeno, 14 chips (1 oz) 3
Original, 14 chips (1 oz) 3
Sea salt & malt vinegar, 14 chips (1 oz)....3

Nabisco

Air crisps potato chips, original,
 22 chips (1 oz) 2
Potato air crisps, barbecue,
 22 crisps (1 oz)....................................2
Potato air crisps, sour cream & onion,
 22 crisps (1 oz)....................................2

Pringles

BBQ, 14 pieces (1 oz)..............................4
Cheez ums, 14 pieces (1 oz) 4
Fat free BBQ, 15 pieces (1 oz)..................1
Fat free original, 15 pieces (1 oz).............1
Fat free sour cream & onion, 15 pieces
 (1 oz)...1
Light crisps original, 16 pieces (1 oz)........3
Original, 14 pieces (28 g) 4
Pizza-licious, 14 pieces (1 oz) 4
Ranch, 14 pieces (1 oz) 4
Ridges BBQ, 12 pieces (1 oz) 4
Ridges Cheddar & sour cream, 12 pieces
 (1 oz)..4
Ridges original, 12 pieces (1 oz) 4
Right BBQ, 16 pieces (1 oz) 3
Right ranch, 14 pieces (1 oz) 3
Right sour cream & onion, 16 pieces
 (1 oz)..3
Salt & vinegar, 14 pieces (1 oz)................4
Sour cream' onion,14 pieces (1 oz) 4

Ruffles

Baked Ruffles Cheddar & sour cream,
 9 (1 oz) 2
Baked Ruffles regular, 9 (1 oz) 2
Buffalo style, 11 (1 oz) 4
Cheddar & sour cream, 11 (1 oz) 4
Flamin' hot, 12 (1 oz)..............................4
Flavor rush big BBQ & Cheddar,
 12 (1 oz)..4
Flavor rush zesty sour cream & onion,
 15 (1 oz)..4
French onion, 11 (1 oz) 4
KC masterpiece mesquite B.B.Q.,
 11 (1 oz)..4
Original, 12 (1 oz)....................................4

P

Potato chips, Ruffles (con't)

Reduced fat regular, 16 (1 oz)..................3
The works, 12 (1 oz) 4

Ruffles Wow
Cheddar & sour cream, 15 (1 oz) 1
Original, 17 (1 oz)....................................1

Terra
Blues potato chips, 1 oz 3
Cinnamon spiced sweet potato chips,
   1 oz..3
Jalapeno sweet potato chips, 1 oz............3
Mesquite BBQ sweet potato chips, 1 oz ...3
Nacho cheese sweet potato chips, 1 oz 3
Salsa sweet potato chips, 1 oz.................3
Spiced sweet potato chips, 1 oz 3
Spiced taro chips, 1 oz 3
Sweet potato chips, 1 oz 3
Terra chips, 1 oz 3
Yukon gold barbecue potato chips, 1 oz ...3
Yukon gold onion & garlic potato chips,
   1 oz..3
Yukon gold potato chips, 1 oz..................3
Yukon gold salt & vinegar potato chips,
   1 oz..3
Yukon gold yogurt & green onion potato
   chips, 1 oz...3

Tostitos Wow Original, 6 (1 oz) 2

Potato flakes
Betty Crocker
Butter & herb mix, prepared, ½ cup 4
Butter & herb mix, reduced-fat recipe,
   prepared, ½ cup 3
Chicken and herb mix, prepared, ½ cup....3
Chicken and herb mix, reduced-fat
   recipe, prepared, ½ cup.........................2
Four cheese mix, prepared, ½ cup 3
Four cheese mix, reduced-fat recipe,
   prepared, ½ cup 2
Hearty beef mix, prepared, ¾ cup 4
Potato buds mix, prepared, ⅔ cup 4
Potato buds, reduced-fat recipe,
   prepared, ⅔ cup....................................3
Roasted chicken mix, prepared, ¾ cup 4
Roasted garlic mix, prepared, ½ cup 3

Roasted garlic mix, reduced-fat recipe,
   prepared, ½ cup 3
Sour cream & chives mix, prepared,
   ½ cup 3
Sour cream & chives mix, reduced-fat
   recipe, prepared, ½ cup........................2

Hungry Jack
Complete mashed potatoes, ½ cup 2
Flakes, prepared, ½ cup...........................4
Idaho mashed potatoes, flakes, ⅓ cup 1
Idaho mashed potatoes, flakes,
   prepared, ½ cup 3
Idaho mashed potatoes, granules,
   2 Tbsp 1
Idaho mashed potatoes, granules,
   prepared, ½ cup 3
Mashed potatoes with brown gravy,
   prepared, ⅐ recipe.................................4
Mashed potatoes with chicken gravy,
   prepared, ⅐ recipe................................4

Martha White
Spud flakes instant mashed potatoes,
   mix, ⅓ cup...1
Spud flakes instant mashed potatoes,
   prepared, 1 serving................................4

Potato mixes, flavored
Betty Crocker
Au gratin mix (5¼ oz & 21 oz), low-
   fat recipe, prepared, ½ cup....................2
Au gratin mix (5¼ oz & 21 oz),
   prepared, ½ cup 3
Au gratin mix (9 oz), low-fat recipe,
   prepared, ½ cup 2
Au gratin mix (9 oz), prepared, ½ cup 3
Broccoli au gratin (homestyle) mix,
   low-fat recipe, prepared, ½ cup 2
Broccoli au gratin (homestyle) mix,
   prepared, ½ cup 3
Cheddar & bacon mix, low-fat recipe,
   prepared, ½ cup 2
Cheddar & bacon mix, prepared, ½ cup....3
Cheddar & sour cream mix, prepared,
   ½ cup 3

P

Cheddar cheese (homestyle) mix,
prepared, ½ cup 2
Cheesy scalloped (homestyle) mix,
prepared, ½ cup 3
Cheesy scalloped (homestyle), low-fat
recipe, prepared, ½ cup.........................2
Chicken & vegetable mix, low-fat recipe,
prepared, ⅔ cup...................................2
Chicken & vegetable mix, prepared,
⅔ cup...3
Hash browns mix, prepared, ½ cup 4
Julienne mix, prepared, ½ cup 3
Ranch mix, prepared, ½ cup 3
Scalloped mix (5 oz & 20 oz), low-fat
recipe, prepared, ⅔ cup 2
Scalloped mix (5 oz & 20 oz), prepared,
½ cup 4
Scalloped mix (8¼ oz), low-fat recipe,
prepared, ⅔ cup....................................2
Scalloped mix (8¼ oz), prepared,
½ cup 3
Sour cream 'n chive mix, prepared,
½ cup 3
Three cheese mix, low-fat recipe,
prepared, ½ cup 2
Three cheese mix, prepared, ½ cup 3
Twice baked Cheddar & bacon mix,
low-fat recipe, prepared, ⅔ cup.............3
Twice baked Cheddar & bacon mix,
prepared, ⅔ cup....................................5

Hungry Jack

Au gratin mix, ½ cup 2
Au gratin mix, prepared, ⅛ recipe 3
Cheddar & bacon mix, ½ cup 2
Cheddar & bacon mix, prepared,
⅛ recipe 3
Cheesy scalloped mix, ½ cup 2
Cheesy scalloped mix, prepared,
⅛ recipe 3
Creamy scalloped mix, ½ cup 2
Creamy scalloped mix, prepared,
⅛ recipe 3
Sour cream & chives mix, ½ cup 2
Sour cream & chives mix, prepared,
⅛ recipe 4

Williams

Potatoes w/ butter herb mix, ⅓ cup 1
Potatoes w/ Parmesan roasted garlic,
⅓ cup 1
Potatoes w/ smokey Cheddar mix,
⅓ cup 1
Potatoes w/ SW Herb mix, ⅓ cup 1

Potato pancakes
Hungry Jack

Potato pancake mix, 2 Tbsp 0
Potato pancake mix, prepared, ⅛ recipe ...2

Potatoes, hash brown
Ore-Ida

Country style hashbrowns, 1 cup 1
Southern style hashbrowns, ⅔ cup 1

Schwan's

Hash brown IQF shreds, 3 oz 1
Hash browns, 1 pattie (85 g) 1

Potatoes, mashed
Ore-Ida Mashed potatoes, prepared,
⅔ cup...3

Preserves
Clearbrook Farms

Bitter-sweet orange marmalade, 1 Tbsp....0
California apricot, 1 Tbsp 1
California peach, 1 Tbsp 1
Cranberry-orange, 1 Tbsp 1
Michigan black cherry, 1 Tbsp 1
Michigan damson plum, 1 Tbsp 1
Michigan red tart cherry, 1 Tbsp 1
Northwest strawberry, 1 Tbsp 1
Oregon black raspberry, 1 Tbsp 1
Oregon blackberry, 1 Tbsp.......................1
Oregon boysenberry, 1 Tbsp....................1
Oregon red raspberry, 1 Tbsp 1
Triple fruit, 1 Tbsp 1
Wild Maine Blueberry, 1 Tbsp 1

E.D.Smith Triple Fruits

Apricot deluxe, 1 Tbsp.............................1
Apricot spread, 1 Tbsp 1
Citrus breeze spread, 1 Tbsp...................1
Grape spread, 1 Tbsp 1
Raspberry deluxe, 1 Tbsp.........................1

P

Preserves, E.D. Smith Triple Fruits (con't)

Raspberry spread, 1 Tbsp 1
Strawberry deluxe, 1 Tbsp 1
Strawberry spread, 1 Tbsp 1
Tropical spread, 1 Tbsp............................1
Wildberry spread, 1 Tbsp.........................1

Harry & David

Apricot preserves, 1 Tbsp.........................1
Bing cherry preserves, 1 Tbsp...................1
Blackberry preserves, 1 Tbsp....................1
Blackberry seedless preserves, 1 Tbsp.......1
Marionberry, 1 Tbsp 1
Orange marmalade, 1 Tbsp.......................1
Peach preserves, 1 Tbsp...........................1
Raspberry seedless preserves, 1 Tbsp........1
Strawberry preserves, 1 Tbsp 1

Smucker's

Apricot, 1 Tbsp 1
Apricot, low sugar, 1 Tbsp 1
Apricot-pineapple, 1 Tbsp.........................1
Blueberry, 1 Tbsp 1
Cherry, 1 Tbsp...1
Grape, low sugar, 1 Tbsp 1
Orange marmalade, low sugar, 1 Tbsp......1
Pineapple, 1 Tbsp....................................1
Plum, 1 Tbsp 1
Peach, 1 Tbsp 1
Red raspberry, 1 Tbsp..............................1
Red raspberry, low sugar, 1 Tbsp 1
Strawberry, 1 Tbsp 1
Strawberry banana, 1 Tbsp.......................1
Strawberry, low sugar, 1 Tbsp 1

Pretzels

Bachman

Fat free thins pretzels, 11 (28 g) 2
Thin 'n right pretzels, 12 (30 g) 2

EXPRESSnacks Yogurt pretzels,

7 pieces (40 g) 4

Hanover Sourdough soft pretzels, 1

(61 g) 3

Harmony Yogurt pretzels, ⅓ cup..............3

Harry & David

Honey mustard, ½ cup 2
Nuggets wild'n spicey, 15 (28 g) 2

Harry's

Everything, 1 (24 g) 2
Hard & crunchy, 1 (26 g) 2
Honey mustard, fat free, 1 oz....................2
Nuggets, 14 nuggets (30 g) 2
Nuggets, 20 nuggets (42 g) 3
Sourdough pretzels, 1 (26 g).....................2
Sourdough pretzels, fat free, 1 (24 g) 2
Spicy ranch, fat free, 1 oz 2
Whole wheat honeys, 1 pretzel (24 g) 2

Lance

Fat free pretzels, 9 (35 g) 3
Pretzels, 7 (28 g) 2
Pretzels, 9 (35 g) 3

Nabisco Pretzel air crisps, original,

23 crisps (1 oz)..2

Schwan's Soft stuffed pretzels w/

cheese, 3 pieces (75 g)............................4

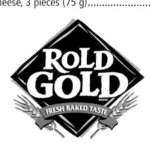

Rold Gold

Cheddar cheese flavored tiny twists,
16 pieces (1 oz)......................................2
Classic sticks, 48 pieces (1 oz) 2
Classic thin twists, 9 pieces (1 oz)............2
Classic tiny twists, 17 pieces (1 oz) 2
Fat free thins, 12 pieces (1 oz) 2
Fat free tiny twists, 18 pieces (1 oz) 2
Hard sourdough, 15 pieces (1 oz).............2
Honey mustard bite-size pretzels,
12 pieces (1 oz)....................................2
Honey mustard flavored tiny twists,
16 pieces (1 oz)....................................2
Parmesan herb bite-size pretzels,
12 pieces (1 oz).....................................2

Rods, 3 pieces (1 oz) 2
Snack mix, ¾ cup 4
Sourdough nuggets, 12 pieces (1 oz)........2

Superpretzel
Soft pretzel bites with ⅐ salt pak,
5 (53 g) 3
Soft pretzel bites without added salt,
5 (53 g) 3
Soft pretzel with ⅙ salt pak, 1 (64 g) 3
Soft pretzels without added salt, 1 (64 g) ..3

Superpretzel Softstix Cheese filled
soft pretzel sticks, Cheddar, 2 (50 g) 3

Tropical Nut & Fruit
Mini pretzels, 1 oz 2
Mustard pretzels, ½ cup 3
Pretzel gems, 1 oz 2

Weight Watchers Oat bran pretzels,
1 serving (42 g) 3

Prunes
Dole Pitted, ¼ cup 2

Sunsweet
Lemon essence prunes, 1½ oz 1
Orange essence prunes, 1½ oz.................1
Pitted prunes, 1½ oz 1

Tropical Nut & Fruit Pitted prunes,
¼ cup 2

Prune juice
Sunsweet Prune juice, 8 fl oz 3

Puddings
Jell-O Americana
Custard dessert, prepared with
2% reduced fat milk, ½ cup 3
Rice pudding (fat free), prepared with
2% reduced fat milk, ½ cup 3
Tapioca pudding (fat free), prepared
with 2% reduced fat milk, ½ cup...........3

Jell-O Cook & Serve
Banana cream, prepared with 2%
reduced fat milk, ½ cup 3
Butterscotch, prepared with 2%
reduced fat milk, ½ cup 3
Chocolate fudge, prepared with 2%
reduced fat milk, ½ cup 3
Chocolate, prepared with 2% reduced
fat milk, ½ cup 3
Coconut cream, prepared with 2%
reduced fat milk, ½ cup 3
Flan, prepared with 2% reduced fat
milk, ½ cup 3
Lemon, prepared with 2% reduced
fat milk, ½ cup 3
Milk chocolate, prepared with 2%
reduced fat milk, ½ cup 3
Vanilla, prepared with 2% reduced
fat milk, ½ cup 3

Jell-O Fat Free Instant
Chocolate, prepared with skim milk,
½ cup 3
Devil's food, prepared with skim milk,
½ cup 3
Vanilla, prepared with skim milk,
½ cup 3
White chocolate, prepared with skim
milk, ½ cup 3

Jell-O Fat Free Pudding Snacks
Chocolate, 1 (113 g) 2
Chocolate/vanilla swirls, 1 (113 g) 2
Devil's food, 1 (113 g)..............................2
Rocky road, 1 (113 g)...............................2
Tapioca, 1 (113 g)....................................2
Vanilla, 1 (113 g) 2

Jell-O Fat Free Sugar Free Instant
Banana, prepared with skim milk,
½ cup 1
Butterscotch, prepared with skim milk,
½ cup 1
Chocolate fudge, prepared with skim
milk, ½ cup 2
Chocolate, prepared with skim milk,
½ cup 2

Vanilla, prepared with skim milk,
½ cup 1

White chocolate, prepared with skim
milk, ½ cup 1

Jell-O Instant
Banana cream, prepared with 2%
reduced fat milk, ½ cup 3

Butterscotch, prepared with 2%
reduced fat milk, ½ cup 3

Chocolate fudge, prepared with 2%
reduced fat milk, ½ cup 3

Chocolate, prepared with 2% reduced
fat milk, ½ cup 3

Coconut cream, prepared with 2%
reduced fat milk, ½ cup 4

French vanilla, prepared with 2%
reduced fat milk, ½ cup 3

Lemon, prepared with 2% reduced
fat milk, ½ cup 3

Pistachio, prepared with 2% reduced
fat milk, ½ cup 3

Vanilla, prepared with 2% reduced
fat milk, ½ cup 3

Jell-O Pudding Snacks
Chocolate, 1 (113 g) 4

Chocolate marshmallow, 1 (113 g)...........4

Chocolate/vanilla swirls, 1 (113 g) 4

Tapioca, 1 (113 g)..................................4

Vanilla, 1 (113 g)...................................4

Jell-O Fat Free Cook & Serve
Chocolate, prepared with skim milk,
½ cup 3

Vanilla, prepared with skim milk,
½ cup 3

Jell-O Sugar Free Cook & Serve
Chocolate, prepared with 2% reduced
fat milk, ½ cup 2

Vanilla, prepared with 2% reduced
fat milk, ½ cup 2

Kraft Handi-Snacks
Banana, 1 (99 g)....................................3

Butterscotch, 1 (99 g) 3

Chocolate, 1 (99 g) 3

Chocolate (fat free), 1 (99 g) 2

Chocolate fudge, 1 (99 g)......................3

Tapioca, 1 (99 g)...................................3

Vanilla, 1 (99 g)....................................3

Vanilla (fat free), 1 (99 g) 2

Pumpkin
E.D.Smith Pure pumpkin, ½ cup 0

Pumpkin seeds
EXPRESSnacks Pumpkin seed,
shelled, ¼ cup 4

Planters
Pumpkin seeds, 1 package (57 g).............5

Pumpkin seeds, ⅓ cup...........................3

Tropical Nut & Fruit
Pumpkin seeds, roasted, 1 oz...................4

Raw pumpkin seeds, ¼ cup 4

Raisins
Dole California seedless, ¼ cup 2

EXPRESSnacks Yogurt raisins, ¼ cup......3

Harmony
Milk chocolate raisins, 44 pieces
(40 g) 3

Yogurt raisins, 30 raisins (41 g)................4

Tropical Nut & Fruit
Dark raisins, ¼ cup 2

Monukka raisins, ¼ cup 2

Raisins, ¼ cup 2

Sulphured gold raisins, ¼ cup..................2

Raspberries
Dole Raspberry, 1 cup 0

Ravioli
Di Giorno
Four cheese ravioli, 1 cup........................8

Italian sausage ravioli in green bell
pepper pasta, 1¼ cups..........................7

Light cheese ravioli, 1 cup 6

Sun-dried tomato ravioli, 1⅓ cups 8

Louise's Rosetto
Beef ravioli, 9 pieces (130 g) 5

Cheese ravioli, 9 pieces (127 g) 5

Homestyle cheese ravioli, 9 pieces
(127 g) 5

R

Rosetto

Beef ravioli, 9 pieces (124 g) 5
Cheese and broccoli ravioli, 4 pieces
　(146 g) 5
Cheese ravioli, 9 pieces (127 g) 5
Chicken and herb ravioli, 9 pieces (125 g) ..4
Sausage ravioli, 9 pieces (123 g)..............5

Relishes

Claussen Sweet pickle relish, 1 Tbsp 0
Del Monte

Hamburger relish, 1 Tbsp.........................0
Hot dog relish, 1 Tbsp 0
Sweet pickle relish, 1 Tbsp 0
Green Giant Corn relish, 1 Tbsp.............0
Harry & David

Calico corn relish, ¼ cup 2
Country cranberry relish, ¼ cup 4
Jalapeno relish, 2 Tbsp 1
Pepper & onion relish, 2 Tbsp 1
Heinz

Hot dog relish, 1 Tbsp 0
India relish, 1 Tbsp.................................0
Sweet relish, 1 Tbsp 0
Old El Paso Jalapeno relish, 1 Tbsp 0

Rice

Budget Gourmet

Oriental rice with vegetables, 1 serving
　(148 g) 5
Rice pilaf with green beans, 1 serving
　(141 g) 5
Faraon

E-z cook rice, uncooked, ¼ cup 4
Long grain rice, uncooked, ¼ cup.............3
Freezer Queen Family Side Dish

　Rice & broccoli au gratin, 1 cup.............3
Green Giant

Cheesy rice & broccoli, frozen,
　1 package (283 g) 6
Rice medley, frozen, 1 package
　(283 g) 5
Rice pilaf, frozen, 1 package (283 g) 4
White & wild rice, frozen, 1 package
　(283 g) 6

Health Valley

Cantonese style, ½ cup 2
Chicken flavored, ½ cup 2
Rice Primarera, ½ cup 2
Shitake vegetable, ½ cup.........................3
Thai style, ½ cup.....................................2
Lipton Rice & Sauce

Beef flavor, prepared, ½ cup 4
Cajun style, prepared, ½ cup 4
Cajun style with beans, prepared,
　½ cup 5
Cheddar broccoli, prepared, ½ cup...........5
Chicken & Parmesan risotto, prepared,
　½ cup 4
Chicken broccoli, prepared, ½ cup...........4
Chicken flavor, prepared, ½ cup 5
Creamy chicken, prepared, ½ cup 5
Herb & butter, prepared, ½ cup................5
Mushroom, prepared, ½ cup....................4
Original long grain & wild rice,
　prepared, ½ cup 4
Pilaf, prepared, ½ cup 4
Rice medley, prepared, ½ cup 4
Scampi style, prepared, ½ cup 4
Spanish, prepared, ½ cup 4
Teriyaki, prepared, ½ cup 4
Oriental stir-fry, prepared, ⅓ cup..............4
Roasted chicken, prepared, ⅓ cup............4
Salsa-style, prepared, ⅓ cup 3
Southwestern chicken flavor, prepared,
　⅓ cup...4
Minute

Enriched pre-cooked boil-in-bag long
　grain white rice, prepared, 1 cup 4
Instant enriched long grain white rice,
　prepared, 1 cup 3
Instant enriched premium long grain
　white rice, prepared, 1 cup 3
Instant whole grain brown rice,
　prepared, ⅔ cup...................................3
Long grain & wild rice seasoned with
　herbs, prepared, 1 cup 4

R

Old El Paso
Cheesy Mexican rice, prepared,
⅓ package 6
Spanish rice, 1 cup 3
Spanish rice, prepared, ⅓ package 6

Riceland Rice 'N Easy
Broccoli & cheese, dry mix, 2½ oz 6
Broccoli & cheese, prepared, 1 cup...........7
Chicken, dry mix, 2 oz 4
Chicken, prepared, 1 cup 5
Long grain & wild rice, dry mix, 2 oz 3
Long grain & wild rice, prepared, 1 cup 4
Long grain rice, cooked, ¾ cup 3
Long grain rice, uncooked, ¼ cup...........3
Medium grain rice, cooked, ¾ cup 3
Medium grain rice, uncooked, ¼ cup.......3
Natural brown rice, cooked, ¾ cup 3
Natural brown rice, uncooked, ¼ cup 3
Perfected rice, cooked, 1 cup 3
Perfected rice, uncooked, ¼ cup............3
Saffron yellow rice, dry mix, 2 oz 3
Saffron yellow rice, prepared, 1 cup 4

Sunsun Long grain rice, uncooked,
¼ cup 3

Tyson Chicken fried rice, 2½ cups 9

Rice bars, crisp
Estee Smart Treats
Sugar free chocolate crunch, 1 (19 g) 1
Sugar free chocolate chip, 1 (19 g)...........1
Sugar free old fashioned vanilla, 1
(19 g) 1
Sugar free peanut butter crunch, 1
(19 g) 1

Hain Pure Foods
Chewy caramel flavor, 1 (27 g) 2
Double chocolate flavor, 1 (27 g) 2
Peanut butter crunch flavor, 1 (27 g) 2

Little Debbie Marshmallow crispy
bars, 1 (35 g) 3

NutraBreak
Crisp rice bar, plain, 1 piece (22 g) 2
Crisp rice bar, plain, 1 piece (37 g) 3
Crisped rice bars with chocolate chips,
1 piece (22 g).........................2

Crisped rice bars with marshmallow
pieces, 1 piece (22 g) 2

Rice beverages
Hain Pure Foods
Cinnamon flavor, 8 fl oz 3
Original flavor, 8 fl oz.............................2

Rice cakes
Estee
Sugar free banana nut, 5 mini rice
cakes (16 g) 1
Sugar free cinnamon spice, 5 mini rice
cakes (16 g) 1
Sugar free Granny Smith apple, 5 mini
rice cakes (16 g) 1
Sugar free mixed berry, 5 mini rice
cakes (16 g) 1
Sugar free peanut butter crunch, 5 mini
rice cakes (16 g) 1

Hain Pure Foods
Apple cinnamon flavor, mini, 6 rice
cakes (16 g) 1
Barbeque flavor, 37 ringers (28 g) 2
Devils food flavor, mini, 5 rice cakes
(15 g) 1
Honey nut flavor, mini, 6 rice cakes
(16 g) 1
Mild Cheddar flavor, 37 ringers (28 g) 2
Peanut butter crunch, mini, 5 rice cakes
(14 g) 1
Plain, mini, 8 rice cakes (16 g) 1
Ranch flavor, mini, 6 rice cakes (16 g) 2
Strawberry cheesecake flavor, mini,
5 rice cakes (15 g) 1

Quaker Oats
Banana nut rice cakes, 1 (13 g)................1
Chocolate crunch rice cakes, 1 (15 g) 1
Cinnamon streusel rice cakes, 1 (14 g) 1
Crispy mini's banana nut, 8 (16 g) 1
Crispy mini's Cheddar cheese rice
snacks, 9 (15 g) 2
Crispy mini's honey nut rice snacks,
8 (16 g) 1
Crispy mini's rice snacks – apple
cinnamon, 8 (16 g) 1

R

Crispy mini's rice snacks – BBQ flavored,
  10 (16 g) 2
Crispy mini's rice snacks – caramel
  corn, 7 (15 g) 1
Crispy mini's rice snacks – chocolate,
  7 (15 g) 1
Crispy mini's sour cream & onion rice
  snacks, 10 (16 g) 2
Plain rice cake, 1 (9 g)...................1

Rice mixes, flavored
Betty Crocker
  Cheddar & broccoli rice mix, prepared,
    1 cup......................................5
  Chicken herb rice mix, prepared, 1 cup.....5
  Creamy herb risotto mix, prepared,
    1 cup......................................6
  Garden vegetable pilaf mix, prepared,
    1 cup......................................4
  Herb rice & barley medley mix, ⅓ cup 3
  Long grain & wild rice pilaf mix,
    prepared, 1 cup 3
  Southwestern rice mix, prepared, 1 cup....4
Durkee
  Fried rice, dry mix, 1 Tbsp 1
  Fried rice, prepared, 1 cup 6
Golden Grain Near East
  Long grain and wild rice mix, 2 oz 3
  Mediterranean black bean & rice pilaf,
    2½ oz.....................................4
  Spanish rice pilaf mix, 2½ oz 4
Golden Grain Near East
Creative Grains
  Chicken & herbs, 2½ oz...................4
  Creamy Parmesan, 2½ oz 4
  Roasted garlic, 2 oz 3
  Roasted pecan & garlic, 2 oz 4
Zatarain's New Orleans Style
Rice Mixes
  Dirty rice mix, 3 Tbsp 3
  Gumbo mix, 2 Tbsp..........................1
  Jambalaya mix, 3 Tbsp 3

Rolls
Pillsbury
  Crescents, 1 (28 g)...................3
  Crescents, grands!, 1 (73 g).....................6
  Crescents, reduced fat, 1 (28 g) 2
  Dinner rolls, wheat, 1 (40 g) 2
  Dinner rolls, white, 1 (40 g) 2
  Hot roll mix, baked, ¼ cup 3
  Schwan's French dinner rolls, 1 (51 g).....2

Roux
  Tony Chachere's Roux mix, 1 tsp..........0

Salads
  Dole Italian blend, 3 oz..............0
Dole Classic
  Cole slaw, 3 oz.......................0
  Iceberg salad, 3 oz...................0
Dole Complete
  Caesar, 3½ oz.........................4
  Lowfat Caesar, 3½ oz..............1
  Lowfat herb ranch, 3½ oz.......................1
  Lowfat raspberry romaine, 3½ oz............1
  Lowfat zesty Italian, 3½ oz....................1
  Oriental, 3½ oz.......................3
  Romano, 3½ oz 4
  Spinach bacon, 3½ oz 4
  Sunflower ranch, 3½ oz 4
Dole Lunch for One
  Caesar, 5¾ oz........................7
  Classic ranch, 7 oz...................9
  Lowfat Caesar, 6 oz 2
  Lowfat Italian, 7 oz...................2
Dole Special Blends
  American blend, 3 oz...........................0
  European blend, 3 oz 0
  French blend, 3 oz 0
  Romaine blend, 3 oz 0
  Green Giant Three bean salad,
    canned, ½ cup......................1
Progresso
  Olive salad (drained), 2 Tbsp 1
  Pepper salad (drained), 2 Tbsp.................0

S

Salad mixes
Betty Crocker Suddenly Salad
Caesar, low-fat recipe, prepared, ¾ cup....3
Caesar, prepared, ¾ cup 3
Classic pasta, prepared, ¾ cup 4
Classic pasta, reduced-fat recipe,
  prepared, ¾ cup....................................4
Garden Italian 98% fat free, ½ cup 2
Ranch & bacon, low-fat recipe,
  prepared, ¾ cup....................................4
Ranch & bacon, prepared, ¾ cup 3
Roasted garlic Parmesan, prepared,
  ¾ cup..3
Roasted garlic Parmesan, prepared,
  ¾ cup..4

Kraft
Classic ranch pasta salad with bacon,
  prepared, ¾ cup....................................8
Creamy Caesar pasta salad, prepared,
  ¾ cup..8
Garden primavera pasta salad, prepared,
  ¾ cup..5
Herb and garlic pasta salad, prepared,
  ¾ cup..6
Italian pasta salad (97% fat free),
  prepared, ¾ cup....................................4
Parmesan peppercorn pasta salad,
  prepared, ¾ cup....................................9

Salami
Boar's Head
Abruzzese, hot & sweet, 1 oz...................3
Beef salami, 2 oz 3
Cooked salami, 2 oz................................4
Hard salami, 1 oz....................................3
Head cheese – square, 2 oz 2
Hot sopressala grande, 1 oz 3
Jellied tongue loaf, 2 oz 3
Natural casing genoa salami, 2 oz 5
Sopressala grande, 1 oz 3
Hormel Pillow Pack Genoa salami,
  2 oz..6
Louis Rich Turkey salami cooked, 2 oz.....3

Oscar Mayer
Salami beef machiaeh brand, 2 slices
  (46 g) 3
Salami cotto, beef, 1 slice (28 g) 2
Salami cotto, made with chicken, beef
  and pork, 1 slice (28 g) 2
Salami for beer, 2 slices (46 g) 3
Salami genoa, 3 slices (27 g) 3
Salami, hard, 3 slices 3

Salmon
Demings
Pink salmon, ¼ cup 2
Red sockeye Alaska salmon, ¼ cup 3
Double "Q"
Pink Alaska salmon, ¼ cup 2
Red sockeye salmon, ¼ cup.....................3
Lascco
Oven roasted salmon, 2 oz 2
Premium nova sliced smoked salmon,
  2 oz..1
Smoked salmon snack bits, 2 oz..............1
Nathan's Smoked salmon, 2 oz..............1
Ocean Beauty
Florentine salmon roulade, 4 oz 4
Honey-garlic salmon burger, 1 burger
  (3.2 oz)..2
Lemon dill salmon burger, 1 burger
  (3.2 oz)..1
Mediterranean salmon roulade, 4 oz 5
Salmon burger fillet, 1 burger (3.2 oz)......2
Salmon fajita, 8 oz..................................2
Rite
Gravlax salmon, 2 oz 2
Nova salmon bits, ¼ cup 3
Nova salmon spread, 2 Tbsp....................1
Smoked Atlantic salmon, 2 oz 2
Smoked pastrami salmon, 2 oz 2
Smoked premium salmon, 2 oz 2

Salsa
Chi-Chi's
Salsa con queso, 2 Tbsp 2
Salsa hot, 2 Tbsp 0
Salsa medium, 2 Tbsp 0

S

Salsa mild, 2 Tbsp 0
Salsa verde medium, 2 Tbsp 0
Salsa verde mild, 2 Tbsp 0

Guiltless Gourmet

Roasted red pepper salsa, 2 Tbsp 0
Southwestern grill salsa, 2 Tbsp 0

Harry & David

Apple/pear salsa, 2 Tbsp 0
Black bean salsa, 2 Tbsp 1
Cactus salsa, 2 Tbsp................................0
Chipotle salsa, 2 Tbsp 0
Chunky peach salsa, 2 Tbsp.....................0
Spicy garlic salsa, 2 Tbsp 0
Zippy raspberry salsa, 2 Tbsp 0

LaTortilla Factory

Fire roasted green tomato & cilantro
   salsa, mild fresh refrigerated, 2 Tbsp......0
Fire roasted roma tomato salsa, mild
   fresh refrigerated, 2 Tbsp 0
Medium salsa, best of festival Sonoma
   County, 2 Tbsp....................................0
Mild salsa, best of festival Sonoma
   County, 2 Tbsp....................................0

Naturally Fresh Picante salsa sauce,
   2 Tbsp 0

Newman's Own

Bandito salsa – hot, 2 Tbsp 0
Bandito salsa - medium, 2 Tbsp 0
Bandito salsa - mild, 2 Tbsp.....................0
Peach salsa, 2 Tbsp 0
Pineapple salsa, 2 Tbsp 0
Roasted garlic salsa, 2 Tbsp.....................0

Old El Paso

Green chili salsa, 2 Tbsp...........................0
Homestyle salsa, medium, 2 Tbsp.............0
Homestyle salsa, mild, 2 Tbsp 0
Salsa verde, 2 Tbsp 0
Thick 'n chunky salsa, extra mild,
   2 Tbsp 0
Thick 'n chunky salsa, hot, 2 Tbsp 0
Thick 'n chunky salsa, medium, 2 Tbsp 0
Thick 'n chunky salsa, mild, 2 Tbsp...........0
Preciosa Picante salsa,1 Tbsp 0

Taco Bell Home Originals

Salsa con queso, medium, 2 Tbsp.............1
Salsa con queso, mild, 2 Tbsp 1
Thick 'n chunky salsa, hot, 2 Tbsp 0
Thick 'n chunky salsa, medium, 2 Tbsp 0
Thick 'n chunky salsa, mild, 2 Tbsp...........0

Salt substitutes
Nu-Salt

Salt substitute, ⅛ tsp 0
Salt substitute, 1 packet (1 g) 0

Sandwiches
Amy's

Broccoli & cheese in a pocket sandwich,
   1 (4½ oz) 6
Cheese pizza in a pocket sandwich,
   1 (4½ oz) 6
Mediterranean vegetables in a pocket
   sandwich, 1 (4½ oz) 4
Mexican tamale in a pocket sandwich,
   1 (4½ oz) 5
Roasted vegetables in a pocket
   sandwich, 1 (4½ oz) 4
Soy cheeze veggie pizza in a pocket
   sandwich, 1 (4½ oz) 6
Spinach feta in a pocket sandwich,
   1 (4½ oz) 5
Vegetable pie in a pocket sandwich,
   1 (5 oz)..6
Vegetarian pizza in a pocket sandwich,
   1 (4½ oz) 5

Healthy Choice Meals To Go

Chicken and broccoli, 1 (6.1 oz)...............6
Ham and cheese with broccoli, 1
   (6.1 oz)..7
Italian style meatball, 1 (6.1 oz)...............6
Philly beef steak, 1 (6.1 oz) 6

Lean Pockets

Chicken broccoli supreme, 1 piece
   (128 g) 6
Chicken fajita, 1 piece (128 g) 5
Chicken Parmesan, 1 piece (128 g)...........6
Ham & Cheddar, 1 piece (128 g) 6
Meatballs & mozzarella, 1 piece (128 g)...6

S

Philly steak & cheese, 1 piece (128 g) 6
Reduced fat pepperoni pizza deluxe,
1 piece (128 g)....................................6
Turkey & ham with Cheddar, 1 piece
(128 g) 6
Turkey, broccoli & cheese, 1 piece (128 g) ..5

Morningstar Farms
Breakfast sandwich – muffin, pattie,
cheese, scramblers, frozen, 1 (171 g)......5
Breakfast sandwich, frozen (muffin,
pattie, scramblers), 1 (146 g)..................4
Schwan's Grilled chicken sandwich,
1 (91 g) 4

Sandwiches, packaged
Oscar Mayer Lunchables
Deli-Carryouts
Chicken/Cheddar – low fat, 1 (6½ oz) 8
Chicken/turkey/Swiss, 1 (6½ oz) 11
Ham/Swiss, 1 (10 oz) 9
Ham/turkey/Cheddar, 1 (6.2 oz)..............11
Turkey/Cheddar, low fat, 1 (6 oz)..............7
Turkey/Cheddar, low fat, 1 (8.7 oz)...........7

Sardines
Sol-Mex Sardines with tomato sauce,
drained, ¼ cup 2
Underwood Fancy sardines in
mustard sauce, 1 can (106 g) 4

Sauces
Boar's Head Brown sugar & spice
ham glaze & cooking sauce, 2 Tbsp 2
Durkee Famous sandwich & salad
sauce, 1 Tbsp 2
Faraon Mexican sauce, 2 Tbsp 0
Giorgio Portabella mushroom sauce,
¼ cup 1
House of Tsang
Bangkok padang sauce, 1 Tbsp 1
Classic stir fry sauce, 1 Tbsp 1
Korean teriyaki sauce, 1 Tbsp...................1
Saigon sizzle sauce, 1 Tbsp......................1
Spicy brown bean sauce, 1 tsp.................0
Szechuan spicy stir fry, 1 Tbsp.................0

Jackaroo
Buffalo wing sauce, 2 Tbsp......................2
Gold sauce, 2 Tbsp..................................1
Honey mustard sauce, 2 Tbsp 4
Meat sauce, 2 Tbsp 1
Naturally Fresh Cajun sauce, 2 Tbsp 1
PA Dutchman Portabella mushroom
sauce, ¼ cup 1
Progresso Lobster, ½ cup......................2
San-J
All purpose szechuan hot & spicy
sauce, 1 tsp..0
All purpose Thai peanut stir-fry &
dipping sauce, 2 Tbsp 1
Cracked pepper sauce, 2 Tbsp..................1
Lemon pepper sauce, 2 Tbsp....................1
Peanut pepper sauce, 2 Tbsp 1
SJ grilling marinade & barbecue sauce,
2 Tbsp 1
Tomato pepper sauce, 2 Tbsp...................1
Taco Bell Home Originals
The restaurant hot sauce, 1 tsp..............0
Trappey's Louisiana hot sauce, 1 tsp.......0

Sauerkraut
Boar's Head Sauerkraut, 2 Tbsp.............0
Claussen Saurkraut, ¼ cup.....................0
Del Monte
Bavarian style sauerkraut, 2 Tbsp.............0
Sauerkraut, 2 Tbsp.................................0

Sausages
Boar's Head
Breakfast sausage – tube, 2 oz 5
Breakfast sausage, link, 2 (43 g) 4
Hot smoked sausage, 1 (91 g)..................8
Kielbasa, 2 oz..3
Mortadella (plain), 2 oz...........................4
Mortadella w/ pistachio nuts, 2 oz 5
Rico picante Spanish style sausage,
2 oz..4
Smoked sausage natural casing,
1 (130 g) 11

S

Butterball
Fat free polska kielbasa, 2 oz 1
Fat free smoked sausage, 2 oz 1
Turkey polska kielbasa, 2 oz 1
Turkey smoked sausage, 2 oz....................3
Hebrew National Beef polish
   sausage, 1 (85 g).....................................7
Hormel Little Sizzlers
Brn 'n serve sausage links, 3 (60 g) 6
Brn 'n serve sausage patties, 2 (50 g).......5
Pork sausage H&S, cooked, 3 (50 g) 6
Sausage link, cooked, 3 (50 g) 6
Sausage patties, cooked, 2 (50 g)..............6
Lance
Hot sausage, 1 (25 g)................................2
Jumbo hot sausage, 1 (40 g)....................3
Louis Rich
Turkey polska kielbasa, 2 oz 2
Turkey sausage (hot and original),
   2½ oz 3
Turkey smoked sausage, 2 oz....................2
Oscar Mayer
Pork sausage link, cooked, 2 (48 g) 5
Smokies links sausage, 1 (43 g) 4
Smokies sausage, little, made with
   pork & turkey, 6 (57 g) 5
Smokies, beef, 1 (43 g) 3
Smokies, cheese, a pork, beef & cheese
   product, 1 (43 g) 4
Smokies, little cheese, a pork, turkey
   & cheese product, 6 (57 g) 5
Summer sausage (thuringer cervelat),
   2 slices (46 g)..4
Summer sausage, beef (thuringer
   cervelat), 2 slices (46 g) 4
Perdue
Fresh sweet Italian turkey sausage,
   cooked, 1 (79 g) 4
Roasted garlic, Romano cheese &
   parsley chicken sausage – link, cooked,
   1 (79 g) 4
Roasted garlic, Romano cheese &
   parsley chicken sausage-rope, cooked,
   1 (56 g) 3

Sweet Italian chicken sausage with
   fennel – link, cooked, 1 (79 g) 4
Sweet Italian chicken sausage with
   fennel – rope, cooked, 1 (56 g) 3
Wampler Foods
Breakfast turkey sausage, 2 links
   (68 g) 3
Fresh hot Italian turkey sausage,
   1 serving (91 g).....................................4
Fresh sweet Italian turkey sausage,
   1 serving (91 g).....................................4

Scallops
Fishery Products Breaded scallops,
   9 (84 g) 5
Sea Cuisine Breaded scallops, 9
   (84 g) 5

Scones
Health Valley
Fat free healthy scones, blueberry,
   1 scone (60 g) 3
Fat free healthy scones, cranberry
   orange, 1 scone (60 g) 3
Fat free healthy scones, raisin
   cinnamon, 1 scone (60 g)......................3

Seasonings
Accent Flavor enhancer, ⅛ tsp 0
Chef Paul Prudhomme's
Seasoning Blends
Blackened redfish magic, ¼ tsp................0
Blackened steak magic, ¼ tsp...................0
Herbal pizza & pasta magic, ¼ tsp 0
Hot & sweet pizza & pasta magic,
   ¼ tsp..0
Magic barbecue seasoning, ¼ tsp 0
Magic salt free seasoning, ¼ tsp...............0
Magic seasoning salt, ¼ tsp 0
Meat magic, ¼ tsp...................................0
Pork & veal magic, ¼ tsp 0
Poultry magic, ¼ tsp 0
Seafood magic, ¼ tsp 0
Vegetable magic, ¼ tsp............................0
Chi-Chi's Seasoning mix, 1 tsp................0

S

Durkee

Buffalo wings, garlic & herb, mix,
2½ tsp 0

Buffalo wings, garlic & herb, prepared,
3 wing halves as served (85 oz).............5

Buffalo wings, hot, 1½ Tbsp 0

Buffalo wings, hot, prepared, 3 wing
halves as served (85 oz)........................5

Buffalo wings, mild, mix, 1⅓ Tbsp............0

Buffalo wings, mild, prepared, 3 wing
halves (85 oz) 5

Buffalo wings, screaming hot, mix,
1½ Tbsp...0

Buffalo wings, screaming hot, prepared,
3 wing halves as served (85 oz).............5

Cajun wings, prepared, 3 wing halves
as served (85 g) 5

Shrimp scampi seasoning, 2 Tbsp.............1

Durkee Pasta Gourmet Cajun wings,
dry mix, 1 Tbsp.....................................0

French's

Enchilada seasoning, mix, 2 tsp 0

Enchilada seasoning, prepared,
1 enchilada (136 oz) 6

Kitchen Bouquet, 1 tsp 0

Knorr Pot roast (sauerbraten) recipe
mix, 1 Tbsp 1

Lawry's

Garlic powder, ¼ tsp...............................0

Garlic salt, ¼ tsp 0

Lemon pepper, ¼ tsp...............................0

Salt-free 17, ¼ tsp 0

Seasoned pepper, ¼ tsp 0

Seasoned salt, ¼ tsp 0

Spices & seasonings for chili, 1 Tbsp 1

Spices & seasonings for fajitas, 2 tsp........0

Taco spices & seasonings, 2 tsp 0

Old El Paso

Burrito seasoning mix, 2 tsp 0

Chili seasoning mix, 1 Tbsp 0

Enchilada sauce mix, 2 tsp 0

Fajita seasoning mix, 1 tsp 0

Shake 'N Bake

Barbecue chicken or pork, as packaged,
⅛ packet (12 g).....................................1

Buffalo wings, as packaged, ⅟₁₀ packet
(10 g) 1

Classic Italian chicken or pork, as
packaged, ⅛ packet (10 g) 1

Country mild recipe, as packaged,
⅛ packet (8 g) 1

Extra crispy recipe for chicken, as
packaged, ⅛ packet (15 g) 1

Extra crispy recipe for pork, as
packaged, ⅛ packet (15 g) 1

Home style flour recipe for chicken,
as packaged, ⅛ packet (11 g)................1

Honey mustard chicken or pork, as
packaged, ⅛ packet (12 g) 1

Hot & spicy chicken or pork, as
packaged, ⅛ packet (10 g) 1

Original recipe for chicken, as
packaged, ⅛ package (10 g)...................1

Original recipe for fish, as packaged,
¼ packet (19 g) 2

Original recipe for pork, as packaged,
⅛ packet (11 g) 1

Tangy honey chicken or pork, as
packaged, ⅛ packet (12 g) 1

Shake 'N Bake Perfect Potatoes

Crispy Cheddar, as packaged, ⅙ packet
(7 g) 1

Herb and garlic, as packaged, ⅙ packet
(7 g) 0

Home fries, as packaged, ⅙ packet
(7 g) 0

Parmesan peppercorn, as packaged,
⅙ packet (7 g) 1

Savory onion, as packaged, ⅙ packet
(7 g) 0

Taco Bell Home Originals

Chicken fajita seasoning mix, 1 Tbsp........0

Taco seasoning mix, 2 tsp 0

S

Tony Chachere's
Lite Creole seasoning, ¼ tsp....................0
More spice seasoning, ¼ tsp 0
More spice, less salt, ¼ tsp.....................0
Salt free Creole seasoning, ¼ tsp 0

Williams
Beef stew seasoning, 2 tsp......................0
Cajun chili seasoning, 2 tsp 0
Cajun taco seasoning, 1 tsp.....................0
Chili seasoning, 1 tsp 0
Chili seasoning w/ onion, 2 tsp 0
Country brown gravy mix, 2 tsp...............1
Country chicken gravy mix, 1 Tbsp 1
Country gravy w/ sausage, 1 Tbsp............1
Meatloaf seasoning, 2 tsp 0
Nonfat country gravy, 1 Tbsp 1
Pork chop gravy mix, 1⅓ Tbsp 0
Sloppy Joe seasoning, 1 tsp.....................0
Spaghetti sauce seasoning, 2 tsp 0
Spicy wings seasoning, 3 Tbsp 1
Taco seasoning, 1 Tbsp............................0
Tex-mex chili, 2 tsp 0
Turkey gravy, 1 Tbsp................................1
White chili seasoning, 1 Tbsp...................0

Seasoning bags
Durkee
Roasting bag, BBQ chicken, mix,
  2½ tsp 1
Roasting bag, BBQ chicken, prepared,
  3 oz 6
Roasting bag, BBQ spare ribs, mix,
  2 tsp...0
Roasting bag, BBQ spare ribs, prepared,
  5 oz 6
Roasting bag, cajun fish, mix, 2 tsp..........0
Roasting bag, cajun fish, prepared, 3 oz ...3
Roasting bag, pot roast, mix, 2 tsp..........0
Roasting bag, pot roast, prepared, 5 oz 5
Roasting bag, sweet & sour chicken,
  mix, 1 Tbsp 1
Roasting bag, sweet & sour chicken,
  prepared, 1 breast with sauce (140 g)....0

French's
Roasting bag, pot roast, mix, 2 tsp...........0
Roasting bag, pot roast, prepared, 5 oz....5
Williams
Chicken bag 'n bake, 1 Tbsp 0
Pot roast bag 'n bake, 1 Tbsp...................0

Seitan
Lightlife
Marinated in barbecue sauce, 4 oz...........3
Marinated in teriyaki sauce, 4 oz 3

Sesame mix
Planters Sesame nut mix, 1 oz................4

Sesame seeds
Tropical Nut & Fruit
Brown natural sesame seeds, ¼ cup.........6
Raw hulled sesame seeds, ¼ cup 5

Sesame sticks
EXPRESSnacks Honey sesame sticks,
  ⅓ cup 3

Shells, stuffed
Rosetto Stuffed shells, 2 pieces (138 g) ...5

Sherbet
Breyers All Natural
Natural Orange, ½ cup.............................3
Natural Rainbow, ½ cup...........................3
Natural Raspberry, ½ cup 3

Shortening
Jewel Shortening, 1 Tbsp 3
Snowdrift
Shortening, 1 Tbsp...................................3
Shortening, 1 Tbsp...................................3

Shrimp
Lascco Shrimp cocktail, 4 oz...................2
Schwan's
Breaded fantail shrimp, 4 (112 g).............5
Gourmet medium P&D shrimp, 16
  (112 g) 3
Oven-ready breaded shrimp, 7 pieces
  (85 g) 5

S

Sloppy Joe sauce
Del Monte
Hickory flavor, ¼ cup................................1
Original recipe, ¼ cup 1
Green Giant Sloppy joe sandwich
sauce, ¼ cup 1
Hormel Not-so-sloppy-Joe sauce,
¼ cup 1

Snack chips
Lance
Hot fries, 44 pieces (25 g) 3
Onion rings, 44 (25 g) 3

Snack mixes
Chex Mix
Bold party blend, ½ cup 3
Bold party blend (single serve),
1 pouch (49 g) 4
Cheddar cheese, ½ cup 3
Cheddar cheese (single serve),
1 pouch (49 g) 5
Hot 'n spicy, ⅔ cup 3
Hot 'n spicy (single serve), 1 pouch
(49 g) 4
Nacho fiesta, ⅔ cup................................2
Nacho fiesta (single serve), 1 pouch
(49 g) 4
Peanut lovers, ½ cup...............................3
Peanut lovers (single serve), 1 pouch
(46 g) 5
Traditional, ⅔ cup 3
Traditional (single serve), 1 pouch
(49 g) 4
EXPRESSnacks
Cajun hots, ¼ cup....................................4
Oriental rice snacks, ⅔ cup 2
Gardetto's
Deluxe snak-ens, ½ cup...........................4
Ranch snak-ens, ½ cup 4
Harmony Cajun mix, ¼ cup 4
New York Style Snack mix, original,
1 oz...2

Tropical Nut & Fruit
After hours, 1 oz......................................4
Bartender's blend, 30 g 4
Cajun harvest, 1 oz 4
Capitol mix, 1 oz 4
Checkmate, 1 oz 4
Cinnamon splendor, 30 g.........................2
Convention mix, ⅓ cup 4
Country club, 1 oz....................................5
Festival mix, 1 oz 3
Firecracker hot & spicy, ½ cup.................4
French quarter, 1 oz 4
Neptune's choice, 1 oz 4
Oriental delight, 1 oz 4
Pasta prime, 1 oz 4
Rise 'n shine, ⅓ cup 3
Rocky top, 15 g 2
Salty dog, 1 oz 4
Sesame nut mix, 1 oz...............................4
Student mix, 1 oz 4
Sweet & salty, 1 oz 4
Sweet Caroline, 1 oz 4

Snack sticks
Tropical Nut & Fruit
Cheddar sesame stix, 1 oz.......................4
Garlic sesame stick, 1 oz 4
Honey mustard onion stick, 1 oz..............4
Honey roasted sesame stick, 1 oz 4
Hot cajun corn sticks, 28 g 3
Oat bran sticks, 1 oz 4
Poppy onion sticks, 1 oz 3
Sesame bread sticks, 24 pieces (28 g) 3
Sesame stick, taco, 1 oz 4
Sesame sticks, 1 oz 4

Snacks
Amy's
Cheese pizza snacks, frozen, 5-6 pieces....4
Spinach feta snacks, frozen, 5-6 pieces.....4
Baked Bugles
Cheddar cheese, 1½ cups 3
Original, 1½ cups 3
Original (single serving), 1 pouch
(40 g) 4

Bugles

Chili con queso, 1⅓ cups..........................4
Nacho cheese, 1⅓ cups............................4
Nacho cheese (single serving),
   1 pouch (25 g) 3
Original, 1⅓ cups 4
Original (single serving), 1 pouch
   (43 g) 6
Ranch, 1⅓ cups.......................................4
Smokin BBQ, 1⅓ cups..............................4
Sour cream & onion, 1⅓ cups...................4

Chester's Fries

Flamin' hot, 1 oz 3
Salsa, 1 oz 3

Combos

Cheddar cheese cracker, 1 bag
   (48.2 g) 6
Cheddar cheese pretzel, 1 bag (51 g) 6
Nacho cheese pretzel, 1 bag (51 g)..........5
Pepperoni pizza, 1 bag (48.2 g) 6
Pizzeria pretzel, 1 bag (51 g) 5

Frito-Lay

Funyuns, 13 (1 oz) 3
Munchos, 16 (1 oz) 4

Harry & David

Cajun fried green peas, ¼ cup 2
Fried green peas, ¼ cup 2
Wasabi peas, ¼ cup 2

Kellogg's Snack Ums Baked Snacks

Big boomin' pops, 1 cup...........................2
Big rollin' froot loops, 1¼ cups 2
Rice krispies treats krunch, 1 cup.............3

Kraft Handi-Snacks

Cheez'n breadsticks, 1 (31 g) 3
Cheez'n crackers, 1 (27 g) 3
Cheez'n pretzels, 1 (29 g) 2
Nacho stix'n cheez, 1 (31 g) 3

Lance

Buffalo wing chips, 22 (28 g)...................4
Honey mustard chips, 25 (28 g) 4

Sun Chips

French onion, 10 (1 oz) 3
Harvest Cheddar, 11 (1 oz) 3
Original, 11 (1 oz)....................................3

Sweet Rewards

Blueberry w/ drizzle, 1 (37 g) 2
Double fudge supreme, 1 (32 g)...............2
Raspberry (variety pack only), 1 (37 g) 2
Strawberry w/ drizzle, 1 (37 g).................2

Tropical Nut & Fruit Rice snacks,

⅔ cup..2

Weight Watchers

Apple chips, 1 serving (21 g) 1
Strawberry snacks, 1 serving (14 g)..........1

Snow peas

LaChoy Snow pea pods, 3 oz 0

Soft drinks

7-Up

7-Up cherry, 1 cup 2
7-Up diet, 1 cup 0
7-Up diet cherry, 1 cup.............................0
7-Up regular, 1 cup..................................2

A&W

Cream soda, 1 cup....................................2
Diet cream soda, 1 cup 0
Root beer, 1 cup 2

Barq's

Diet French vanilla crème soda, 8 fl oz 0
Diet red crème soda, 8 fl oz......................0
Diet root beer, 8 fl oz...............................0
French vanilla crème soda, 8 fl oz 2
Red crème soda, 8 fl oz............................2
Root beer, 8 fl oz 2

Canada Dry

Club soda, 8 fl oz.....................................0
Collins mixer, 8 fl oz................................2
Cranberry ginger ale, 8 fl oz 2
Diet cranberry ginger ale, 8 fl oz..............0
Diet tonic water, 8 fl oz............................0
Ginger ale, 8 fl oz....................................2
Seltzer, 8 fl oz..0
Tonic water, 8 fl oz...................................2
Citra, 8 fl oz 2

Coca-Cola

Caffeine free Coca-Cola classic, 8 fl oz 2
Caffeine free diet Coke, 8 fl oz.................0
Cherry Coke, 8 fl oz..................................2

Soft drinks,
Coca-Cola (con't)

	POINTS
Coca-Cola classic, 8 fl oz	2
Diet cherry Coke, 8 fl oz	0
Diet Coke, 8 fl oz	0

Country Time

Cranberry-raspberry lemonade, prepared, 8 fl oz	2
Lemonade, 8 fl oz	2
Lemonade, prepared, 8 fl oz	1
Lemonade, prepared, sugar free, 8 fl oz	0
Pink lemonade, prepared, 8 fl oz	1
Pink lemonade, prepared, sugar free, 8 fl oz	0
Raspberry lemonade, prepared, 8 fl oz	2
Strawberry lemonade, prepared, 8 fl oz	2
Strawberry lemonade, prepared, sugar free, 8 fl oz	0
Wildberry lemonade, prepared, 8 fl oz	2

Crush Orange, 8 fl oz ... 2

Crystal Light

Cranberry breeze, 8 fl oz	0
Cranberry breeze, prepared, 8 fl oz	0
Fruit punch, 8 fl oz	0
Fruit punch, prepared, 8 fl oz	0
Iced tea decaffeinated, prepared, 8 fl oz	0
Iced tea, prepared, 8 fl oz	0
Kiwi-strawberry, 8 fl oz	0
Lemon tea, 8 fl oz	0
Lemonade, 8 fl oz	0
Lemonade, prepared, 8 fl oz	0
Lemon-lime, prepared, 8 fl oz	0
Orange-strawberry-banana, 8 fl oz	0
Passion fruit-pineapple, prepared, 8 fl oz	0
Peach tea, 8 fl oz	0
Peach tea, prepared, 8 fl oz	0
Pineapple-orange, prepared, 8 fl oz	0
Pink lemonade, 8 fl oz	0
Pink lemonade, prepared, 8 fl oz	0
Raspberry ice, 8 fl oz	0
Raspberry ice, prepared, 8 fl oz	0
Raspberry tea, 8 fl oz	0
Raspberry tea, prepared, 8 fl oz	0
Strawberry-kiwi, 8 fl oz	0
Strawberry-orange-banana, 8 fl oz	0
Watermelon-strawberry, prepared, 8 fl oz	0

Dr. Pepper

	POINTS
Caffeine free diet, 8 fl oz	0
Caffeine free regular, 8 fl oz	2
Diet, 8 fl oz	0
Regular, 8 fl oz	2

Fanta

Grape, 8 fl oz	2
Orange, 8 fl oz	2

Fresca, 8 fl oz ... 0

Fruitworks

Apple raspberry, 12 fl oz	3
Guava berry, 12 fl oz	3
Orange juice conc., 8 fl oz	2
Passion orange, 12 fl oz	3
Peach papaya, 12 fl oz	3
Pink lemonade, 12 fl oz	3
Strawberry melon, 12 fl oz	3
Tangerine citrus, 12 fl oz	3

Hawaiian Punch Fruit juicy red, 8 oz ... 3

Health Valley

Ginger ale,1 bottle (355 ml)	2
Old fashioned root beer, 1 bottle (355 ml)	2
Sarsaparilla root beer, 1 bottle (355 ml)	2

Hershey's Chocolate, 8 fl oz ... 2

Hires

Cream soda, 8 fl oz	2
Diet cream soda, 8 fl oz	0
Diet root beer, 8 fl oz	0
Root beer, 8 fl oz	2

IBC

Black cherry, 8 fl oz	2
Cream soda, 8 fl oz	2
Diet root beer, 8 fl oz	0
Root beer, 8 fl oz	2

Kool-Aid

Black cherry, mix, prepared with sugar and water, 8 fl oz	2
Cherry, sugar-sweetened mix, prepared, 8 fl oz	1
Cherry, mix, prepared with sugar and water, 8 fl oz	2
Cherry, prepared, sugar free, 8 fl oz	0

Grape berry splash, sugar-sweetened mix, prepared, 8 fl oz 1

Grape berry splash, mix, prepared with sugar and water, 8 fl oz 2

Grape, sugar-sweetened mix, prepared, 8 fl oz..1

Grape, mix, prepared with sugar and water, 8 fl oz..2

Grape, prepared, sugar free, 8 fl oz 0

Kickin' kiwi-lime, sugar-sweetened mix, prepared, 8 fl oz.....................................1

Kickin' kiwi-lime, mix, prepared with sugar and water, 8 fl oz 2

Lemonade, sugar-sweetened mix, prepared, 8 fl oz....................................1

Lemonade, mix, prepared with sugar and water, 8 fl oz 2

Lemonade, sugar-sweetened mix, prepared, sugar free, 8 fl oz...................0

Lemon-lime, mix, prepared with sugar and water, 8 fl oz 2

Mano-o-mango berry, sugar-sweetened mix, prepared, 8 fl oz.............................1

Man-o-mango-berry, mix, prepared with sugar and water, 8 fl oz 2

Oh yeah orange pineapple, sugar-sweetened mix, prepared, 8 fl oz 1

Oh yeah orange-pineapple, mix, prepared with sugar and water, 8 fl oz...2

Orange, sugar-sweetened mix, prepared, 8 fl oz.....................................1

Orange mix, prepared with sugar and water, 8 fl oz..2

Piña-pineapple, sugar-sweetened mix, prepared, 8 fl oz.....................................1

Piña-pineapple, mix, prepared with sugar and water, 8 fl oz 2

Pink lemonade, mix, prepared with sugar and water, 8 fl oz 2

Raspberry, sugar-sweetened mix, prepared, 8 fl oz.....................................1

Raspberry, mix, prepared with sugar and water, 8 fl oz 2

Roarin' raspberry-cranberry, sugar-sweetened mix, prepared, 8 fl oz 1

Roarin' raspberry-cranberry, mix, prepared with sugar and water, 8 fl oz...2

Scary blackberry ghoul-aid, mix, prepared with sugar and water, 8 fl oz...2

Slammin' strawberry-kiwi, sugar-sweetened mix, prepared, 8 fl oz 1

Slammin' strawberry-kiwi, mix, prepared with sugar and water, 8 fl oz...2

Soarin' strawberry lemonade, sugar-sweetened mix, 8 fl oz...........................1

Soarin' strawberry lemonade, mix, prepared with sugar and water, 8 fl oz...2

Soarin' strawberry lemonade, prepared, sugar free, 8 fl oz 0

Strawberry, sugar-sweetened mix, prepared, 8 fl oz 1

Strawberry, mix, prepared with sugar and water, 8 fl oz 2

Strawberry-raspberry, sugar-sweetened mix, prepared, 8 fl oz.............................1

Strawberry-raspberry, mix, prepared with sugar and water, 8 fl oz.................2

Tropical punch, sugar-sweetened mix, prepared, 8 fl oz.....................................1

Tropical punch, mix, prepared with sugar and water, 8 fl oz 2

Tropical punch, prepared, sugar free, 8 fl oz..0

Watermelon-cherry, sugar-sweetened mix, prepared, 8 fl oz.............................1

Watermelon-cherry, mix, prepared with sugar and water, 8 fl oz 2

Kool-Aid Bursts

Cherry, 1 (200 ml) 2

Grape, 1 (200 ml) 2

Great bluedini, 1 (200 ml) 2

Kickin' kiwi-lime, 1 (200 ml) 2

Oh yeah orange-pineapple, 1 (200 ml) 2

Slammin' strawberry-kiwi, 1 (200 ml).......2

Tropical punch, 1 (200 ml).......................2

S

Soft drinks (con't)   POINTS

Kool-Aid Splash
Blue raspberry, 8 fl oz 2
Cherry, 8 fl oz..2
Grape berry punch, 8 fl oz.......................2
Kiwi-strawberry, 8 fl oz 2
Tropical punch, 8 fl oz 2
Watermelon, 8 fl oz 2

Mello Yello
Diet Mellow Yello, 8 fl oz.........................0
Mello Yello, 8 fl oz 2

Minute Maid
Black cherry, 8 fl oz.................................2
Blueberry, 8 fl oz.....................................2
Diet orange, 8 fl oz..................................0
Fruit punch (carbonated), 8 fl oz..............2
Grape, 8 fl oz..2
Orange, 8 fl oz..2
Peach, 8 fl oz...2
Pineapple, 8 fl oz.....................................2
Strawberry, 8 fl oz...................................2

Mountain Dew
Caffeine free, 12 fl oz..............................3
Diet, 12 fl oz 0
Diet caffeine free, 12 fl oz 0
Regular, 12 fl oz 3

Mr. Pibb
Diet Mr. Pibb, 8 fl oz 0
Mr. Pibb, 8 fl oz......................................2

Mug
Cream, 12 fl oz..3
Diet cream, 12 fl oz 0
Diet root beer, 12 fl oz 0
Root beer, 12 fl oz...................................3

Pepsi
Caffeine free, 12 fl oz..............................3

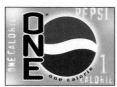

Diet, 12 fl oz 0

POINTS

Diet caffeine free, 12 fl oz 0
Diet caffeine free, military, 12 fl oz...........0
Diet, military, 12 fl oz..............................0

Pepsi one, 12 fl oz 0
Regular, 12 fl oz 3
Wild cherry, 12 fl oz 3
Wild cherry, diet, 12 fl oz.........................0

Schweppes
Bitter lemon, 8 fl oz.................................2
Club soda, 8 fl oz....................................0
Collins mixer, 8 fl oz................................2
Diet ginger ale, 8 fl oz.............................0
Ginger ale, 8 fl oz 2

Slice
Cherry lime, 12 fl oz................................3
Cherry spice, 12 fl oz...............................3
Diet lemon-lime, 12 fl oz..........................0
Diet orange, 12 fl oz................................0
Dr. Slice, 12 fl oz.....................................3
Fruit punch, 12 fl oz.................................4
Grape, 12 fl oz...4
Lemon-lime, 12 fl oz................................3
Orange with caffeine, 12 fl oz...................3
Orange without caffeine, 12 fl oz..............4
Pineapple, 12 fl oz...................................4
Red, 12 fl oz..4
Slice cola, 12 fl oz....................................3
Slice cola, diet, 12 fl oz 0
Strawberry, 12 fl oz..................................3

Sprite
Diet Sprite, 8 fl oz...................................0
Sprite, 8 fl oz..2

Squeezit
Berry B. Wild, 1 (200 ml) 2
Blue raspberry, 1 (200 ml) 2
Chucklin' cherry, 1 (200 ml).....................2

S

Grumpy grape, 1 (200 ml) 2
Rockin' red puncher, 1 (200 ml) 2
Strawberry, 1 (200 ml) 2
Tropical punch, 1 (200 ml)......................2

Squeezit 100
Apple, (200 ml)......................................2
Berry, 1 (200 ml) 2
Grape, 1 (200 ml) 2
Punch, 1 (200 ml) 2

Squirt
Squirt diet, 8 fl oz 0
Squirt diet ruby red, 8 fl oz....................0
Squirt regular, 8 fl oz.............................2
Squirt ruby red, 8 fl oz 2

Storm
Storm, 12 fl oz......................................3
Storm light, 12 fl oz..............................0

Sundrop
Cherry Sundrop, 8 fl oz..........................2
Sundrop diet, 8 fl oz 0
Sundrop regular, 8 fl oz.........................3

Sunkist Orange, 8 fl oz......................3
Surge, 8 fl oz 2
Tab, 8 fl oz.....................................0
Tahitian treat, 8 fl oz 2

Tang
Mango, prepared, 8 fl oz 2
Orange pineapple, prepared, 8 fl oz 2
Orange, prepared, 8 fl oz.......................2
Orange, prepared, sugar free, 8 fl oz 0

Vernors
Diet, 8 fl oz 0
Regular, 8 fl oz 2

Waist Watcher
Diet black cherry, 12 fl oz 0
Diet caffeine free cola, 12 fl oz 0
Diet citrus frost, 12 fl oz........................0
Diet cream, 12 fl oz 0
Diet ginger ale, 12 fl oz.........................0
Diet lemon up, 12 fl oz..........................0
Diet orange, 12 fl oz 0
Diet raspberry ginger ale, 12 fl oz 0
Diet root beer, 12 fl oz 0

Welch's Grape, 8 fl oz 3
Wink, 8 fl oz...................................2

Sorbets
Ben & Jerry's
Devil's food chocolate, ½ cup 3
Doonesberry, ½ cup 3
Lemon swirl, ½ cup................................2
Purple passion fruit, ½ cup......................3

Dreyer's
Boysenberry, ½ cup................................3
Chocolate, ½ cup...................................3
Lemon, ½ cup 3
Mango, ½ cup 3
Peach, ½ cup...3
Raspberry, ½ cup 3
Strawberry, ½ cup..................................2

Edy's
Boysenberry, ½ cup................................3
Chocolate, ½ cup...................................3
Lemon, ½ cup 3
Mango, ½ cup 3
Peach, ½ cup...3
Raspberry, ½ cup 3
Strawberry, ½ cup..................................2

Haagen-Dazs
Chocolate, ½ cup...................................2
Mango, ½ cup, ...2
Orange, ½ cup.......................................2
Orchard peach, ½ cup 3
Raspberry, ½ cup 2
Strawberry, ½ cup..................................2
Zesty lemon, ½ cup................................2

Soup mixes
Hain Pure Foods
Black bean, 1.9 oz 3
Cheddar broccoli, 1.1 oz.........................3
Chicken noodle, .8 oz.............................2
Chicken vegetable, 1 oz 2
Country mushroom, 1.2 oz 3
Lentil, 1.8 oz 3
Navy bean, 1.3 oz..................................2
Potato leek, 1 oz....................................2

S

Soup mixes,
Hain Pure Foods (con't)   POINTS

Split pea, 1.8 oz 3
Sweet corn chowder, 1 oz........................2
Tomato herb, .9 oz..................................1

Harry & David
Chicken chili, ¼ cup 2
Fajita chili, ¼ cup 2
Harvest vegetable soup, 6 Tbsp.................2
Potato corn chowder, ½ cup 2
Seafood corn chowder, ¼ cup 1
Split pea soup, ¼ cup...............................2
Tomato rice soup, 4 Tbsp..........................2

Health Valley
Chicken flavored noodles with
  vegetables, ½ cup................................2
Corn chowder with tomatoes, ½ cup........1
Creamy potato with broccoli, ⅓ cup.........1
Fat free pasta Italiano, ⅓ cup 2
Fat free pasta Mediterranean, ½ cup........2
Garden split pea with carrots, ⅓ cup........2
Lentil with couscous, ⅓ cup.....................2
Spicy black bean with couscous, ⅓ cup 2
Zesty black bean with rice, ⅓ cup 1

Health Valley Fat Free
Pasta marinara, ½ cup 2
Pasta Parmesan, ½ cup 2

Knorr
Black bean soup in cup, 1 package
  (53 g) 3
Chicken flavor noodle savory soup
  mix, 3 Tbsp 1
Corn chowder soup in cup, 1 package
  (36 g) 3
Cream of broccoli soup and recipe mix,
  3 Tbsp 1
Cream of spinach soup and recipe mix,
  2 Tbsp 1
Creamy chicken flavored savory soup
  with rice, 3 Tbsp 2
French onion soup and recipe mix,
  2 Tbsp 1
Hearty chicken flavored noodle,
  1 package (30 g) 2
Hearty lentil soup, 1 package (57 g).........3

Hot and sour soup mix, 2 Tbsp 1
Leek soup and recipe mix, 2 Tbsp 2
Mediterranean style minestrone savory
  soup mix, 3 Tbsp 2
Navy bean soup, 1 package (38 g) 2
Roasted garlic herb soup & recipe mix,
  3 Tbsp 2
Split pea soup, 1 package (43 g)...............2
Spring vegetable soup and recipe mix,
  2 Tbsp 0
Tomato beef flavor (oxtail) soup &
  recipe mix, 2 Tbsp................................1
Tomato with basil soup and recipe mix,
  3 Tbsp 2
Vegetable soup mix, 2 Tbsp 1
Vegetarian vegetable soup in cup,
  1 package (45 g) 3

Lipton Cup a Soup
Broccoli & cheese, 1 envelope (16 g)........1
Chicken broth, 1 envelope (6 g) 0
Chicken broth with pasta, 1 envelope
  (13 g) 1
Chicken noodle with white meat,
  1 envelope (13 g) 1
Chicken vegetable flavor, 1 envelope
  (14 g) 1
Cream of chicken, 1 envelope (17 g) 1
Cream of mushroom, 1 envelope
  (15 g) 1
Creamy chicken vegetable, 1 envelope
  (19 g) 2
Green pea, 1 envelope (21 g) 1
Hearty chicken noodle, 1 envelope
  (16 g) 1
Ring noodle, 1 envelope (14 g) 1
Spring vegetable, 1 envelope (13 g) 1

Lipton Kettle Creations
Soup Secrets
Chicken flavor 'n onion with long
  grain and wild rice, ¼ cup.....................2
Chicken flavor with pasta and beans,
  ¼ cup...2
Country chicken flavor with pasta and
  herbs, ¼ cup 2

Homestyle lentil with bow tie pasta,
¼ cup 2

Lipton Recipe Secrets
Beefy mushroom, 1½ Tbsp 1
Beefy onion, 1 Tbsp 1
Fiesta herb with red pepper, 1⅓ Tbsp 1
Garlic mushroom, 1⅓ Tbsp 0
Golden onion, 1⅔ Tbsp..........................1
Onion, 1 Tbsp 0
Onion-mushroom, 1⅔ Tbsp 1
Savory herb with garlic, 1 Tbsp 0
Vegetable, 1⅔ Tbsp 0

Lipton Soup Secrets
Chicken noodle, 3 Tbsp 2
Extra noodle, 3 Tbsp 2
Noodle soup with real chicken broth,
2 Tbsp 1
Ring-o-noodle, 2 Tbsp 2
Spiral pasta soup, 3 Tbsp.........................1

Williams
Bean soup, ¼ cup 2
Minestrone soup, 3 Tbsp 1
Potato soup w/ potatoes, ⅓ cup...............3
Tortilla soup, 3 Tbsp 1
Vegetable soup (inc. veg.), 3 Tbsp.............1

Soups, canned, condensed
Cape Cod Premium New England
style clam chowder, ½ cup 1

Campbell's Healthy Request
Bean with ham and bacon, ½ cup.............2
Chicken noodle, ½ cup 1
Chicken vegetable, ½ cup........................1
Chicken with rice, ½ cup 1
Cream of broccoli, ½ cup 1
Cream of celery, ½ cup............................1
Cream of chicken, ½ cup 1
Cream of chicken and broccoli, ½ cup 2
Cream of mushroom, ½ cup 1
Hearty vegetable and pasta, ½ cup 1
Minestrone, ½ cup 1
Tomato, ½ cup.......................................2
Vegetable, ½ cup....................................1
Vegetable beef, ½ cup.............................1

Chincoteague
Chesapeake bay cream of crab soup,
1 cup..5
Crab & Cheddar soup, ½ cup 2
Manhattan clam chowder, ½ cup 2
New England clam chowder, ½ cup..........2
Premium clam bisque, ½ cup 2
Premium corn chowder, ½ cup 2
Premium lobster bisque, ½ cup 2
Premium shrimp bisque, ½ cup 1
Shrimp bisque, ½ cup..............................2

Snow's
New England clam chowder, ½ cup..........2
New England corn chowder, ½ cup 2

Soup, canned, ready-to-eat
Campbell's
98% fat free cream of mushroom,
1 cup..2
98% fat free New England clam
chowder, 1 cup......................................2
Bean and ham, 1 cup..............................3
Chicken and pasta with roasted garlic,
1 cup..2
Chicken and rice, 1 cup 2
Chicken vegetable, 1 cup.........................2
Chicken with egg noodles, 1 cup..............2
Country mushroom rice, 1 cup 1
Country vegetable, 1 cup.........................2
Creamy potato with roasted garlic,
1 cup..4
Fiesta vegetable, 1 cup............................2
Grilled chicken with sundried tomatoes
& mushrooms, 1 cup...............................2
Italian chicken with vegetables, 1 cup 2
New England clam chowder, 1 cup 2
Old world minestrone, 1 cup....................2
Oriental noodles with vegetables, 1 cup ...1
Roasted chicken with white and wild
rice, 1 cup...2
Savory lentil, 1 cup 2
Split pea with ham, 1 cup 3
Tomato garden, 1 cup 1
Tuscany style minestrone, 1 cup...............4
Vegetable beef, 1 cup 2

S

Campbell's Healthy Request (Canada)

Hearty bean & vegetable, 1 serving
(250 ml)..2
Herbed chicken noodle, 1 serving
(250 ml)..2
Italian style minestrone, 1 serving
(250 ml)..2
New England clam chowder, 1 serving
(250 ml)..2
Vegetable beef with barley, 1 serving
(250 ml)..2

Campbell's Healthy Request (United States)

Chicken noodle, 1 cup..............................2
Chicken vegetable, 1 cup..........................2
Creamy potato with roasted garlic,
1 cup...2
Hearty chicken corn chowder, 1 cup 2
Hearty chicken rice, 1 cup........................2
Hearty country vegetable, 1 cup................2
Hearty vegetable, 1 cup 1
Hearty vegetable beef, 1 cup 2
New England clam chowder, 1 cup 2
Split pea with ham, 1 cup 3
Tomato ravioli with vegetable, 1 cup........3

Campbell's Simply Home

Chicken & pasta, 1 cup 1
Chicken noodle, 1 cup..............................1
Chicken with white & wild rice, 1 cup 2
Country vegetable soup, 1 cup..................2
Minestrone, 1 cup....................................2
Vegetable beef with pasta, 1 cup..............2
Vegetable garden, 1 cup 2

Campbell's Soup to Go

Chicken rice soup, 1 can (305 g) 3
Garden vegetable, 1 can (305 g)...............2
Hearty chicken noodle, 1 can (305 g) 2
Minestrone, 1 can (305 g) 2
Vegetable beef with pasta, 1 can (305 g)...2

Chincoteague Vegetable red crab
soup, 1 cup 2

Hain Pure Foods

Black bean, 1 cup 1
Chicken noodle soup, 1 cup......................3
Chicken noodle soup, no salt added,
1 cup...2
Chunky tomato, 1 cup...............................2
Cream of mushroom, 1 cup 3
Minestrone, 1 cup.....................................2
Mushroom barley, 1 cup...........................2
Vegetarian lentil, 1 cup 3
Vegetarian split pea, 1 cup.......................1
Wild rice, 1 cup 2

Health Valley

99% fat free chicken noodle soup,
1 cup...2
99% fat free chicken rice soup, 1 cup.......2
Fat free 14 garden vegetable soup,
1 cup...1
Fat free 5 bean vegetable soup, 1 cup 2
Fat free black bean vegetable soup,
1 cup...1
Fat free country corn & vegetable,
1 cup...1
Fat free lentil & carrot soup, 1 cup 1
Fat free minestrone soup, 1 cup 1
Fat free pasta bolognese soup, 1 cup 1
Fat free pasta cacciatore soup, 1 cup 1
Fat free pasta fagioli soup, 1 cup 2
Fat free pasta Romano soup, 1 cup 1
Fat free pasta rotini soup, 1 cup...............1
Fat free split pea & carrot soup, 1 cup......1
Fat free super broccoli carotene soup,
1 cup...1
Fat free vegetable barley soup, 1 cup 1
Fat free, tomato vegetable soup, 1 cup.....1
Organic black bean soup, 1 cup 2
Organic black bean soup, no salt, 1 cup ...2
Organic lentil soup, 1 cup........................1
Organic lentil soup, no salt, 1 cup 1
Organic minestrone soup, 1 cup...............1
Organic minestrone soup, no salt, 1 cup...1
Organic mushroom barley soup, 1 cup 1
Organic mushroom barley soup, no salt,
1 cup...1

S

Organic potato leak soup, 1 cup 1
Organic potato leak soup, no salt, 1 cup...1
Organic split pea soup, 1 cup 1
Organic split pea soup, no salt, 1 cup.......1
Organic tomato soup, 1 cup 1
Organic tomato soup, no salt, 1 cup.........1
Organic vegetable soup, 1 cup.................1
Organic vegetable soup, no salt, 1 cup.....1

Hormel Micro Cup Soups

Bean & ham soup, 1 cup 3
Beef vegetable, 1 cup..............................2
Broccoli cheese w/ ham, 1 cup................4
Chicken & rice, 1 cup 2
Chicken noodle, 1 cup.............................2
New England clam chowder, 1 cup 3
Potato cheese w/ ham, 1 cup...................5

Progresso

Basil rotini tomato, 1 cup 2
Bean & ham, 1 cup 3
Beef barley, 1 cup 2
Beef minestrone, 1 cup 2
Beef noodle, 1 cup...................................3
Cheese & herb tortellini tomato, 1 cup 3
Chickarina, 1 cup.....................................3
Chicken & wild rice, 1 cup 2
Chicken barley, 1 cup 2
Chicken broth, 1 cup................................1
Chicken minestrone, 1 cup......................2
Chicken noodle, 1 cup.............................2
Chicken rice with vegetables, 1 cup 2
Chicken vegetable, 1 cup.........................2
Creamy Cheddar chicken, 1 cup 5
Creamy tomato garlic, 1 cup....................3
Escarole in chicken broth, 1 cup..............0
French onion, 1 cup 1
Green split pea, 1 cup..............................3
Hearty black bean, 1 cup.........................3
Hearty chicken & rotini, 1 cup.................2
Hearty penne in chicken broth, 1 cup 1
Herb & rotini vegetable, 1 cup.................1
Herb & shell minestrone, 1 cup 2
Homestyle chicken with vegetables,
    1 cup..2

Lentil, 1 cup ....
Macaroni & bean, 1 cup..........................
Manhattan clam chowder, 1 cup..............2
Minestrone, 1 cup...................................2
Minestrone Parmesan, 1 cup 2
New England clam chowder, 1 cup 4
Oregano penne Italian style vegetable,
    1 cup..2
Peppercorn penne vegetable, 1 cup..........2
Potato broccoli & cheese, 1 cup 4
Potato ham & cheese, 1 cup 4
Roasted chicken garden herb, 1 cup.........1
Roasted chicken Italiano, 1 cup................2
Roasted chicken rotini, 1 cup...................2
Roasted garlic & lentil, 1 cup...................2
Roasted potato garlic, 1 cup....................4
Southwestern style corn chowder, 1 cup...4
Spicy chicken & penne, 1 cup...................2
Split pea with ham, 1 cup 3
Tomato basil, 1 cup..................................2
Tomato vegetable Italiano, 1 cup 1
Tortellini in chicken broth, 1 cup 1
Turkey noodle, 1 cup 2
Turkey rice with vegetable, 1 cup 2
Vegetable, 1 cup......................................1
Vegetarian vegetable, 1 cup 1
Zesty herb tomato, 1 cup.........................2

Progresso 99% Fat Free

Beef barley, 1 cup 2
Beef vegetable, 1 cup..............................3
Chicken noodle, 1 cup.............................2
Chicken rice with vegetables, 1 cup 2
Creamy chicken broccoli, 1 cup................2
Lentil, 1 cup 2
Minestrone, 1 cup...................................1
New England clam chowder, 1 cup 2
Roasted chicken with Italian style
    vegetables, 1 cup 2
Roasted chicken with wild rice, 1 cup.......2
Split pea, 1 cup 3
Tomato garden vegetable, 1 cup..............2
Vegetable, 1 cup......................................1
White Cheddar potato, 1 cup...................2

Soups, ready-to-eat
Amy's
Organic black bean vegetable soup,
  1 cup 1
Organic cream of mushroom soup,
  1 serving (14.1 oz)..................................1
Organic cream of tomato soup,
  1 serving (14½ oz)..................................1
Organic lentil soup, 1 serving (14½ oz) 2
Organic minestrone soup, 1 serving
  (14.1 oz) 1
Organic no chicken noodle soup,
  1 serving (14.1 oz)..................................2
Snow's Authentic New England clam
  chowder, 1 cup 4
Snow's Healthy Values Authentic
  New England clam chowder, 1 cup 2

Soy beverage
Hain Pure Foods
Original flavor, 8 fl oz...............................1
Vanilla flavor, 8 fl oz 2
Health Valley
Fat free, fat soy moo non-dairy soy
  drink, 1 cup..2
Low fat, soy moo non-dairy soy drink,
  1 cup 2
WestSoy
Café westbrae mocha, 1 cup 3
Café westbrae, coffee, 1 cup....................3
Drink plain, 1 cup 2
Lite plain, 1 cup 2
Lite vanilla, 1 cup 3

Soy cheese
Galaxy Foods
Feta veggie slices (alternative), 1 slice
  (19 g) 1
Garden herb topping, 2 tsp 0
Veggie American sandwich slices
  (alternative), 1 slice (19 g) 1
Veggie blue cheese sandwich slices
  (alternative), 1 slice (19 g) 1
Veggie Caeser Parmesan sandwich
  slices (alternative), 1 slice (19 g)............1

Veggie Cheddar and pepper Jack cheese
  (alternative), 1 oz 1
Veggie Cheddar cheese (alternative),
  1 oz...1
Veggie Cheddar sandwich slices
  (alternative), 1 slice (19 g) 1
Veggie cream cheese, garden vegetable,
  1 oz...1
Veggie cream cheese, honey-nut, 1 oz......1
Veggie cream cheese, strawberry, 1 oz 1
Veggie low fat cream cheese alternative,
  rich & creamy, 1 oz 1
Veggie low fat mild Cheddar cheese
  (alternative), 1 oz 1
Veggie low fat mozzarella cheese, 1 oz 1
Veggie mozzarella cheese
  (alternative), 1 oz 1
Veggie mozzarella sandwich slices
  (alternative), 1 slice (19 g) 1
Veggie Parmesan mozzarella Romano
  cheese (alternative), 1 oz 1
Veggie pepper Jack slices (alternative),
  1 slice (19 g) 1
Veggie provolone slices (alternative),
  1 slice (19 g) 1
Veggie Swiss sandwich slices
  (alternative), 1 slice (19 g) 1
Veggie topping, 2 tsp...............................0
Galaxy Foods Monterey Veggie
  Monterey Jack and Cheddar cheese
  (alternative), 1 oz 1
SoyaKaas
Mild Cheddar style, 1 oz...........................2
Mozzarella style, 1 oz 2

Soy milk
Galaxy Foods
Low fat chocolate veggie milk, 1 cup 3
Low fat veggie mix, 1 cup 2
Sun Soy
Chocolate soymilk, 1 cup 3
Creamy original soymilk, 1 cup 1
Vanilla soymilk, 1 cup 2

S

Vitasoy

Carb supreme (shelf), 8 fl oz.....................3
Cream original, refrigerated, 8 fl oz..........2
Creamy original, 8 fl oz 3
Enriched original, shelf, 8 fl oz 2
Enriched vanilla, shelf, 8 fl oz 3
Light cocoa, 8 fl oz 2
Light original, 8 fl oz................................1
Light vanilla, 8 fl oz 2
Rich chocolate, refrigerated, 8 fl oz 3
Rich cocoa (shelf), 8 fl oz 3
Soy milk, unsweetened, 8 fl oz 2
Vanilla delite, 8 fl oz 3

Soy nuts

Tropical Nut & Fruit Soybeans, 1 oz.....4

Soy sauce

House of Tsang

Dark soy sauce, 1 Tbsp 0
Ginger flavored soy sauce, 1 Tbsp 0
Light soy sauce, 1 Tbsp 0
Low sodium ginger flavored soy sauce,
  1 Tbsp 0
Low sodium soy sauce, 1 Tbsp 0

San-J

Organic whole soybean shoyu
  naturally brewed soy sauce, 1 Tbsp 0
Organic whole soybean tamari wheat
  free soy sauce, 1 Tbsp 0
Reduced sodium tamari natural soy
  sauce, 1 Tbsp 0
Reduced sodium tamari organic wheat
  free soy sauce, 1 Tbsp 0
Tamari premium soy sauce, 1 Tbsp 0

Soy yogurt

Galaxy Foods

Low fat veggie yogurt, apple pie, 6 oz......4
Low fat veggie yogurt, blueberry, 6 oz......4
Low fat veggie yogurt, peach, 6 oz 4
Low fat veggie yogurt, raspberry, 6 oz......4
Low fat veggie yogurt, strawberry, 6 oz....4
Low fat veggie yogurt, vanilla, 6 oz..........4

Spinach

Boston Markets Creamed spinach,
  1 serving (140 g) 5
Budget Gourmet Spinach au gratin,
  1 serving (141 g) 4

Del Monte

Chopped spinach, ½ cup 0
Spinach, no salt added, ½ cup 0
Spinach, whole leaf, ½ cup 0

Green Giant

Creamed spinach, frozen, ½ cup 2
Cut leaf spinach, frozen, ¾ cup 0
Cut leaf spinach, frozen, ½ cup...............0

Green Giant Harvest Fresh Spinach,
  frozen, ½ cup 0
Hanover Cut leaf spinach, 1 cup.............0

Stouffer's

Creamed spinach, ½ cup 4
Spinach souffle, ½ cup 3

Sports drinks

All Sport

Black citrus, 8 fl oz 1
Blue ice, 8 fl oz......................................1
Cherry slam, 8 fl oz.................................1
Fruit punch, 8 fl oz..................................1
Grape, 8 fl oz 1
Lemon-lime, 8 fl oz..................................1
Orange, 8 fl oz..1
Raspberry burst, 8 fl oz 1
Watermelon, 8 fl oz 1

Gatorade

Citrus cooler, 8 fl oz 1
Cool blue raspberry, 8 fl oz......................1
Fruit punch, 8 fl oz..................................1
Lemon ice, 8 fl oz 1
Lemon lime, 8 fl oz 1
Mandarina, 8 fl oz 1
Orange, fl 8 oz..1
Strawberry kiwi, 8 fl oz 1
Tropical burst, 8 fl oz 1

Gatorade Fierce

Fierce berry, 8 fl oz.................................1
Fierce grape, 8 fl oz 1

S

Sports drinks,
Gatorade Fierce (con't) POINTS

Fierce lime, 8 fl oz.................................1
Fierce melon, 8 fl oz.............................1

Gatorade Frost

Alpine snow, 8 fl oz.............................1
Glacier freeze, 8 fl oz..........................1
Riptide rush, 8 fl oz.............................1

Powerade

Arctic shatter, 8 fl oz..........................1
Dark downburst, 8 fl oz.......................1
Fruit punch, 8 fl oz.............................1
Green squall, 8 fl oz............................1
Jagged ice, 8 fl oz...............................1
Lemon-lime, 8 fl oz.............................1
Mountain blast, 8 fl oz........................1
Orange tangerine, 8 fl oz......................1

Torq

Grape, 12 fl oz....................................5
Orange, 12 fl oz..................................5
Wild berry, 12 fl oz 5

Spreads
Best Foods

Dijonnaise creamy mustard, 1 tsp 0
Sandwich spread, 1 Tbsp.......................1

Ferrero Nutella, 2 Tbsp...........................4

Galaxy Foods

Veggie low fat honey butter spread,
  1 Tbsp 1
Veggie low fat spread, 1 Tbsp..................1

Hellmann's

Dijonnaise creamy mustard, 1 tsp 0
Sandwich spread, 1 Tbsp.......................1

Imperial Seasoning Spreads

Garlic & herb, 1 Tbsp 3
Parmesan & herb, 1 Tbsp........................3

Kraft

Reduced fat sandwich spread, 1 Tbsp.......1
Sandwich spread, 1 Tbsp........................1

Oscar Mayer Sandwich spread, 2 oz......3
Wish-Bone Spread, 2 Tbsp.....................1

Spreadable fruit
Clearbrook Farms

Bitter-sweet orange marmalade, 1 Tbsp....1
California apricot, 1 Tbsp 1

POINTS

Cranberry-orange, 1 Tbsp 1
Michigan red tart cherry, 1 Tbsp..............1
Northwest strawberry, 1 Tbsp 1
Oregon blackberry, 1 Tbsp 1
Oregon red raspberry, 1 Tbsp...................1
Peach-ginger, 1 Tbsp..............................1
Triple berry, 1 Tbsp................................1
Wild Maine blueberry, 1 Tbsp 1

E.D.Smith No Sugar Added

Apricot spread with sucralose, 1 Tbsp 0
Blueberry spread with sucralose, 1 Tbsp ...0
Five fruit spread with sucralose, 1 Tbsp 0
Midnight raspberry spread with
  sucralose, 1 Tbsp 0
Strawberry spread with sucralose,
  1 Tbsp...0

E.D.Smith Triple Fruits Lemon

spread, 1 Tbsp.......................................1

Harry & David

Tart cherry fruit spread, 1 Tbsp 1
Triple berry fruit spread, 1 Tbsp...............1

Polaner All Fruit

Apricot, 1 Tbsp 1
Blueberry, 1 Tbsp 1
Grape, 1 Tbsp..1
Raspberry, 1 Tbsp..................................1
Strawberry, 1 Tbsp 1

Smucker's Light Fruit Spreads

Apricot, 1 Tbsp 0
Blackberry (seedless), 1 Tbsp 0
Boysenberry, 1 Tbsp 0
Grape, 1 Tbsp 0
Orange marmalade, 1 Tbsp......................0
Red raspberry, 1 Tbsp.............................0
Strawberry, 1 Tbsp 0

Smucker's Simply Fruit

Apple butter, 1 Tbsp...............................1
Apricot, 1 Tbsp 1
Blackberry (seedless), 1 Tbsp 1
Black cherry, 1 Tbsp 1
Black raspberry (seedless), 1 Tbsp............1
Blueberry, 1 Tbsp 1
Grape, 1 Tbsp..1

S

Orange marmalade, 1 Tbsp......................1
Peach, 1 Tbsp 1
Red raspberry, 1 Tbsp..............................1
Red raspberry (seedless), 1 Tbsp 1
Strawberry, 1 Tbsp 1
Strawberry (seedless), 1 Tbsp...................1

Squash
Del Monte Zucchini with Italian style
  tomato sauce, ½ cup 0

Steak sauce
A1
Bold & spicy, 1 Tbsp................................0
Steak sauce, 1 Tbsp.................................0
Sweet and tangy, 1 Tbsp 1
Thick 'n hearty, 1 Tbsp............................1
Dawn Fresh Steak sauce, ¼ cup 0
Heinz
57 sauce, 1 Tbsp 0
Traditional steak sauce, 1 Tbsp 0
Lea & Perrins
HP steak sauce, 1 Tbsp............................0
Steak sauce sweet 'n spicy, 1 Tbsp 1
Traditional steak sauce, 1 Tbsp 1

Stews
Austex Original beef stew, 1 cup.............8
Castleberry's
Brunswick stew, chicken & beef,
  canned, 1 cup 6
Original beef stew, 1 cup........................8
Dinty Moore
Beef stew, 1 cup 4
Chicken stew, 1 cup 5
Meatball stew, 1 cup................................6
Turkey stew, 1 cup 3
Dinty Moore American Classics
Beef stew, 1 bowl (283 g) 6
Dinty Moore Microwave Cups
Beef stew, 1 cup 3
Chicken stew, 1 cup 4
Hearty burger stew, 1 cup 5
Turkey stew, 1 cup 2

Hormel Microcup Meals Beef stew,
  1 cup..3
Strawberries
Dole Strawberries, 8................................0
Schwan's Strawberries, frozen,
  1¼ cups..1
Tropical Nut & Fruit Dried
  strawberries, ½ cup 2
Strawberry drink
Hershey's Strawberry drink, 1 box 4
Stuffing
Kellogg's Crouettes Stuffing mix,
  1 cup..2
Stove Top
Chicken flavor, prepared with
  margarine, ½ cup 4
Cornbread, prepared with margarine,
  ½ cup 4
For beef, prepared with margarine,
  ⅓ cup 4
For pork, prepared with margarine,
  ½ cup 4
For turkey, prepared with margarine,
  ½ cup 4
Long grain & wild rice, prepared with
  margarine, ½ cup 4
Lower sodium chicken flavor, prepared
  with margarine, ½ cup 4
Mushroom & onion, prepared with
  margarine, ½ cup 4
San Francisco style, prepared with
  margarine, ½ cup 4
Savory herbs, ½ cup................................4
Traditional sage flavor, prepared with
  margarine, ½ cup 4
Stove Top Flexible Serve
Chicken flavor, prepared with margarine,
  ½ cup 4
Cornbread flavor, prepared with
  margarine, ½ cup 4
Homestyle herb, prepared with
  margarine, ½ cup 4

S

Stove Top Microwave

Chicken flavor, prepared with
margarine, ½ cup 4
Homestyle cornbread, prepared with
margarine, ½ cup 4

Sugar

Sugar in the Raw

Turbinado sugar from natural cane,
1 packet (5 g)..0
Turbinado sugar from natural cane,
1 tsp..0

Sugar substitutes

EQUaL.
SWEETENER

Equal Sweetener, 1 packet (1 g) 0
Natrataste Sugar substitute,
1 packet (1 g)..0
Sans Sucre Cinnamon sugar
substitute, ½ tsp....................................0
Sweet Magic Sugar substitute,
1 packet (0.6 g).....................................0

Sweet 'N Low

Brown granulated sugar substitute,
¹⁄₁₀ tsp...0
Granulated sugar substitute, ¹⁄₁₀ tsp..........0
Granulated sugar substitute, 1 packet
(1 g) 0
Low calorie sugar substitute tablets,
1 tablet (15 mg) 0
Zero-cal liquid sweetener, 10 drops
(0.6 g) 0
Sweet One Granulated sugar substitute,
1 packet (1 g)..0

Sunflower seeds

EXPRESSnacks Sunflower seeds,
salted, ¼ cup 4
Frito-Lay Sunflower seeds, 3 Tbsp..........4

Lance

Sunflower seeds, in shell, ½ cup 3
Sunflower seeds, in shell, 1 package
(53 g) 4
Sunflower seeds, shelled, ¼ cup...............4

Planters

Dry roasted sunflower kernels, ¼ cup.......4
Dry roasted sunflower kernels,
1 package (49 g) 7
Oil roasted honey roasted sunflower
kernels, ¼ cup 4
Sunflower seeds, ¾ cup 4
Sunflower seeds, 1 package (21 g)...........3
Sunflower seeds, 1 package (25 g)...........4
Sunflower seeds, 1 package (28 g)...........4
Sunflower seeds, 1 package (43 g)...........7
Sunflower seeds, 1 package (46 g)...........7

Tropical Nut & Fruit

In-shell sunflower seeds, 1 oz 0
Sunflower seeds, 1 oz 5
Sunflower seeds, raw, 1 oz 3

Sweet and sour sauce

Contadina Sweet & sour sauce with
pineapple, 2 Tbsp 1

House of Tsang

Sweet & sour concentrate, 1 tsp 0
Sweet & sour stir fry sauce, 1 Tbsp...........1
Kraft Sweet 'n sour sauce, 2 Tbsp 1
Naturally Fresh Sweet & sour sauce,
2 Tbsp 2
San-J Fruit juice & honey sweetened
sweet & sour stir-fry, dipping &
marinade, 2 Tbsp 1

Sweet potatoes

Green Giant Candied sweet potatoes,
frozen, ¾ cup.......................................5
Rosetto Sweet potatoes with
candied sauce packet, 5 pieces with
sauce (148 g) 3

Sweet roll

Lance

Pecan twirls, 2 pieces (57 g) 5
Swiss rolls, 1 (35 g)................................4

s

You'll Love This Little Dish.
And This Little Number: *3 POINTS*®!

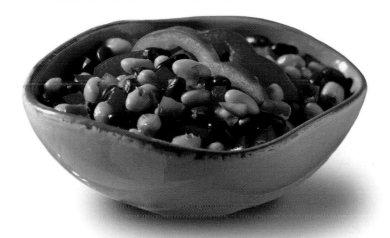

White and Black Bean Salad.

Who says food that's good for you can't taste good too? Equal® sweetener lets you enjoy mouthwatering recipes without the additional calories of sugar.
Enjoy the recipe below and visit **www.equal.com** for other great tasting Equal recipes such as refreshing fruit smoothies, rich cheesecakes and delicious fruit pies.

White and Black Bean Salad — EQUAL® www.equal.com

1	cup finely chopped red onions
2	cloves garlic, minced
2	tablespoons olive oil or vegetable oil
1/3	cup red wine vinegar
1/4	cup chopped red pepper
1/4	cup chopped green pepper
2	tablespoons minced parsley
1	teaspoon Equal® for Recipes *or* 3 packets Equal® sweetener *or* 2 tablespoons Equal® Spoonful™
1/4	teaspoon salt
1/4	teaspoon pepper
1	can (15 ounces) great northern beans, rinsed, drained
1	can (15 ounces) black beans, rinsed, drained
	Red and green pepper rings

◆ SAUTE onions and garlic in oil until crisp-tender in medium skillet; remove from heat and cool until warm.
◆ STIR vinegar, peppers, parsley, **Equal®**, salt and pepper into onions.
◆ POUR onion mixture over combined beans in a bowl; mix well.
◆ GARNISH with pepper rings.

Makes 8 servings (about 1/2 cup each).

Nutrition information per serving:
174 cal., 9 g pro., 27 g carb., 4 g fat, 0 mg chol., 78 mg sodium, 8 g fiber

Sweet roll (con't) POINTS

Little Debbie Pecans spinwheels, 1
(28 g) 2
Morton
Honey buns, 1 (2.3 oz) 6
Mini honey buns, 1 (1.3 oz) 4
Pillsbury
Apple cinnamon rolls with icing,
1 (44 g) 3
Caramel rolls, 1 (49 g)............................4
Cinnamon raisin rolls with icing,
1 (49 g) 4
Cinnamon rolls with icing, 1 (44 g) 3
Cinnamon rolls with icing, reduced fat,
1 (44 g) 3
Orange sweet rolls with icing, 1
(49 g) 4
Pillsbury Grands!
Caramel rolls, 1 (100 g)...........................7
Cinnamon rolls with butter cream icing,
1 (99 g) 8
Cinnamon rolls with cream cheese icing,
1 (99 g) 7
Cinnamon rolls with icing, 1 (99 g) 7
Cinnamon rolls with icing, reduced fat,
1 (99 g) 6
Schwan's
Freezer to oven caramel rolls, 1 roll with
caramel (96 g).....................................7
Freezer to oven cinnamon rolls, 1 roll
wth icing (92 g) 6

Syrups
Golden Griddle
Cinnamon flavor syrup, 4 Tbsp.................5
Syrup, 4 Tbsp...4
Hershey's
Chocolate malt syrup, 1 pouch (56 g) 3
Chocolate syrup, 2 Tbsp 2
Genuine chocolate flavored lite syrup,
2 Tbsp 1
Special dark chocolate syrup, 2 Tbsp 2
Strawberry syrup, 2 Tbsp 2
Hershey's Chocolate Shoppe
Sundae syrup, chocolate cherries
jubilee, 2 Tbsp 2

POINTS

Sundae syrup, fat free double
chocolate, 2 Tbsp.................................2
Karo
Dark corn syrup with refiners' syrup,
2 Tbsp 2
Light syrup, 2 Tbsp.................................2
Pancake syrup, 4 Tbsp 5
Maple Mountain Sugar free syrup,
2 oz..0
Nesquik
Chocolate syrup, 2 Tbsp 2
Strawberry syrup, 2 Tbsp 2
Pillsbury Hungry Jack
Butter maple, ¼ cup 4
Butter maple lite, ¼ cup..........................2
Regular, ¼ cup 4
Regular lite, ¼ cup..................................2
Smucker's Sugar free breakfast
syrup, ¼ cup 1
Smucker's Guilt Free Chocolate
flavored syrup, 2 Tbsp 2
Vermont Maid
Lite syrup, ¼ cup 2
Syrup, ¼ cup 4

Tabouli
Golden Grain Near East Taboule
wheat salad mix, 1 oz...........................1
Tribe of Two Sheiks Tabouli, 2 Tbsp.....0

Taco sauce
Chi-Chi's Taco sauce, 1 Tbsp 0
Heinz
Mild taco sauce, 1 packet (9 g) 0
Taco sauce, hot, 1 packet (9 g) 0
Old El Paso
Taco sauce, hot, 1 Tbsp 0
Taco sauce, medium, 1 Tbsp 0
Taco sauce, mild, 2 Tbsp 0
Pancho Villa Taco sauce, mild, 1 Tbsp.....0
Taco Bell Home Originals
Taco sauce, medium, 2 Tbsp 0
Taco sauce, mild, 2 Tbsp 0

Taco seasonings
Hain Pure Foods Taco seasoning
   mix, 2 tsp..0
Old El Paso
   Cheesy taco seasoning mix, 1 Tbsp 0
   Taco seasoning mix, 2 tsp 0
   Taco seasoning mix, 40% less sodium,
      2 tsp..0
   Taco seasoning mix, mild, 2 tsp 0

Taco Shells
Chi-Chi's
   White corn taco shells, 2 (35 g) 4
   Yellow corn taco shells, 2 (35 g) 4
Old El Paso
   Mini taco shells, 7 (31 g)........................3
   Regular taco shells, 3 (32 g) 3
   Soft taco shells, 1 (34 g)..........................2
   Soft taco shells (shelf stable), 2 (50 g)......3
   Super size taco shells, 2 (37 g)................4
   White corn taco shells, 3 (32 g) 3
Pancho Villa Taco shells, 3 (34 g)...........3
Taco Bell Home Originals Taco
   shells, 3 (32 g).......................................3

Tahini
Tribe of Two Sheiks Sesame tahini,
   2 Tbsp 1

Tamales
Hormel
   Beef tamales, canned, 2 (142 g)...............3
   Chicken tamales, 2 (142 g) 3
   Hot-spicy beef tamales, canned, 2
      (142 g)..3
   Jumbo beef tamales, 2 (198 g)................4
Old El Paso Tamales in chili gravy,
   3 tamales in chili gravy (206 g) 7

Tangerines
Dole Tangerines, 2 1

Tapioca
Minute Tapioca, as packaged, 1½ tsp......0

Tart shells
Oronoque Orchards 3" tart shell,
   ready to bake, 1 shell (28 g) 4

Tartar sauce
   Tartar sauce, 2 Tbsp 2
   Tartar sauce, low fat, 2 Tbsp 1
Hellmann's
   Tartar sauce, 2 Tbsp 2
   Tartar sauce, low fat, 2 Tbsp 1
Kraft
   Fat free tartar sauce, 2 Tbsp 1
   Natural lemon & herb flavor tartar
      sauce, 2 Tbsp 4
   Tartar sauce, 2 Tbsp 3
Naturally Fresh Tartar sauce, 2 Tbsp 4

Tea
General Foods
   English breakfast creme, prepared,
      8 fl oz...2
   English raspberry creme decaffeinated,
      prepared, 8 fl oz 2
   English raspberry creme, prepared,
      8 fl oz...2
   Island orange creme, prepared, 8 fl oz......2
   Viennese cinnamon creme
      decaffeinated, prepared, 8 fl oz 2
   Viennese cinnamon creme, prepared,
      8 fl oz...2
Lipton
   Cal-free iced team mix – lemon, 1 Tbsp....0
   Diet iced tea mix – decaffeinated,
      1 Tbsp...0
   Diet iced tea mix – tea & lemonade,
      1 Tbsp...0
   Diet iced tea mix – lemon, 1 Tbsp............0
   Diet iced tea mix – raspberry, 1 Tbsp........0
   Diet iced tea mix – peach, 1 Tbsp 0
   Sugar sweetened iced tea mix – lemon,
      1½ Tbsp...2
   Unsweetened iced tea mix, 1½ Tbsp 0
   Unsweetened iced tea mix –
      decaffeinated, 1½ Tbsp 0
Nestea
   100% decaf tea iced tea mix, 2 tsp..........0
   100% tea iced tea mix, 2 tsp...................0
   Cool from Nestea, 8 fl oz 2

T

Diet cool from Nestea, 8 fl oz 0
Diet lemon iced tea, 8 fl oz......................0
Herb tea lemon bliss iced tea mix,
  1 Tbsp 0
Herb tea orange spice iced tea mix,
  1 Tbsp 0
Lemon & sugar iced tea mix, 2 Tbsp........2
Lemon iced tea, 8 fl oz............................2
Lemon iced tea mix, 2 tsp 0
Lemon iced teaser ice tea mix, ⅛ tub.......0
Lemonade tea iced tea mix, 2 Tbsp 2
Peach iced tea, 8 fl oz.............................2
Raspberry iced tea, 8 fl oz 2
Sugar free decaf iced tea mix, 2 tsp 0
Sugar free iced tea mix, 2 tsp 0
Sun tea iced tea mix, 1 tsp 0
Sweet iced tea, 8 fl oz.............................1
Unsweetened iced tea, 8 fl oz..................0

Snapple

Cactus tea, 8 fl oz...................................2
Caffeine free tea, 8 fl oz..........................2
Diet lemon tea, 8 fl oz 0
Diet lemon tea, 1 can (11½ fl oz)..............0
Diet peach tea, 8 fl oz.............................0
Diet raspberry tea, 8 fl oz........................0
Ginseng tea, 8 fl oz.................................2
Green tea, 8 fl oz....................................2
Just plain tea, unsweetened, 8 fl oz 0
Lemon sun tea, 8 fl oz 2
Lemon tea, 8 fl oz...................................2
Lemon tea, 1 can (11½ fl oz)....................3
Lemonade iced tea, 8 fl oz 2
Lightning – ginseng black tea, 8 fl oz.......2
Mint tea, 8 fl oz......................................2
Moon – green tea, 8 fl oz........................2
Peach sun tea, 8 fl oz..............................2
Peach tea, 8 fl oz....................................2
Peach tea, 1 can (11½ fl oz) 3
Raspberry tea, 8 fl oz..............................2
Raspberry tea, 1 can (11½ fl oz) 3
Sweet tea, 8 fl oz....................................2
Vitasoy Green tea chai, 8 fl oz.................2

Tempeh
Lightlife

Barbecue marinated grille, 1 (78 g) 3
Lemon marinated grille, 1 (78 g)..............3
Organic garden vege, 4 oz.......................4
Organic soy, 4 oz 4
Organic three grain, 4 oz.........................4
Organic wild rice, 4 oz 4
Tamari marinated grille, 1(78 g)...............3

Teriyaki sauce
San-J All purpose teriyaki seasoning
  & marinade, 1 Tbsp...............................0

Toast
Burns & Ricker

Garlic crispini, 5 pieces (30 g)..................2
Seeds & spices crispini, 5 pieces (30 g).....2
Sesame crispini, 5 pieces (30 g) 2

New York Style

Coffee break toast, blueberry, 1 oz...........3
Coffee break toast, cinnamon, 1 oz..........3
Coffee break toast, French vanilla, 1 oz 3

Regina

Garlic Parmesan panetene, 5 pieces
  (28 g) 3
Roasted garlic panetene, 5 pieces
  (28 g) 3

Toaster pastries
Flavor Kist

Toast'em pop-up, frosted wild berry,
  1 (52 g) 4
Toast'em pop-ups, frosted blueberry,
  1 (52 g) 4
Toast'em pop-ups, frosted brown
  sugar cinnamon, 1 (52 g) 4
Toast'em pop-ups, frosted cherry, 1
  (52 g) 4
Toast'em pop-ups, frosted chocolate
  fudge, 1 (52 g) 4
Toast'em pop-ups, frosted strawberry,
  1 (52 g) 4

T

Health Valley

Low-fat tart, baked apple, 1 (40 g)...........3
Low-fat tart, blueberry, 1 (40 g)...............3
Low-fat tart, chocolate, 1 (40 g)...............3
Low-fat tart, raspberry, 1 (40 g)...............3
Low-fat tart, red cherry, 1 (40 g)..............3
Low-fat tart, strawberry, 1 (40 g)..............3

Kellogg's Poptarts

Apple cinnamon, 1 pastry (52 g)...............5
Blueberry, 1 pastry (52 g) 4
Brown sugar cinnamon, 1 pastry (50 g)....5
Frosted blueberry, 1 pastry (52 g)............4
Frosted brown sugar cinnamon,
   1 pastry (50 g) 5
Frosted chocolate vanilla crème,
   1 pastry (52 g) 4
Frosted grape, 1 pastry (52 g) 4
Frosted raspberry, 1 pastry (52 g) 4
Frosted s'mores, 1 pastry (52 g) 4
Frosted strawberry, 1 pastry (52 g) 4
Frosted wild berry, 1 pastry (54 g)............4
Frosted wild magicburst, 1 pastry (52 g)...4
Frosted wild tropical blast, 1 pastry
   (54 g) 4
Frosted wild watermelon, 1 pastry
   (54 g) 4
Low fat frosted brown sugar cinnamon,
   1 pastry (50 g) 4
Low fat frosted chocolate fudge,
   1 pastry (52 g) 4
Low fat frosted strawberry, 1 pastry
   (52 g) 4
Low fat strawberry, 1 pastry (52 g) 4
Strawberry 1 pastry (52 g)....................4

Kellogg's Pop-Tarts Pastry Swirls

Apple cinnamon, 1 pastry (62 g)..............6
Cheese, 1 pastry (62 g) 6
Strawberry, 1 pastry (62 g) 6

Kellogg's Pop-Tarts Snack-Stix

Frosted berry, 1 pastry (52 g) 4
Frosted strawberry, 1 pastry (52 g)...........4

Pillsbury

Cheese & egg, 1 (47 g) 5
Cheese, egg & bacon, 1 (47 g)................5
Cheese, egg & ham, 1 (47 g) 5
Cheese, egg & sausage, 1 (47 g) 5
Western style, 1 (47 g) 4

Pillsbury Toaster Strudel

Apple, 1 (54 g) 4
Blueberry, 1 (54 g) 4
Caramel apple, 1 (54 g)......................4
Cherry, 1 (54 g) 4
Chocolate, 1 (54 g) 5
Cinnamon, 1 (54 g) 4
Cream cheese, 1 (54 g) 5
Cream cheese & cherry, 1 (54 g) 5
Cream cheese & strawberry, 1 (54 g)........5
Cream cheese & strawberry, 1 (54 g)........5
Raspberry, 1 (54 g) 4
Strawberry, 1 (54 g) 4
Wildberry, 1 (54 g) 5

Weight Watchers

Blueberry, 1 serving (52 g)...................4
Cherry, 1 serving (52 g) 4
Strawberry, 1 serving (52 g).................4

Tofu

Azumaya

Extra firm, 2.8 oz............................2
Firm, 2.8 oz.................................2
Lite extra firm, 2.8 oz.......................1
Lite silken, 3.2 oz...........................1
Silken, ⅕ block (91 g) 1

Nasoya

5 spice tofu, ¼ block (85 g)...................2
Enriched firm tofu, ⅕ block (79 g)............1
Enriched silken tofu, ⅕ block (91 g) 1
Extra firm tofu, ⅕ block (91 g)...............2
Firm tofu, ⅕ block (91 g)....................2
Garlic onion tofu, ¼ block (85 g) 2
Silken tofu, ⅙ block (90 g) 1
Soft tofu, ⅕ block (91 g) 2

T

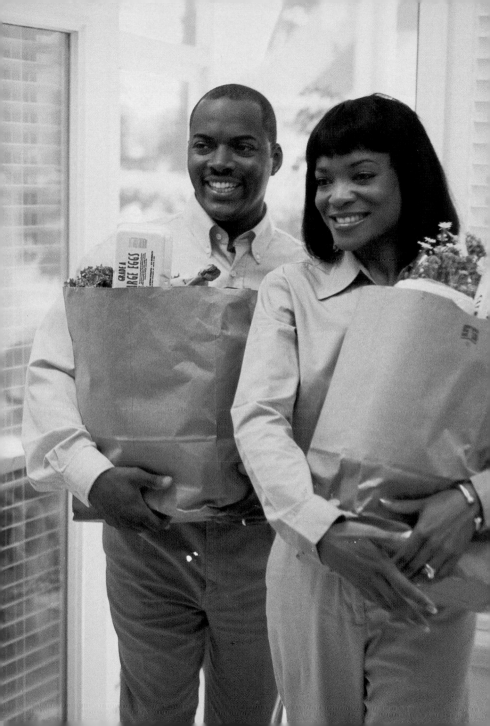

Tomatoes

Chi-Chi's Diced tomatoes & green
chilies, ¼ cup 0

Chiquita Tomato, 1 medium (148 g) 1

Claussen Tomatoes, halves, 1 oz 0

Contadina

Crushed tomatoes in tomato puree,
¼ cup 0

Crushed tomatoes with Italian herbs,
¼ cup 0

Crushed tomatoes with roasted garlic,
¼ cup 0

Diced tomatoes, ½ cup...........................1

Diced tomatoes with Italian herbs,
½ cup 1

Diced tomatoes with roasted garlic,
½ cup 1

Diced tomatoes with sauteed onions,
½ cup 1

Italian style stewed tomatoes w/ garlic,
oregano & basil, ½ cup 1

Peeled whole tomatoes, ½ cup 0

Stewed tomatoes w/ onions, celery
& green peppers, ½ cup 1

Del Monte

Chunky tomatoes, chili style, ½ cup...........0

Chunky tomatoes, pasta style, ½ cup 1

Crushed tomatoes with garlic, ½ cup 1

Crushed tomatoes, Italian recipe, ½ cup ...0

Crushed tomatoes, original recipe,
½ cup 1

Diced tomatoes, ½ cup...........................0

Diced tomatoes with basil, garlic &
oregano, ½ cup 1

Diced tomatoes with garlic & onion,
½ cup 1

Diced tomatoes with green pepper
& onion, ½ cup 0

Diced tomatoes with jalapenos,
½ cup 0

Diced tomatoes, no salt added, ½ cup......0

Stewed, Cajun recipe, ½ cup...................0

Stewed, Italian recipe, ½ cup 0

Stewed, Mexican recipe, ½ cup 0

Stewed, original recipe, ½ cup 0

Stewed, original recipe, no salt added,
½ cup 0

Tomato wedges, ½ cup 0

Whole tomatoes peeled in juice, ½ cup 0

Old El Paso Tomatoes & green chillies,
¼ cup 0

Progresso

Crushed tomatoes, ¼ cup.......................0

Italian style tomatoes, peeled, ½ cup 0

Whole tomatoes, peeled, ½ cup 0

Tomato juice
Campbell's

Healthy Request tomato juice, 1 cup 1

Low sodium tomato juice, 1 cup 1

Tomato juice, 1 serving (243 g) 1

Del Monte

Tomato juice from concentrate, 8 fl oz......1

Tomato juice not from concentrate,
8 fl oz...................................1

Tomato paste
Contadina

Italian paste – tomato paste product
with Italian seasonings, 2 Tbsp 1

Italian paste – tomato paste product
with roasted garlic, 2 Tbsp 1

Italian paste – tomato paste product
with tomato pesto, 2 Tbsp.....................1

Tomato paste, 2 Tbsp 0

Tomato puree
Contadina Tomato puree, ¼ cup 0

Progresso

Tomato puree, ¼ cup 0

Tomato puree, thick style, ¼ cup 0

Tomato sauce
Contadina

Italian style tomato sauce, ¼ cup..............0

Tomato paste – 100% tomatoes, 2 Tbsp...0

Tomato sauce, ¼ cup 0

Tomato sauce – extra thick & zesty,
¼ cup 0

Tomato sauce – garlic and onion,
¼ cup 0

Tomato sauce (con't)   POINTS

Del Monte
Sauce, tomato, ¼ cup 0
Sauce, tomato no salt added, ¼ cup 0
Faraon Tomato sauce, ¼ cup 0
Progresso Tomato sauce, ¼ cup 0

Toppings
E.D.Smith
Blueberry fruit topping, 2 Tbsp 1
Cherry fruit topping, 2 Tbsp 1
Strawberry, cranberry, blackberry fruit
   topping, 2 Tbsp 1

Harry & David
Lemon curd, 1 Tbsp 1
Raspberry chipotle sauce, 1 Tbsp 1
Raspberry honey cream, 1 Tbsp 1
Raspberry sauce, 1 Tbsp 1
Vanilla honey cream, 1 Tbsp 1

Hershey's
Shell topping, chocolate, 2 Tbsp 6
Shell topping, chocolate fudge, 2 Tbsp 5
Shell topping, cookies 'n' crème, 2 Tbsp ...5
Shell topping, krackel, 2 Tbsp 5
Shell topping, peanut, 2 Tbsp 6

Hershey's Chocolate Shoppe
Fat free caramel, 2 Tbsp 2
Fat free hot fudge topping, 2 Tbsp 2
Sprinkles candy coated milk chocolate,
   2 Tbsp 3
Sprinkles Reese's peanut butter and
   milk, 2 Tbsp 4
Sprinkles York mint chocolate, 2 Tbsp 4

Kraft
Artificially flavored butterscotch, 2 Tbsp ...3
Caramel, 2 Tbsp 2
Chocolate flavored, 2 Tbsp 2
Hot fudge, 2 Tbsp 3
Pineapple, 2 Tbsp 2
Strawberry, 2 Tbsp 2

Smucker's Guilt Free Hot fudge
   topping, 2 Tbsp 2
Smucker's Light Hot fudge topping,
   2 Tbsp 1

POINTS

Toppings, whipped

Cool Whip, Whipped Topping (KRAFT)

Cool Whip
Extra creamy whipped topping, 2 Tbsp 1
Free whipped topping, 2 Tbsp 0
Lite whipped topping, 2 Tbsp 0
Whipped topping, 2 Tbsp 1
Dream Whip Whipped topping mix,
   prepared as directed, 2 Tbsp 0
Estee Sugar free whipped topping mix,
   2 Tbsp 0
Kraft Whipped light cream, 2 Tbsp 0
Kraft Free Fat free whipped topping,
   2 Tbsp 0

Tortellini/Tortelloni
Di Giorno
Beef and roasted garlic tortellini, 1 cup 8
Lemon chicken tortelloni in cracked
   black pepper pasta, 1 cup 6
Mozzarella garlic tortelloni, 1 cup 6
Pesto tortelloni, 1 cup 6
Portabello mushroom tortelloni, 1 cup......6
Three cheese tortellini, ¾ cup..................5
Rosetto Cheese tortellini, 1¼ cups 6

Tortillas

LaTortilla Factory

LaTortilla Factory
13" low fat/fiber boost wrap flour
   tortillas, 1 (110 g)................................5
13" roma wrap flour tortillas, 1
   (110 g) 6

T

Lite Goes Luscious

COOL 'N TROPICAL TREAT   Prep: 5 minutes

Nonfat yogurt, any flavor
Lowfat granola
COOL WHIP LITE or FREE Whipped Topping, thawed
DOLE® Pineapple Chunks, drained

ALTERNATE layers of yogurt, granola, whipped topping and pineapple chunks in glass or small bowl. Top with whipped topping.

99% fat free burrito size flour tortillas, 1 (71 g) 2

99% fat free whole wheat soft taco size flour tortillas, 1 (51 g) 1

100% fat free soft taco size flour tortillas, 1 (51 g)............1

Family pack white corn tortillas, 2 (59 g) 2

Flour tortillas burrito size, 1 (56.7 g) 3

Flour tortillas soft taco size, 1 (42½ g) 2

King size 98% fat free/preservative free yellow corn tortillas, 2 (66 g) 2

Preservative free Tamayo family burrito size flour tortillas, 1 (68 g) 3

Preservative free Tamayo family traditional flavor tortillas, 1 (54 g) 3

Preservative free Tamayo family whole wheat low carb/high fiber flour tortillas, 1 (36 g) 1

Saben como hecha a mano! taste like hand made! Bigger & thicker white corn tortillas, 1 (51 g) 2

Senor Miguel homemade flour tortillas, 1 (51 g) 3

Whole wheat garlic & herb flour tortillas, 1 (36 g)............1

Whole wheat large size flour tortillas, 1 (62 g) 1

Whole wheat original size flour tortilla, 1 (36 g) 1

Whole wheat taco flavor flour tortillas, 1 (36 g) 1

LaTortilla Factory WrapArounds

Chile & lime, 1 (75 g) 4

Garlic & herb, 1 (75 g) 4

Spinach flavor, 1 (75 g) 4

Sun dried tomato, 1 (75 g) 4

Mission

Burrito size 98% fat free flour tortillas, 1 (67 g) 3

Burrito size flour tortillas, 1 (71 g) 5

Fajita size 98% fat free flour tortillas, 1 (33 g) 1

Fajita size flour tortillas, 1 (33 g)............2

Garden spinach herb mission wraps, 1 (83 g) 5

Reduced fat classic mission wraps, 1 (83 g) 4

Soft taco size 96% fat free whole wheat tortillas, 1 (51 g) 3

Soft taco size 98% fat free flour tortillas, 1 (50 g)............2

Soft taco size flour tortillas, 1 (50 g) 3

Southwestern chili mission wraps, 1 (83 g) 5

Sundried tomato basil mission wraps, 1 (83 g) 5

White corn tortillas, 2 (56 g)............2

Yellow corn tortillas, 2 (56 g)............2

Zesty garlic herb mission wraps, 1 (83 g) 5

Old El Paso

Flour tortillas, 1 (41 g) 3

Flour tortillas (shelf stable), 1 (41 g) 3

Flour tortillas, low fat, 1 (41 g) 2

Tortilla chips

Boston's Baked tortilla chips, low fat, 13 (30 g) 2

Doritos

3D's cooler ranch, 27 (1 oz)............3

3D's jalapeno Cheddar, 33 (1 oz) 3

3D's nacho cheesier, 27 (1 oz) 3

Baja picante, 12 (1 oz) 3

Cooler ranch, 12 (1 oz)............3

Flamin' hot, 11 (1 oz)............3

Nacho cheesier, 11 (1 oz) 3

Salsa verde, 12 (1 oz) 3

Smokey red BBQ, 12 (1 oz) 3

Sonic sour cream, 11 (1 oz) 3

Spicy nacho, 12 (1 oz) 3

Taco supreme, 12 (1 oz) 3

Toasted corn, 13 (1 oz)............3

Doritos Wow Nacho cheese, 11 (1 oz)...2

Guiltless Gourmet

Chili lime tortilla chips, 18 (1 oz) 2

Mucho nacho tortilla chips, 16 (1 oz) 2

T

Organic blue corn tortilla chips, 6 (1 oz) ...2
Red corn tortilla chips, 18 (1 oz) 2
Spicy black bean tortilla chips, 15 (1 oz) ...2
Sweet white corn tortilla chips, 6
(1 oz)...2
Unsalted yellow corn tortilla chips,
6 (1 oz)...2
Yellow corn tortilla chips, 6 (1 oz) 2

Harry's
Blue tortilla chips, 1 oz...........................3
Guacamole chips, 1 oz 3
Harry's Rio Grande Tortilla chips, 1 oz..3
Jax Restaurant style tortilla chips,
6 (28 g) 3
Lance White corn round tortillas, 33
(35 g) 4

Nabisco Air Crisps
Tortilla nacho chips, 24 crisps (1 oz) 3
Tortilla original chips, 24 crisps (1 oz) 3

Santitas
100% white corn, 9 (1 oz).......................3
Restaurant style chips, 9 (1 oz) 3

Tostitos
Baked bite size, 20 (1 oz) 2
Baked bite size Cheddar quesadilla,
19 (1 oz)..2
Baked bite size salsa & cream cheese,
16 (1 oz)..2
Baked original, 9 (1 oz) 2
Bite size, 15 (1 oz) 3
Crispy rounds, 13 (1 oz) 3
Restaurant style, 6 (1 oz).........................3
Restaurant style hint of lime, 6 (1 oz).......3
Santa Fe gold, 7 (1 oz) 3

Tostada shells
Old El Paso Tostada shells, 3 (32 g) 3

Trail mix
EXPRESSnacks
Carob chip trail mix, ¼ cup 3
Yogurt chip trail mix, ¼ cup.....................3
Harmony Tropical trail mix, ¼ cup 3

Harry & David
Rice cracker trail mix, ½ cup.....................2
Wasabi trail mix, ½ cup............................2

Planters
Trail mix apple cranberry crunch, 3 Tbsp ...3
Trail mix caramel nut crunch, 3 Tbsp 3
Trail mix flamin' cajun crunch, ⅓ cup 3
Trail mix fruit & nut mix, 3 Tbsp...............3
Trail mix, Caribbean crunch nuts,
sesame sticks and fruit, 3 Tbsp 3
Trial mix nuts & chocolate mix, 3 Tbsp 4
Trial mix nuts, seeds & raisins, 3 Tbsp.......4

Tuna
Ocean Beauty
Ahi tuna fajitas, 8 oz................................2
Southwest tuna burger, 1 burger
(3.2 oz)..2
Tuna burger, 100% fat free, 1 burger
(3.2 oz)..2
Tuna burger, 98% fat free, 1 burger
(3.2 oz)..2
Progresso Solid tuna in olive oil
(drained), ¼ cup 4

StarKist
Chunk light in pure vegetable oil, 2 oz 3
Chunk light in pure vegetable oil,
1 can (76 g) 3
Chunk light in spring water, 2 oz 1
Chunk light in spring water, 1 can
(76 g) 2
Chunk white in spring water, 2 oz............1
Low sodium chunk light tuna in spring
water, 2 oz 1
Low sodium chunk light tuna in spring
water, 1 can (76 g) 1
Low sodium chunk white tuna in pure
distilled water, 2 oz 1
Low sodium chunk white tuna in pure
distilled water, 1 can (76 g) 2
Solid white albacore in spring water,
2 oz (56 g) 2
Solid white albacore in spring water,
1 can (79 g) 2
Tuna salad, 1 kit (99 g) 4

T

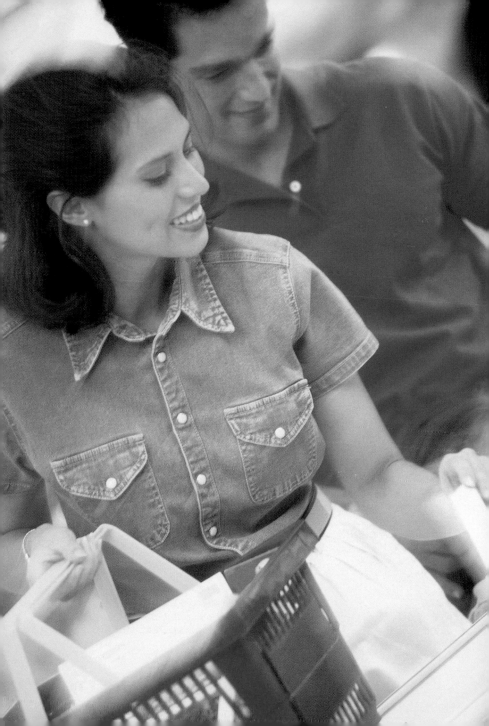

Tuna (con't)

StarKist Gourmet's Choice
Tuna fillet solid light tuna in olive oil,
2 oz..4
Tuna fillet solid light tuna in spring
water, 2 oz...1

StarKist Select
Hickory smoke fillets chunk light tuna
in spring water, 2 oz 1
Prime light fillets in spring water, 1 can
(79 g) 2
Prime light fillets in spring water,
2 oz..1

Turkey
Hormel
Chunk turkey, 2 oz 2
Chunk white turkey, 2 oz..........................1

Louis Rich
Breast of turkey, hickory smoked,
1 slice (56 g) 1
Breast of turkey, honey roasted,
1 slice (56 g) 1
Breast of turkey, oven roasted, 1 slice
(56 g) 1
Breast of turkey, rotisserie flavor, 1 slice
(56 g) 1
Ground turkey, 4 oz 5
Hickory smoked breast of turkey, 2 oz 1
Honey roasted breast of turkey, 2 oz 1
Oven roasted breast of turkey, 2 oz..........1
Rotisserie flavor breast of turkey, 2 oz......1
Turkey breast & white turkey, oven
roasted, 2 oz 1
Turkey nuggets, 4 (92 g) 7
Turkey patties, 1 (85 g).............................5
Turkey patties, white, 1 (113 g) 4
Turkey sticks, 3 (85 g) 6
Perdue Breast tenderloins, 3 oz...............2

Shady Brook Farms
Homestyle Italian turkey meatballs,
3 (85 g) 3
Homestyle oven roasted carved turkey
breast, ½ cup (70 g) 1
Homestyle peppered carved turkey
breast, ½ cup 1

OnlyOne boneless turkey tenderloins,
½ tenderloin (85 g)................................2
OnlyOne turkey breast for London broil,
1 (85 g) 2
OnlyOne turkey cutlets, 1 (85 g)...............2

Wampler Foods
98% fat free turkey breast tenders, 4 oz...3
99% fat free ground turkey breast, 4 oz ...3
99% fat free turkey breast steaks, 4 oz 2
Boneless turkey breast roast, 4 oz............4
Homestyle turkey burgers, 1 (85 g)...........4
Lean ground turkey, 4 oz 4
Mesquite flavor turkey burgers, 1
(85 g) 4
Seasoned turkey burgers, 1 (85 g)............4
Turkey breast half, 4 oz 4

Turkey, deli
Boar's Head
All natural turkey breast, 2 oz..................1
Baby maple glazed honey coat turkey,
2 oz..1
Cajun style oven roasted smoked
breast of turkey, 2 oz 1
Cracked pepper mill smoked turkey
breast, 2 oz...1
Deli dinners ovengold turkey single
(skin on), 3 oz 2
Golden oven roasted turkey breast
skin on, 2 oz 1
Golden oven roasted turkey breast
skinless, 2 oz 1
Hickory smoked turkey breast 32%
lower sodium, 2 oz 2
Maple glazed honey coat cured turkey
breast, 2 oz...1
Mesquite wood smoked breast of turkey
skinless, 2 oz 1
Our premium 25% lower sodium
turkey – skin on, 2 oz 1
Our premium 25% lower sodium
turkey – skinless, 2 oz...........................1
Ovengold roast breast of turkey –
skinless, 2 oz...1

T

Turkey, deli, Boar's Head (con't) POINTS

Ovengold roast breast of turkey –
skin on, 2 oz 1
Pastrami seasoned turkey breast, 2 oz......1
Salsalito roasted breast of turkey, 2 oz....1

Perdue
Golden browned turkey breast, 2 oz.........1
Hickory smoked turkey breast, 2 oz 1
Honey smoked turkey breast, 2 oz............1

Wampler Foods
4 diamond Cajun style turkey breast
(deli), 2 oz 1
5 diamond brown sugar turkey breast
(deli), 2 oz 1
5 diamond hickory smoked netted
turkey breast (deli), 2 oz 1
5 diamond honey roasted turkey breast
(deli), 2 oz 1
5 diamond Italian style herb turkey
breast (deli), 2 oz 1
5 diamond oil browned turkey breast
(deli), 2 oz 1

Turnovers
Pillsbury
Apple, 1 (57 g) 4
Cherry, 1 (57 g) 4
The Fillo Factory Apple, 5 pieces
(142 g) 5

V

Vegetable juice

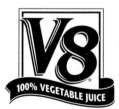

V8
Low sodium V8, 6 fl oz.............................0
V8, 6 fl oz 0
V8 juice calcium enriched, 6 fl oz.............0

POINTS

Vegetable side dishes, frozen
Budget Gourmet New England recipe
vegetables, 1 serving (141 g).................5

Green Giant
Green bean casserole, ⅔ cup...................2
Vegetable alfredo, ¾ cup 1
Vegetables teriyaki, 1¼ cups 2

Green Giant Pasta Accents
Alfredo, 2 cups 4
Creamy Cheddar, 2⅓ cups 5
Garden herb, 2 cups...............................4
Garlic, 2 cups 5
Primavera, 2¼ cups 6
Three cheese, 2 cups 6
White Cheddar, 1¾ cups 6

Vegetable side dishes, shelf stable
House of Tsang
Hong Kong sweet & sour, ½ cup 3
Szechuan hot & spicy, ½ cup 1
Tokyo teriyaki, ½ cup 2

Vegetables in sauce, frozen
Freezer Queen Family Side Dish
Broccoli, pasta, cauliflower & carrots
in cheese sauce, ⅔ cup 2

Vegetables, mixed
Del Monte
Mixed vegetables, ½ cup..........................0
Mixed vegetables NSA, ½ cup 0
Peas and carrots, ½ cup 1

Green Giant
Broccoli, cauliflower & carrots in
cheese flavored sauce, frozen, ⅔ cup.....1
Garden medley vegetables, canned,
½ cup 0
Mixed vegetables, canned, ½ cup 1
Mixed vegetables, frozen, ¾ cup 1
Sweet peas & carrots, canned, ½ cup.......0
Sweet peas with tiny pearl onions,
canned, ½ cup.....................................0

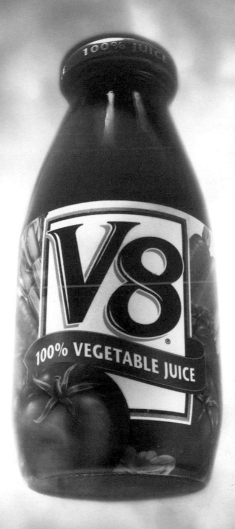

ZERO *POINTS*''
A FULL SERVING OF VEGETABLES'

GO AHEAD, PINCH YOURSELF.

*Per 6 oz. serving. ©2000 CSC

Vegetables, mixed (con't)   POINTS

Green Giant Select American Mixtures
Broccoli, carrots & cauliflower, frozen, ⅔ cup 0
Broccoli, carrots & water chestnuts, frozen, ⅔ cup 0

Hanover
Broccoli & cauliflower blend, 1 cup 0
Garden medley, ¾ cup 0
Mixed vegetables, ⅔ cup 1
Oriental blend, ¾ cup 0
Succotash, ⅔ cup 1
Vegetables for soup, ⅔ cup 0

Hanover The Gold Line
Petite asparagus blend, ⅔ cup.................1
Petite broccoli blend, ¾ cup 1
Petite green bean blend, ⅔ cup 1
Shoepeg corn & petite peas, ½ cup 1

LeSueur Early peas with mushrooms & pearl onions, canned, ½ cup 1

Schwan's
California blend, 1 cup 0
Fire roasted veg. blend, ¾ cup.................1
Stir fry vegetables, 1 cup 0
Summer garden pasta blend, 1 cup 1
Vegetable stew blend, ⅔ cup 1

Vegetarian meat substitutes

Amy's
California veggie burger, frozen, 1 (2½ oz) 2
Chicago veggie burger, frozen, 1 (2½ oz) 3
Texas veggie burger, frozen, 1 (2½ oz) 2

Gardenburger Original, 2½ oz 2

Lightlife
Gimme Lean, real beef taste, 2 oz 1
Gimme Lean, real sausage taste, 2 oz 1
Lean Italian links, 1 (40 g) 1
Light burgers, 3 oz 1
Meatless light sausages, 2 (68 g) 1
Smart deli jumbos, 1 (76 g) 1
Smart deli sticks, 1 oz 1

POINTS

Smart dogs!, 1 (42 g)................................1
Tofu pups, 1 (42 g)...................................1
Wonderdogs, 1 (42 g) 1

Lightlife Smart Cutlets
Salisbury steak, 4½ oz 2
Seasoned chick'n, 4 oz 2

Lightlife Smart Deli
Country ham style, 3 slices (43 g) 1
Old world bologna style, 3 slices (43 g) 1
Roast turkey style, 3 slices (43 g) 1
Three peppercorn style, 3 slices (43 g) 1

Lightlife Smart Ground
Original, ⅓ cup.......................................1
Taco & burrito, ⅓ cup..............................1

Morningstar Farms
America's original veggie dog, frozen, 1 (57 g) 1
Better 'n burgers, frozen, 1 (78 g) 1
Breakfast links, frozen, 2 (45 g) 1
Breakfast patties, frozen, 1 (38 g) 1
Breakfast patties, refrigerated, 2 (56 g) 2
Breakfast strips, frozen, 2 (16 g) 2
Burger style recipe crumbles, frozen, ⅔ cup...1
Chik nuggets, frozen, 4 (86 g)..................3
Chik nuggets, refrigerated, 4 (86 g)..........3
Chik patties, frozen, 1 (71 g) 3
Garden grille, frozen, 1 (71 g) 2
Garden veggie patties, frozen, 1 (67 g).....1
Garden veggie patties, refrigerated, 1 (100 g) 2
Grillers, frozen, 1 (64 g)...........................3
Ground meatless, frozen, ½ cup 1
Hard rock café all natural veggie burgers, frozen, 1 (85 g)......................3
Harvest burgers Italian style, frozen, 1 (90 g) 2
Harvest burgers original, frozen, 1 (90 g) 2
Harvest burgers recipe crumbles, frozen, ½ cup 1

Harvest burgers southwestern style,
frozen, 1 (90 g) 2

Meatfree buffalo wings, frozen, 5
(85 g) 4

Meatfree burger and cheese style
stuffed sandwich, frozen, 1 (128 g) 6

Meatfree corn dog, frozen, 1 (71 g) 3

Meatfree ham and cheese style stuffed
sandwich, frozen, 1 (128 g) 6

Meatfree mini corn dogs, frozen, 4
(76 g) 4

Meatfree pepperoni pizza style stuffed
sandwiches, frozen, 1 (128 g) 5

Quarter prime, frozen, 1 (96 g) 2

Quarter prime, refrigerated, 1 (96 g) 2

Sausage style recipe crumbles, frozen,
⅔ cup 2

Spicy black bean burger, frozen, 1
(78 g) 1

Spicy black bean burger, refrigerated,
1 (93 g) 2

Vinegar
Heinz
Apple cider vinegar, ½ fl oz 0
Balsamic vinegar, 1 Tbsp 0
Gourmet malt vinegar, 1 Tbsp 0
Premium tarragon vinegar, 1 Tbsp 0
Red wine vinegar, 1 Tbsp 0
Salad vinegar, 1 Tbsp 0
Naturally Fresh
Malt vinegar, ¼ oz 0
Red wine vinegar, ¼ oz 0
White wine vinegar, ½ Tbsp 0
Progresso
Balsamic vinegar, 1 Tbsp 0
Garlic flavored vinegar, 1 Tbsp 0
Red wine flavored distilled vinegar,
1 Tbsp 0
Red wine vinegar, 1 Tbsp 0
White wine vinegar, 1 Tbsp 0
Regina
Balsamic vinegar, 1 Tbsp 0
Red wine vinegar, 1 Tbsp 0

Red wine vinegar with garlic, 1 Tbsp 0
White wine vinegar, 1 Tbsp 0
White wine vinegar with tarragon,
1 Tbsp 0

w

Waffles
Kellogg's
Frozen waffles, low fat homestyle,
2 (70 g) 3
Frozen waffles, strawberry, 2 (70 g) 4
Kellogg's Eggo
Apple cinnamon, 2 (70 g) 4
Banana bread, 2 (70 g) 4
Blueberry, 2 (70 g) 4
Buttermilk, 2 (70 g) 4
Chocolate chip, 2 (70 g) 4
Cinnamon toast, 3 sets of 4 waffles
(92 g) 6
Golden oat, 2 (70 g) 2
Homestyle, 2 (70 g) 4
Low fat nutri-grain, 2 (70 g) 2
Low fat nutri-grain, blueberry, 2 (70 g) 3
Minis homestyle, 3 sets of 4 waffles
(93 g) 6
Nut & honey, 2 (70 g) 5
Nutri-grain, 2 (70 g) 3
Nutri-grain, multi-bran, 2 (70 g) 3
Special K, 2 (58 g) 2
Pillsbury Hungry Jack
Apple cinnamon, 2 (71 g) 5
Blueberry, 2 (71 g) 5
Buttermilk, 2 (68 g) 4
Homestyle, 2 (68 g) 4
Wildberry, 2 (71 g) 5

Walnuts
Tropical Nut & Fruit
Black walnuts, 1 oz 5
Walnut halves, ¼ cup 5
Walnut halves & pieces, ¼ cup 5
Walnut pieces, ¼ cup 5
Walnuts, ¼ cup 5

Y

Water
Dasani, 8 fl oz 0
Naturally Fresh Mountain spring
water, 8 fl oz 0
Propel
Berry, 8 fl oz...0
Lemon, 8 fl oz 0
Orange, 8 fl oz..0

Welsh rarebit
Stouffer's Welsh rarebit, ¼ cup 3

Wheat germ
Kretschmer
Honey crunch wheat germ, 1⅔ Tbsp 1
Toasted wheat bran, ¼ cup 0
Wheat germ (regular), 2 Tbsp 1

Whitefish
Rite Smoked whitefish salad, 2 Tbsp.........2

Wine
Ernest & Julio Gallo
Cabernet sauvignon, ½ cup 2
Café zinfandel, ½ cup 2
Chardonnay, ½ cup 2
Hearty burgundy, ½ cup 2
Malvasia chardonnay, ½ cup 2
Merlot, ½ cup...2
Sauvignon blanc, ½ cup 2
White grenache, ½ cup 2
White zinfandel, ½ cup 2
Gossamer Bay
Cabernet sauvignon (Italy) ('96), ½ cup....2
Chardonnay ('98), ½ cup 2
Merlot ('97), ½ cup 2
Pinot grigio ('98), ½ cup...........................2
Sauvignon blanc ('98), ½ cup 2
White zinfandel ('99), ½ cup......................2
Zinfandel ('98), ½ cup 2

Wine, cooking
Regina
Cooking wine sauterne, 2 Tbsp 0
Cooking wine, burgundy, 2 Tbsp 1
Cooking wine, sherry, 2 Tbsp 1

Worcestershire sauce
A1 Worcestershire sauce, 1 tsp 0
Heinz Worcestershire sauce, 1 tsp............0
Lea & Perrins
Worcestershire sauce, 1 tsp 0
White wine worcestershire sauce,
1 Tbsp 0

Yogurt
Breyers Blended Lowfat
Blueberry, 4.4 oz......................................3
Peach, 4.4 oz...3
Strawberry, 4.4 oz....................................3
Breyers Light
Apple pie a la mode, 8 oz.........................2
Berry banana split, 8 oz 2
Black cherry jubilee, 8 oz.........................2
Blueberries n' cream flavored, 8 oz 2
Cherry bon-bon flavored, 8 oz 2
Cherry vanilla cream flavored, 8 oz 2
Classic strawberry, 8 oz............................2
Key lime pie, 8 oz 2
Lemon chiffon, 8 oz 2
Peaches n' cream flavored, 8 oz...............2
Raspberries n' cream flavored, 8 oz 2
Strawberry cheesecake flavored, 8 oz.......2
Breyers Lowfat
Black cherry, 8 oz.....................................5
Blueberry, 8 oz 5
Mixed berry, 8 oz 5
Peach, 8 oz 5
Pineapple, 8 oz 5
Red raspberry, 8 oz 5
Strawberry, 8 oz 5
Strawberry banana, 8 oz 5
Vanilla, 8 oz 5
Breyers Smooth & Creamy
Apple cobbler, 8 oz 5
Black cherry parfait, 8 oz..........................5
Black cherry parfait, 4.4 oz.......................3
Blueberries 'n cream flavored, 4.4 oz 3

Notes

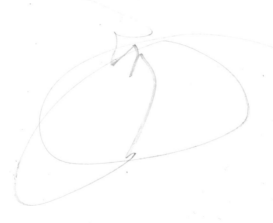

Notes

Notes

Notes